JASMINE HEMSLEY

EAST BY WEST

Simple Ayurvedic Recipes for
Ultimate Mind-Body Balance

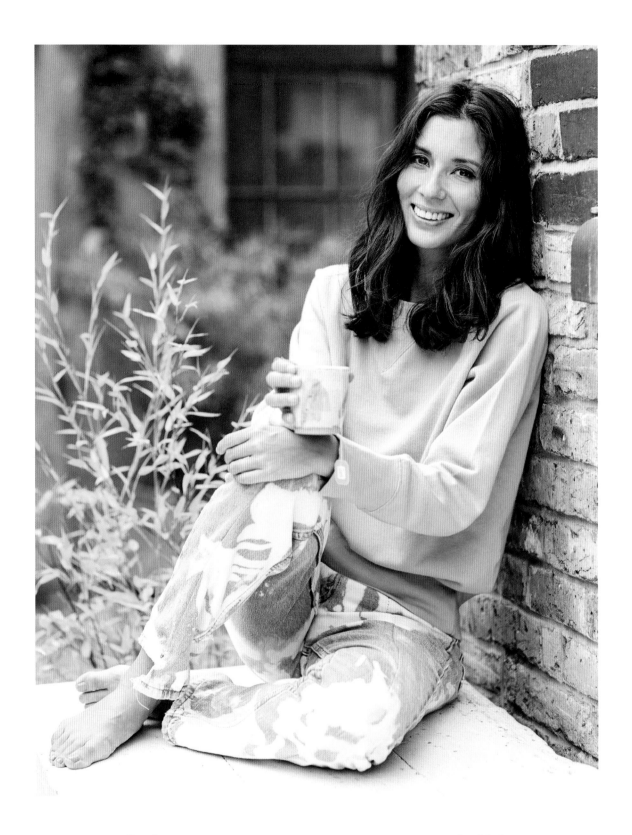

Dedicated to my mum, Evangelina; my partner, Nick; and my great aunt, Joan – for all the love.

JASMINE HEMSLEY

EAST ᴮʸ WEST

Simple Ayurvedic Recipes for
Ultimate Mind-Body Balance

bluebird
books for life

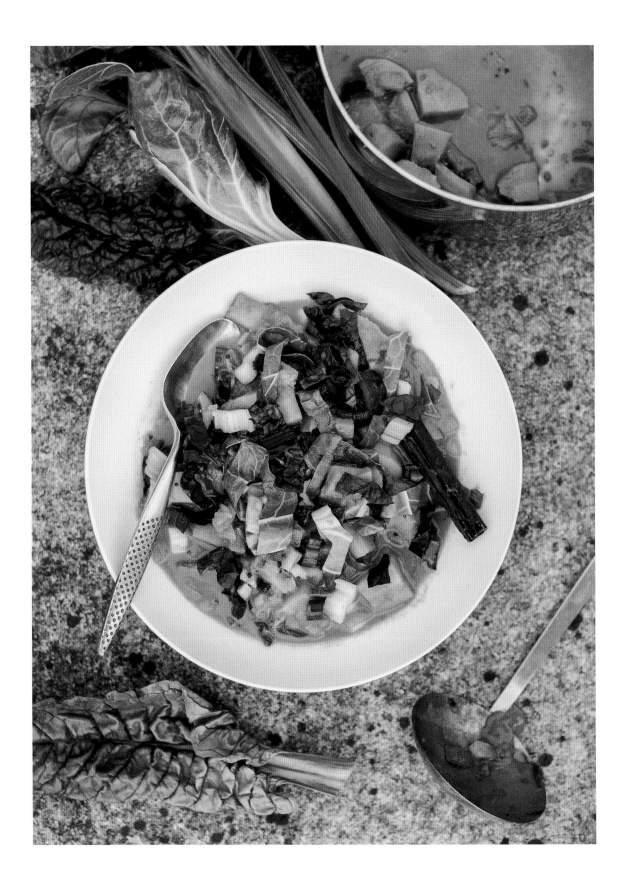

Contents

INTRODUCTION

How I got here

We are not necessarily what we eat. We are what we digest, absorb and assimilate – physically, emotionally and mentally. I have long had a fascination with digestion and the critical role it plays in gut health, not only for our immunity but for the entire health of our mind and body. Enter Ayurveda – the 5,000-year-old ancient holistic system that supports the idea that our vitality, wellbeing and happiness come from a life in balance, and that the secret to maintaining this balance lies in the strength of our Agni, or digestive 'fire' (see page 278). Ayurveda is the 'science of life', revolving around an awareness of your world and how to live according to your personal, physical and emotional needs and attributes.

It is our individual food choices, daily routines and connection to the environment that dictate the balance of the physical, mental and emotional states that we enjoy (or don't enjoy) every day. And it was these 'don't enjoy' days that fuelled my desire to make wellbeing a priority. Seemingly small and often obvious changes had a profound impact on my health. I found that once I understood my wellbeing in this more elemental way – that it is connected to the Ayurvedic qualities of foods, rather than their chemical breakdown – I could let my body, rather than my cravings, dictate what it needs.

Ayurveda enriched my life, giving me a tried-and-tested structure to fall back on and a more intuitive understanding of my changing needs. For the last 15 years I have been exploring and refining my knowledge around how to be well and stay well in manic modern times. I wanted to share this understanding in *East by West*, which is my interpretation of Ayurveda, presented in a way that is accessible for anyone looking to embrace a holistic lifestyle.

MY JOURNEY TO AYURVEDA

I have come a long way from the processed white-bread cheese and ketchup toasties that I lived on in my first year at uni. Add uni nights to a uni diet and you have a digestive system in disarray and the symptoms to match: midday fatigue; lack of concentration; dull complexion; weak hair, skin and nails. When I started modelling full-time after university, it was an awakening – few jobs make you think so much about the effects of food and lifestyle habits on your body. I was a commercial model, so thankfully I never had to suffer measurements, weigh-ins and weight loss. However, during this time I became much more clued up about which foods suited me, and I learned more about nutrition in general. This was the start of my connection to healthy eating and the mind–body balance that would become a passion. When I discovered Ayurveda, the oldest healing system in the world, I was a little late, or a little too early, to the party – it was 2001 and health was all about fitness: punitive gym sessions and restrictive eating programmes, low-fat and low-cal. It wasn't about rest (unless you earned it) and nurturing your body, or understanding the qualities, processes and provenance of foods.

Picking up my first book on Ayurveda was like picking up a book on rocket science in Russian – it was a whole new language, a whole new concept. I dipped and dived through several books, simultaneously absorbing what I could and only taking on board messages that made sense in the light of my own experiences. For example, cooked foods are gently nourishing – think of the soups, stews and porridges given to babies, the elderly and the sick. The advice to eat earlier in the day was also a light-bulb moment. There were the obvious things, too, like eating warm food when you're cold and cooling foods when you're hot. The absolute game-changers were the power of the gut – recently acknowledged in the West as the second brain and centre of immunity – and of course the importance of digestion.

These are the basic principles that informed my lifestyle overhaul. In 2010 I became a food and wellbeing coach and a chef for private clients who were looking for something more to life than calorie-counting, calorie-burning workouts and fat-free meals. Using emerging new science combined with traditional wisdom, the Hemsley + Hemsley philosophy was born of a passion to distil the best health advice.

As my commitment to this field grows, the more I am convinced that the new health rules are actually the old ones – 5,000 years old, in fact. As you'll see from my love and appreciation of food in this cookbook, every meal is an opportunity to fortify your body and boost energy, but at the same time the food you eat is by no means the whole 360. Beyond food there are so many ways we can help our bodies and minds to find balance. If you're stressed and not sleeping well, you will find it hard to digest and get the most out of even the most nutritious food.

EASTERN WISDOM FOR WESTERN WELLBEING

Over the years I have enjoyed yoga and meditation as part of my daily routine, and I have also spent time in India studying with Vaidyas (Ayurvedic practitioners) to get a better understanding of what many in the West would consider esoteric nonsense. I undertook two Panchakarmas – month-long Ayurvedic detoxes far removed from any detox we know in the West. These experiences led me to open my own pop-up cafe called East by West, London's first Ayurvedic restaurant. In the run-up to Christmas, we served hot bowls of dal, lightly spiced desserts and chai teas to cold and curious customers. The food was embraced by everyone – from businessmen to fashionistas, curious foodies to tourists. They loved that I had removed overwhelming choice from their lives for a moment and that they could enjoy simple, delicious Ayurveda-inspired food. At long last, Londoners came to understand that newly popular steaming mugs of 'turmeric latte' are in fact Golden Milk, an ancient nourishing drink, and the now-ubiquitous energy balls are based on the traditional Ayurvedic sweets called ladoos.

I've immersed myself in the subject and grown a lot as a person to get here, but for me this is still the tip of the iceberg. I continue to be inspired, influenced and educated by some of the most remarkable and generous individuals in the Ayurvedic world, people whose knowledge and commitment to this science of life runs so deep. I'm still dancing around the periphery of Western eating and Ayurvedic philosophy, and I hope that my experience and interpretation will fuel your passion for Ayurveda and enrich and empower you on your journey towards true mind–body balance.

How to use this book

First and foremost this is a cookbook – albeit with a difference! – so feel free to flick through the host of breakfast, lunch, supper and snack ideas inspired by my travels. You will begin to feel the vibe of Ayurvedic philosophies through the ingredients, terminology and recipe introductions that tell the story of the recipes and how they came about. Or you can start at the beginning.

My mission with *East by West* is to introduce the way of Ayurveda and impart a deeper understanding of its principles and styles. For example, why milk and sugar, which have become the outcasts of modern health philosophies, can be good and nourishing in their whole form when properly prepared, and why, according to ancient Ayurveda, animal foods such as bone broth and meat have a place in our diet.

I'm looking at the concepts of this age-old Eastern philosophy in their simplest form – enough to get a feel for it and much more than just a flavour for anyone interested. Like all simple techniques, this means learning a new skill and allowing it to become second nature. Remember learning to ride a bike or drive a car? It takes a while to be totally confident and at ease with these, even on the most familiar routes. When you get to know more about new things, they can become very beautiful, which is why strange foods, customs and art can suddenly have so much meaning and appeal. At its simplest, use these recipes to balance your current feelings.

This is also a practical guide to making Eastern philosophy more accessible, taking the reader on a journey to learn healthy principles from a culture that is so different to ours and one that is rich in spiritual and ancient wisdom. More than anything, this book gives an explanation of some of the fundamentals of Ayurveda and offers some easy guidelines for following a more Ayurvedic lifestyle. It goes way beyond simply food, inviting the reader to look at their entire way of life.

Ayurvedic guidelines are designed to enhance your health and wellbeing. Enjoy the first round of learning this new language – you certainly don't need to do everything to enjoy the benefits and it's not an exclusive club. Dip your toes in and try these tips to help you as an individual in your environment – every time you work with Ayurveda, which is working with nature, you experience the benefits of vitality.

If you've ever read or heard anything about Ayurveda you might know about Doshas, or 'body types'. In the West we love to pigeonhole and label, and while knowing your genetic body type is fascinating, even more important is being in tune with your body in the day to day – knowing how to remedy how you are feeling in the moment in order to give your body what it needs. This book helps you understand how the way you are feeling relates to food and your digestion. You'll be relieved to know that while we are all individuals and have individual needs, by supporting our digestive 'fire' we are dealing with our health at its very heart. A well-functioning digestive system is at the centre of optimum health; not only in how we digest and deal with food but also how we digest and deal with life.

THE PARTS OF THE BOOK

This book is split into three parts: Part 1: Introduction, followed by Part 2: The Recipes, then Part 3: Ayurveda Explained, which includes guidance on Doshas, Qualities, Tastes and lifestyle advice from the philosophy of Ayurveda.

The recipes are split into nine sections, beginning with the all-important Morning Milks – potent small meals that that are great for easing you into the day, as well as out of it. These are followed by more substantial Parana (breakfasts), some of which also make good lunches and suppers – look out for the moon signs which indicate what time of day each recipe is suited to. Then come the Sweet Treats – yes, these come before lunch in this book. This is because lunch, which I like to call 'Surya Agni' ('Sun Fire' in Sanskrit) is when your digestion is at its strongest. This is the best time of day to enjoy a main meal, and since sweet foods are the most heavy to digest as well as the most satisfying, in Ayurveda your starter is small and sweet and leaves you feeling just right, rather than eating savoury foods until you're full and then pushing yourself over the edge with pudding! Pick lunch and dinner from the next two sections – Pakti Bowls and Soups and Stews. A cooked meal is considered ideal in Ayurveda, and this book celebrates the soups and stews that make the perfect easy-to-digest supper. As wonderfully homely as they are, sometimes we need some crunch and so my 'Pakti bowls' (Pakti's meanings include 'cooked, dignity, digestion' in Sanskrit) are easy-to-digest hot salads and cooked dishes with plenty of texture. There is also a section for celebratory dishes – the kinds of things you save for entertaining – followed by a section dedicated to condiments and side dishes that can complete or elevate any meal. Last but not least, there's an Apothecary section with medicinal teas and a medicine cabinet full of age-old recipes to support you through anything that doesn't make you feel good.

The recipes are satisfying and nourishing, and are supported by essential information to show how they work together to enhance health and vitality. All the dishes are straightforward and make use of readily available ingredients, from my favourite Ayurvedic classics – including traditional recipes from around the world that already incorporate Ayurvedic principles – to some delicious Indian-inspired dishes and beautiful recipes that I've created to fit the principles. Most recipes suit everyone and can be tweaked to suit individuals – for instance, you'll notice a little icon alongside recipes asking you how you are feeling according to the Doshas (see pages 270–275). To understand whether to add extra ginger for Mum, greens for Dad or fats for someone else, read up on the Doshas in Part 3: Ayurveda Explained.

If you're used to big flavours, the recipes here might seem subtle at first, but that is part of the experience. Ayurvedic cooking doesn't rely on garlic and onion, or sting you with chilli, lemon and vinegar. Too often we use foods (and other stimuli) to distract us from our crazy lives or to kick us out of our fatigue.

Ayurvedic cooking is about following guiding principles rather than rules. It's the ultimate way to know how to balance your inner world with your ever-changing environment. I hope that this book helps you feel more connected, well-rounded and excited about life. Once you can put this knowledge to use intuitively and find your groove, you can step out of it with confidence now and then to fully experience the rich tapestry of life, knowing that Ayurveda has got your back.

The story of Ayurveda

This is a big story to tell, and at every level it is completely fascinating. In this book I look at the essentials of Ayurveda so that we can begin to see the depth and gravitas of this ancient knowledge and how best to begin to understand it, and from there how we can work with it. Sounds a bit complicated already? Yes, that was my first thought when I initially stumbled across this idea, but not so now. Essentially, implementing Ayurveda is like learning a new language, a new way of looking at things that is probably a little different from a more linear Western way of doing things. Trust me, this all begins to make sense when you immerse yourself in this new holistic (which comes from the word 'whole') approach, relearning the fundamentals of health and viewing life through a 360-degree lens.

THE MOST DEVELOPED MEDICAL SYSTEM

Ayurveda is the mother of all healing systems. It developed thousands of years ago to help people sync with nature and thrive in an ever-changing environment. Bringing 5,000 years of human experience to the table since its birthplace in India, it is now practised all over the world. Ayurveda translates as the science or knowledge of life – 'Ayur' meaning life and 'Veda' meaning knowledge in ancient Sanskrit. It's worth noting that Sanskrit is said to to be the oldest, most rich and systematic language, having influenced several Western languages and holding a status in India and across Southeast Asia similar to that of Latin and Greek in the Western world. Ayurveda was passed down as an oral tradition from one generation to the next until it was committed to text in around 1000 BC, in 'the Vedas', which are amongst the world's oldest-existing work of literature.

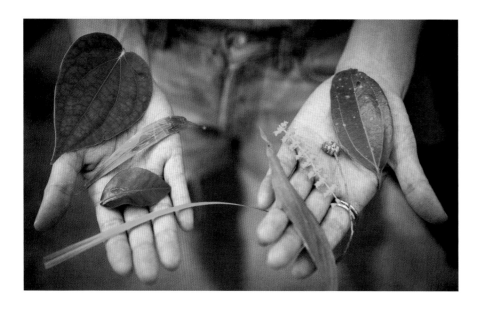

Along with Chinese traditional medicine, with which it shares many similar concepts, Ayurveda is said to be one of the oldest, if not the oldest, and most developed medical system. It was created to help people maintain health and longevity. In some rural parts of India it has been the only healthcare system for thousands of years, even though under British rule Ayurveda was banned in 1835 in favour of European medicine, which is a much more recent phenomenon. Thankfully for us, the poor continued to use the tried-and-tested traditional treatments for their ailments, so Ayurveda survived underground until 1947, when India became a free nation and Ayurveda received full recognition as a medical system.

A PHILOSOPHY FOR LIFE

The principles of this ancient holistic healing system are based on the belief that health and wellbeing depend on a delicate balance between the mind, body and spirit, which are all unified, so therefore being ill in one area affects the others. As opposed to viewing health as simply an absence of disease, Ayurveda defines wellbeing as reaching and maintaining this unique balance. Ayurveda focuses on promoting good health as a proactive method of warding off disease, and working with the principle of 'like increases like', offers a comprehensive approach to treating disease by slowly unravelling the causes of ill health through remedying the imbalances. So just as disease manifests, it can also unwind. Ayurveda is an energetic system that addresses internal imbalances which prevent us from obtaining optimum health and healing. These include how we eat, move and live in our world. Because we are all individuals, Ayurveda works on the idea that no single diet or lifestyle works for everyone ('one man's food is another man's poison', so to speak), but that food, daily routines and how we connect to our environment are essential for maintaining a physically and emotionally balanced state.

Ayurvedic cooking is in itself part of the medicine of wellbeing. The principles of Ayurveda can therefore find a home in everyday food practices, and manifest themselves in meals through ingredients, preparation and the process of eating. In Ayurvedic practice, meals are nutritious, nurturing, wholesome and satisfying. In short, they are comforting, supporting, restoring and revitalising.

A vast treasure trove of knowledge about natural healthcare, Ayurveda encompasses all aspects of your wellbeing, from breathing to digestion, and supporting you from birth to the end of your life. A major principle of Ayurveda is that we, like everything else in the universe, are made up of the same five key Elements (see page 15), the difference being that everyone and everything is its own unique blend. Ayurveda teaches us to work with our constitution by observing who we are, how we feel, what we like and what we are like. Learning and understanding your real nature is the name of the game in life, and from there you can live a truly authentic life that suits you and allows your health – mind, body and spirit – to flourish.

Basic principles of Ayurveda

Ayurveda is the ancient Indian art of living a more healthy, wholesome life. It evolved alongside yoga thousands of years ago. It's difficult to make a plan or map of something that is as deep as it is wide, and this list is by no means exhaustive, but here you can find the basic principles of Ayurveda in a glossary form and see how they relate to each other. Nature is recognised by its characteristics, and these form the language of Ayurveda.

WE ARE ONE

Individual life is part of universal life. We are truly microcosms of the universe and are governed by forces bigger than us: the Sun, the Moon and the wind. Science and Ayurveda tell us that if we break everything down, we are made of the same atoms and energy. Everything around us is a recycling of that energy, and from Ayurveda's perspective we need to harness that energy in its different forms to sustain us.

Metaphorically speaking, we are as a drop in the ocean, and at the same time, as Rumi says, 'You are the entire ocean in a drop.' It stands to reason that outside energies affect us in our day-to-day life. The world operates in a rhythm; for example, the cycles of the Sun, Moon, tides and seasons, and so do we – anything less and we feel the effects of moving in the opposite direction to the forces and life gets tough. Being in sync and going with the flow of nature is the way forward.

THE THREE PSYCHIC ENERGIES FORM THE CIRCLE OF LIFE

Sattva, Rajas and Tamas are the three psychic energies that form the very fabric of creation (or pure consciousness). They interact to create a unique and harmonious flow – the circle of life. Everything that 'is' goes through the process of creation – Rajas (or kinetic energy) signifies birth; Sattva (or potential energy) signifies maintenance; and Tamas (or inertia) signifies destruction. It is born, lives and dies.

When we refer to these three energies in terms of food, it is like the life of an apple: some part of it is ripening, some of it is ripe and then it is overripe – all three are always present. When we apply this understanding to our general diet we want to concentrate on the Sattvic, the 'ripe' foods, as much as possible because these are perfectly developed. This is fresh food, grown naturally, treated naturally and consumed naturally. Rajasic foods, which include onions, garlic, chilli, lemon, tomatoes, aubergine, tea, coffee, meat, eggs and commercial condiments, are very stimulating, just like the sharpness of the underripe apple, and too much of these foods can lead to stress and anxiety. Then there are Tamasic foods such as meat; fried foods; leftovers; reheated, processed, preserved, tinned and refined foods;

junk foods and soft drinks; commercial cakes and pastries; confectionery; and even mushrooms, which are said to have a heavy energy on the body – too much makes you lethargic and mentally dull. Avoiding most Rajasic and Tamasic foods in your day-to-day life makes sense for anyone who is interested in an Ayurvedic diet. However, it is also important to have the other two psychic energies present in our life and in our diet – after all, they are also part of the circle of life, so in this cookbook you will find natural Rajasic and Tamasic foods used in small amounts.

Sattvic, Rajasic and Tamasic are more than just qualities in food – they are a way of life. We can think of Sattvic when waking in the morning at a perfectly balanced time. Rajasic might be the wired person waking too early and relying on stimulants to power through the day. Tamasic would be the one who wakes late and feels lethargic, using junk food to get through. Choosing to do and eat more of the Sattvic things in life helps to make us clear-minded, balanced and spiritually aware.

THE FIVE ELEMENTS ARE THE BUILDING BLOCKS OF LIFE

The three psychic energies form the five Elements – Space, Air, Fire, Water and Earth – the building blocks of life from which everything in the universe is constructed. Since the human body is therefore also a combination of these five Elements, it needs the right amount of the vital nutrients found within each of the Elements for the wellbeing of various parts of the body. Too much or too little of any of these natural nutrients leads to illness. On a subtle level, each human being has a variation of these Elements that's different from any other human being and it's in this way that Ayurveda also recognises our individual needs.

THE THREE DOSHAS REPRESENT MIND–BODY TYPES

The five Elements are categorised into three mind–body types known as Doshas, which describe certain characteristics based on the Elements that they contain. They are: Vata (prominent Air), Pitta (prominent Fire) and Kapha (prominent Earth). Each of us have all three Doshas in varying proportions. Our mind–body health is dependent on our own unique balance. To understand more about the Doshas and how they can be used to great effect in Ayurveda, turn to page 270.

THERE ARE 20 QUALITIES TO ACHIEVE BALANCE

Everything in our physical and mental world can be described as a mixture of 10 pairs of opposites known as the 20 Qualities (see pages 283–284). Ayurveda believes that if we expose ourselves to more of the Qualities that are causing an ailment, it increases or aggravates that ailment. Only an opposite Quality can combat or pacify it and help bring it back into balance.

THE FIVE SENSES RELATE TO SIX TASTES

We are made of the same five Elements as everything else, so our sensory impressions are considered crucial to health in Ayurveda. Just as the food that we select via our Senses creates our bodily tissues, our hearing, touch, sight, taste and smell also determine the quality of our thoughts and emotions. We can therefore use our five Senses: hearing (ears), touch (skin), sight (eyes), taste (mouth) and smell (nose) – which directly correspond to the five Elements of Space, Air, Fire, Water and Earth – to bring balance to ourselves and our three Doshas. We can sense Qualities through our five Senses, to make choices that bring balance to our health.

When it comes to food, one of these Senses is particularly important – that of taste. According to Ayurveda, there are six Tastes (see pages 285–287), which describe the attributes of any food. Since food is made of the same Elements as ourselves, we can determine the correct ratios of different food types to suit us as individuals.

THERE ARE THREE ESSENTIAL FORCES

Prana, linked to Air, is the vital life-force energy that flows through us and all living things; and can be enhanced through freshly prepared foods and other lifestyle practices such as yoga. Tejas is the inner radiance, our courage for life which is responsible for the metabolic processes of the body and is linked to the element of Fire. These together become Ojas – our overall vigour, immunity and strength which is linked to the heart and the element of Water. Foods that are deemed Sattvic are high in Prana.

FOOD IS MEDICINE

It stands to reason that the better the quality of the food, the better the medicine. Just as we are created from the five Elements, so too are foods. Food = Energy. Each food is defined by one of the six Tastes, which helps us to work out which contain the elemental building blocks that we are in need of in our body, and makes it simple for us to get a wide variety of foods to support our growth.

Ayurveda's approach to choosing the right foods for yourself at any given time, can be compared to putting on a jumper when you start to feel cold – you don't think about it and it isn't a big effort – it happens naturally. Many of us don't know how to express what our body needs and even if we do, we might override our biological intuition, simply because we've never been taught to place any importance on it.

Even more powerful than the food we eat is how we eat it, and more powerful than that is how it is digested to boost our digestive fire.

The ancient texts of Ayurveda state that meat is a medicine. Just like other foods, it is only a medicine in the right dose, taken at the right time, prepared in the right way and suitable for the individual. Meat is Rajasic and Tamasic, so although it shouldn't be a staple of your diet or dominate your plate as Sattvic foods should, it can still be part of a healthy diet. While the right amount will both invigorate and ground certain individuals, the same amount can also stress and depress others, so we need to be conscious in both in the sourcing and eating of meat.

HEALTH AND DISEASE ARE TWO SIDES OF THE SAME COIN

Ayurveda is about understanding your food and environment through their Qualities and how they affect us. Disease means dis-ease – not being at ease with oneself. It's our body being out of whack – not communicating with itself and out

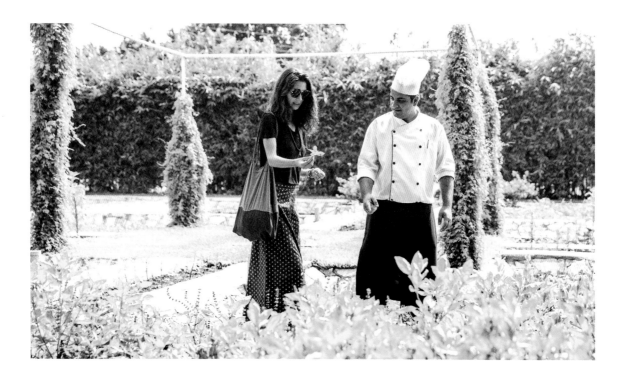

of rhythm with its environment. If we eat too much of the wrong foods, our digestion is hindered and toxins can accumulate.

A SUPPORTIVE LIFESTYLE IS ESSENTIAL

The most important contribution that anyone can make to their overall state of health is managing their everyday lifestyle. It's all about finding your rhythm so you can go with the flow. We have choices in our daily diet and routine, and these ultimately create our body, mind and consciousness. The more we understand these choices, the more we support our continued health and happiness. See more on this in the Living la Vida 'Veda section (see page 288).

Sleep is one of the pillars of Ayurveda, and is considered to be as important as diet in maintaining health and balance in the body. Sleep is the time when the body is able to repair and heal itself. In the East exercise is swapped for rest if you're suffering a cold or feeling rundown – you are already depleted and your body needs energy reserves to fight the infection. In the West we are encouraged to power on through, with the help of some handy pharmacy extras. However without appropriate rest we cannot absorb all the good stuff that we've done for our ourselves – from food through to meditation and movement – and our body won't have the energy to make light work of the not-so-favourable stuff. Make time for yourself and try the cleanse and reset on page 290.

Yoga and Ayurveda evolved at around the same time and complement each other. Yoga is not about flexibility and strength or exercise, as is often portrayed here in the West – like Ayurveda, it is the union of the mind, body and soul, with a focus on health in order to facilitate regular periods of meditation to reach enlightenment.

Ayurveda today

'Without proper nutrition, medicine is of little use... With proper nutrition, medicine is of little need' – Charaka Samhita, an ancient classical text on Ayurveda

Right now, a revolution is happening. A growing number of people are beginning to reject the conveniences and fast pace of modern life in favour of a more natural, more grounded one, where we know the source and environmental impact of the foods that we buy. A new fashion for wellbeing has resulted in practices that were once considered alternative, such as yoga, meditation and mindfulness, becoming mainstream. As quickly as we're moving with the demands of technology there is the same strong pull that seeks a move back to nature, as we struggle with the irony that the more time-saving technology we create, the less time we seem to have.

WHY THE BIG CHANGE?

In the last century the power over our own health – the knowledge of what, when and how we should nourish ourselves – has been lost. In 2002 the World Health Organization (WHO) released a statement saying that the biggest threat to public health is our own lifestyles. In an age where the US, a leading nation with first-world healthcare, lists medical intervention as the third most common cause of death after cancer and heart disease, the big question is: where does that leave us? There are many factors at play, and many seem beyond our control, leaving us feeling dissatisfied and helpless. 'Cured' and 'healed' have become medical words. We are living in a time when most think we cannot 'get well' without the intervention of medicine, surgery and people who have studied allopathy. In an era where the concept of food as medicine is scoffed at and healthcare has become a disease-management system, the fusion of the holistic and considered approach from the East has never been more needed. It's time for us to look at our whole being, not just diet and exercise.

Long before we relied on science, and after we'd pushed back the wilderness and had food to eat as well as shelter, we discovered the optimal way to care for ourselves. A mix of self-care, self-fulfilment and community, all of which we understood had to fit side by side with nature. Slowly, we are seeing the return of this ancient wisdom from cultures all over the world, and with it, Ayurveda.

The Indian traditions of yoga and Ayurveda were first introduced to the rest of the world in the 1960s, encouraging people to live a happy, healthy and conscious lifestyle. As has been the fashion in the West, the physical side of yoga took off in a big way and it has become the myriad brands and branches of yoga that we see today. Meditation and mindfulness, the more spiritual aspects, followed slowly behind, in part because they are harder to market, less tangible to 'prove', too closely linked to religion and sometimes seen as hippyish, backward or self-indulgent. Rather than a tool to prepare you for meditation, yoga became a tool to prepare you for the beach.

Now Ayurveda, 'the knowledge' of individual self-care and growth, completes the circle with the greater end product of benefiting our world. 'Ayur', or 'life', is understood as four parts: the physical body, the mind, the soul and the senses. Compare this to Western medicine, which focuses on the body and only more recently on the mind – we need to get to grips with the idea that everything is connected! The latest research into quantum physics echoes the Ayurvedic principles that we are made of the same elements as everything else in the universe and are moved by the same forces that move the oceans, the winds, the stars and the planets. It stands to reason that outside energies affect our day-to-day life, and so the modern lifestyle of artificial light, 24-hour technology, industrially produced food, global transportation, planet desecration and pollution pushes us out of sync with the natural rhythm of the world. Going with the flow of nature is the smooth way forward, anything less and things get tough. Yoga is described as the practice of Ayurveda, uniting the mind, body and spirit as a powerful system for creating health, nourishment and healing at home. Using ancient wisdom alongside modern tools, we have a tremendous resource to transform ourselves and our environment if we apply it to our daily lives.

Today Ayurveda is still flourishing in India and Sri Lanka and is now practised all over the world, often working in harmony with modern medicine. In the same way that acupuncture was once seen as 'woo woo', because it could not be proven as to why or how it worked, it is now accepted as a valuable 'alternative' or 'complementary' therapy to allopathy. There is actually no greater catalyst to health than beginning to look at your whole life based on Ayurvedic principles. It is the influence behind all natural therapies that we use today: acupuncture, marma therapy, herbalism, homeopathy – we have Ayurveda to thank for all of them.

THE KEY TO OPTIMUM HEALTH

Ayurveda helps me to strike balance in a world where we are constantly thrown around like a yo-yo, and 20 years of living and working in a big city has, for me, emphasised the importance of routine and a stable home. I could not operate as I do without the grounding principles of Ayurveda: from my daily meditations and Sundays spent lying in the park, to the rituals of going to bed early, rising early and eating homemade, well-cooked suppers. While I'm not ready to hang up my high heels just yet, I do everything I can to bring about a balance between my urban habitat and my natural soul, and my first port of call is the food I eat.

Dipping your toes into the pool of Ayurveda might seem intimidating at first, but the good news is that its overall message is simple: Ayurveda recognises above all else the importance of digestion, and that the strength of your digestive fire is key to good health. So if you focus on supporting your digestion with your lifestyle choices you don't have to fixate on food types or study Ayurveda in depth. Balance means taking a holistic approach to life with a self-awareness that enables you stay you on track and bring you back if needs be. Once you reach a balance, you can really start to understand what makes you tick and what doesn't float your boat. This is the starting point of intuitively mastering what you need to do in order to maintain your optimum health.

The golden guidelines

Since every person is uniquely different, as well as ever-changing, Ayurveda is all about natural guidelines, which soon become 'second nature'. Helpfully there are also universal rules: the dos and don'ts of food combining, which we can apply wherever possible to protect our digestive fire, rather than having to be fully in tune with what's going on with you today.

GOLDEN GUIDELINES

How much I'm able to apply these principles to my life varies. When I'm at home and in a routine I'm pretty good at applying them because I've built my home around them; I've organised my life to include them. When I'm travelling, it totally depends on the structure of my days and where I am, so at these times I draw on many other sources of nourishment to keep me balanced, such as meditation, affirmations or positive thinking, or I just enjoy some wild abandonment and go with the flow for a week or two!

The details below will help you to reconnect to your own intuition at your own pace, so that you can eventually be guided by what works for you. That may mean remaining strict on certain points or in certain situations because it makes all the difference to how you feel – for example, caffeine really affects me when I'm working because my job is already very stimulating, but a coffee on holiday leaves me totally chilled. Or it may mean you use the principles more loosely to keep you feeling good in general; for example, every time a healthy choice is available, you take it. Deciding what works for you is just one of the joys of this philosophy.

- Fresh is best – if you have to eat leftovers, make sure they are no older than a day or two and sauté with ginger and black pepper first.
- Avoid caffeine after lunch and avoid it full stop if you're feeling wired.
- Enjoy a balance of Tamasic and Rajasic foods around a central diet of Sattvic foods.
- Don't eat the same foods for more than two meals in a row.
- Don't make a meal out of a meal!
- Reduce the amount of packaged, processed, canned and frozen food in your diet.
- Be moderate and avoid extremes – for instance, too much or too little food.
- Eat the six Tastes in every meal for a well-balanced plate (see pages 285–287).
- Choose foods and lifestyle practices with opposite Qualities to your dominant Dosha (see pages 283–284) to bring or maintain balance.
- Choose organic and local wherever possible, especially for animal products.
- Water quality – go for filtered, distilled or spring water.
- Say yes to real fats and natural sweeteners, according to how you feel on a daily basis.
- Respect the food, the time of day, the seasons and your digestive capability.
- Let vegetables and fruit make up 50 to 60 per cent of your daily food intake.
- You can eat all kinds of foods but minimise those that are not helpful for your

constitution (for example, eat such foods only every 5–7 days or every 2 weeks if your digestion is weak).
– Stay present with your food.
– Cooked foods are easier to digest.
– Stick to warm or hot drinks ('room-temperature' water is too variable, depending on where you live!) – similarly with food, although occasional 'cool' food is okay if it is warmed thoroughly in the mouth.
– Drink milk after simmering it for 15 minutes with water (and spices, if desired) to make it more digestible.
– Stick to freshly made yoghurt and cheese rather than shop-bought yoghurt and mature cheeses.
– Eat legumes, pseudocereals or grains with one of the following spices: ginger, cinnamon, black pepper or turmeric.

FOOD-COMBINING RULES

Exploring the concept of food-combining can be a little daunting at first! When you look at what doesn't go together in Ayurveda it can feel as if you're left with a limited number of options, especially if these combinations have made up your staple diet until now. This is quite typical of a Western diet, but it is only when these incompatabilities are practised together and on a regular basis that you will experience ill-health, so you don't have to be exhaustive with this approach unless your health really needs addressing. There are, of course, times when you have to or want to eat such food combinations, and if your digestive fire is strong you won't feel any immediate ill-effects. In general, if you follow these guidelines you will experience benefits both in the long and short term. This detailed list is also very useful for people who suffer from digestive discomfort sporadically after eating a meal and can't put their finger on what the trigger might be.

WHAT TO AVOID, AT A GLANCE
– Milk and yoghurt in excess. Be sure to prepare milk first by cooking it.
– Wet, green, leafy veggies (like spinach) or salads in excess.
– Pickled or fermented foods in excess.
– Heating honey (always use raw).
– Drinking more than three cups of tea – herbs and spices are powerful!
– Eating more than one source of protein per meal.
– Mixing salt with dairy milk or sour foods (it curdles) – except for ricotta or paneer.
– Mixing equal weights of ghee with honey.
– Mixing milk with fish.
– Eating ice cream, yoghurt or cheese at night.
– Eating sweets and oily food at night.
– Eating heavy sweets and foods early in the morning.
– Eating very sour, salty and pungent things in the afternoon.

So bang goes the cheese plate for dessert, yoghurt with fruit for breakfast, surf 'n' turf, chicken with rice, and sipping on those giant iced fizzy drinks, right? Not so fast … A good digestive fire can handle these incompatabilities, day in and day out; however, it can eventually weaken. Having said that, the body works hard to find balance and we get used to certain food combinations and eating patterns, especially where it has been part of our culture for thousands of years.

But if you suffer digestive discomfort and feel less than your best, Ayurveda could be your saving grace.

You have choices and chances, so take them where possible. As one of my teachers, Gary Gorrow, reminded me:

'The thing to note is that Ayurveda is a very compassionate and accommodating science. It doesn't set out to impose itself upon others but rather prefers to foster innate wisdom, and that is the source of one's guidance along the path of life. Ayurveda will simply seek to harmonise the influence of things – such as if you want to eat cheese, sprinkle black pepper on it, and so on and so forth.'

	DIFFICULT TO DIGEST WITH …	WORKS WELL WITH …
BEANS	Fruit, milk, cheese, yoghurt, eggs, meat, fish	Grains, vegetables, other beans, nuts, seeds
BUTTER + GHEE	Ghee is a better option for most foods	Grains, vegetables, beans, nuts, seeds, meat, fish, eggs, cooked fruit
CHEESE + YOGHURT	Incompatible with each other, as well as with fruit, beans, meat, fish, eggs, milk, hot drinks and nightshades (potato, pepper, tomato, aubergine, cayenne pepper and paprika)	Grains, vegetables
MILK	Salt, or any other food, especially fish.	Milk is best enjoyed alone... except to make rice pudding or porridge, or with dates or almonds
EGGS	Milk, cheese, yoghurt, fruit (especially melons), beans, Kitchari, potatoes, meat, fish	Grains, non-starchy vegetables
FRUITS	Any other food (aside from other fruit). Exceptions: dates with milk, some cooked/dried fruit combinations Melon is best eaten on its own. Banana is best eaten in the afternoon after lunch	Other fruits with similar qualities (such as citrus together, apples with pears, a berry medley, etc.). Choose limes over lemons, especially with tomatoes and cucumber
GRAINS	Fruit	Beans, vegetables, other grains, eggs, meat, fish, nuts, seeds, cheese, yoghurt
VEG	Fruit, milk	Grains, beans, other vegetables, meat, fish, nuts, seeds, eggs. Also with cheese and yoghurt (except nightshade vegetables: pepper, aubergine, potato, tomato)
LEFT-OVERS	Freshly cooked foods	Other leftovers from the same meal, but only on occasion, preferably not more than 24 hours old and first sautéed throughly with ghee and black pepper
RAW FOODS	Cooked foods (especially in large quantities)	Other raw foods, ideally in small quantities. Avoid raw after four, best at lunchtime and in warmer weather

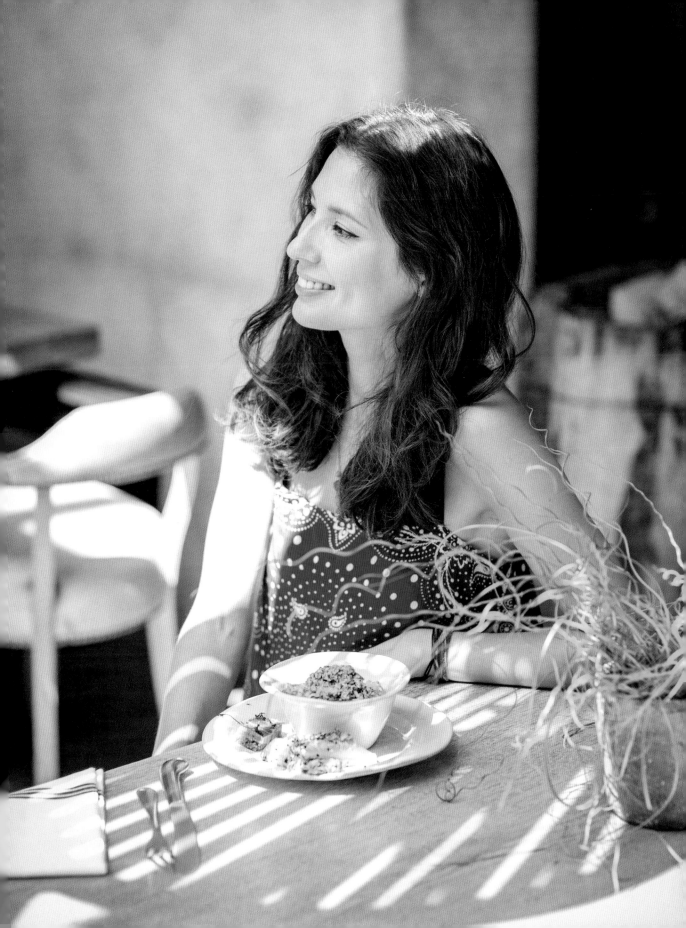

The Ayurvedic pantry

Local foods, fresh from the farm or garden (including quality dairy, see page 32), are always welcome on the plate, but these are not the only foods that deliver energy and nutrition. The following Ayurvedic pantry list sets out all the ingredients you can keep in the cupboard ready to accompany and complement your meals. Most of the ingredients are available at large supermarkets, but you could also try popping into your local Asian shops to learn even more about these foods from the people who eat them daily. Buy the best quality you can afford, avoid precooked or refined versions of these foods, and just because many of these have a long shelf-life, don't leave them hanging around for a lifetime – fresh is best!

Keep variety in your food choices. Some ingredients, such as mung dal and white basmati rice, are easy to digest for all Doshas, and a small amount of spices used medicinally work in your everyday cooking, otherwise try not to overeat any ingredients, so as not to aggravate your Dosha. Check in with yourself – what worked last week when you were in your routine might not be your friend today.

PULSES

A staple in Ayurvedic cooking, pulses offer excellent and affordable vegetarian protein. If prepared properly they are easy to digest. They are usually available dried and in three forms: the whole pulse, and the split pulse either halved with skin on, or halved and with the skin removed. The last is the easist to digest.

The term 'dal' is often used to refer to lentils, or to describe any soup or stew dish containing lentils, but it actually refers to the hulled split version of several pulses. For example, mung dal is the hulled split version of mung beans. As a general rule, all dried pulses require some soaking – from 15 minutes for some split types to overnight for whole. However, red split lentils are the exception as they cook very quickly. Avoid the sachets of precooked or tinned beans and lentils – not only are these less Sattvic, they are also a bit 'windy pops', if you know what I mean! Cooking your own lentils is simple, cheap and fresh.

ADZUKI BEANS

Ruby-red adzuki (also known as aduki beans) are popular in Asian desserts (sometimes as red bean paste), as well as in macrobiotics. They are also considered amongst the most digestible beans, but soak them overnight before cooking. Their astringent and drying qualities make them ideal to balance Kapha and Pitta, however Vata should eat them only occasionally.

BLACK TURTLE BEANS

Satisfying and brimming with protein and fibre, black turtle beans have a rich and earthy flavour that makes stews and soups incredibly comforting. Soak them and spice them up for digestibility.

MUNG BEANS

This little green bean is easy to cook, cheap, versatile and one of the most easily digested legumes. I've used it in the cookbook for dals, sweet soups and even a bread recipe (see page 232). It also has a long history of healing, cleansing and nourishment and is the perfect detox food. Mung dal – hulled split beans – is not as easy to find in supermarkets as the whole green ones with their jackets on, but is worth seeking out at your local Asian store if your digestion is weak. Make sure you soak the whole beans overnight and rinse before cooking. They are filling and satisfying, while being low-calorie and having a diuretic effect. Mung beans have a cooling effect, which makes them perfect for summer.

RED SPLIT LENTILS

A good staple for home as they don't need soaking before cooking, making them perfect for quick dals – especially great if you are an impatient or lazy cook! Throw them in a pot together with spices to make them even easier to digest and you have a delicious meal. Vata types should eat them only occasionally and with plenty of spices and ghee.

BROWN LENTILS

This hassle-free legume is easy to find and cook. It's a cupboard lifesaver that make a great last-minute addition to dinner. They hold their shape even after cooking, so work in salads.

TOOR DAL

Also known as pigeon peas, toor dal has a nutty and sweet flavour. Use it for a comforting bowl of dal, soup or kitchari. It is slightly more difficult to find than some of the other pulses, but worth seeking out to enjoy its different flavour.

URAD DAL

Urad beans have black jackets which come off to reveal a white split bean. Whole urad beans are used in black dal, but take ages to cook and are hard on the digestion so avoid regularly. The split bean is easier to digest especially when soaked, ground and fermented lightly, as in the Dosa recipe on page 80.

CHANA DAL

This is a type of chickpea that has been hulled and split (halved). If you have difficulties telling them apart from yellow split peas, you're not alone! Sometimes they're even sold with the wrong label. Chana dal holds its shape when cooked, which is great for dry curries and to add texture to dishes, and their skin looks more wrinkled than yellow split peas. It is high in fibre, has a low GI, and is used for making your own gram flour (see below). Make sure you soak them overnight or for a couple of hours before cooking.

GRAM FLOUR

Also known as besan, gram flour is from the chana family. You can interchange it with chickpea flour although gram flour is easy to find. This versatile, protein-rich flour is a staple ingredient in Asia and the Middle East. It is a beloved beauty secret in Ayurveda and in India – everything from removing pimples and facial hair to making an invigorating body scrub. It is from the pulse family, so make sure it is cooked well, otherwise it can taste like grass!

WHEAT AND GLUTEN

Traditionally wheat was considered a nourishing food, but modern-day wheat is much higher in gluten (the protein of the wheat) than it has been in previous generations, making it sticky and often leading to inflammation in our systems, which may cause discomfort. Thanks to a wide variety of pseudocereals and pulses, as well as teff and basmati rice that are gentler on your digestion, it's easy to leave wheat and therefore large amounts of gluten, out of these recipes. If you can find ancient varieties of wheat such as einkorn, or even spelt, barley and kamut, which have much lower gluten content, then enjoy them in the traditional Ayurvedic way – which is often as a food in winter when heavier, warmer foods are required to help balance. This book is about finding your optimal balance to achieve optimal health, and if you are lucky to have a robust digestion you should be able to tolerate gluten as part of a varied, Sattvic diet. There's no need to get caught up in the 'Free-from aisle' in the local supermarket – plenty of whole, nutritious foods are free from gluten.

GRAINS AND SEEDS

FLAXSEEDS

Also known as 'linseeds', flaxseeds are oily, slimy and full of fibre. To get all their benefits, grind them fresh when you need them. This makes them better for your wallet and health, especially since they oxidise quickly. High in fibre and oil, these are great for constipation. Since they are mucilaginous and hold moisture, Kapha doesn't need much of these. You can take advantage of their properties for thickening broths, dressings, porridges or drinks.

BASMATI RICE

White basmati is the golden grain of Ayurveda. Brown rice has a higher nutritional value than white but is not as easy to digest. To find out how to cook it, see page 267. Aged basmati rice, available at supermarkets, is even better for all Doshas.

RICE FLOUR

You can make your own from white basmati rice if you have a strong blender or a grinder. Otherwise use a small amount of shop-bought white or brown rice flour – it won't be basmati, so avoid sweet rice flour, which is much stickier and more elastic. Always read the labels before buying!

SATTVIC VS RAJASIC + TAMASIC FOODS

This cookbook is built on fresh, wholesome ingredients considered Sattvic in Ayurveda for their Prana – life-giving goodness (see page 16). Since Rajasic and Tamasic foods also have their place in Ayurveda, small amounts of unprocessed foods in those categories will be found in the recipes – from garlic and onion to meat and mushrooms. Ayurveda recommends avoiding eating leftovers and cooking fresh where possible – you soon get used to cooking the portions that you need. For more notes on how to enjoy food, read the golden guidelines on pages 20–21 and check out the secrets on lively Agni on page 282.

TEFF FLOUR

If you've ever had Ethiopian food, you've probably eaten injera bread, which is made from fermented teff flour. Teff seeds are so tiny (roughly the size of poppy seeds), that they can't be husked, so all of the nutrient-rich benefits are eaten. Teff is gluten-free and high in calcium, fibre, iron and protein. Its flavour is nutty and sweet and a bit chocolatey – making it great for gluten-free baking, especially if mixed with other flours to add extra nutrition and complexity to the taste.

RAGI

A type of millet, ragi is also known as finger millet. It is usually bought as a brown-pinkish flour that has a delicious chocolatey taste and can be used for gluten-free rotis. Because the plant is rarely attacked by pests, it can usually be grown without pesticides. It's light and digestible and its warming qualities can balance Kapha, but aggravate Pitta and Vata when eaten in large amounts. Ragi is a great source of calcium, as well as important amino acids, and it helps with weight control, stabilises blood sugar, lowers cholesterol and aids sleep. Find it at your local Asian store. Unfortunately regular millet and millet flour is not the best substitute for it – buckwheat flour is a closer alternative.

PSEUDOCEREALS

Technically these are not grains but the seeds of fruits, and they are much higher in protein. The most common is quinoa, which you can now buy homegrown in Essex, followed by buckwheat and amaranth (see below). They are available whole or in flour form. It's best to soak whole pseudocereals as you would pulses and grains.

AMARANTH

A sweet, nutty and gluten-free seed, usually used like a grain in breads, porridges and stews. This versatile Aztec staple is high in protein compared to grains. It's perfect for Kapha, but Vata should eat it only occasionally and with a generous drizzle of ghee to balance dryness.

BUCKWHEAT

This nutty and earthy fruit seed is gluten-free. Use it in a similar way to grains. It is the solution to keeping warm and cosy when the temperature drops. Its astringent qualities are ideal for Kapha, but Pitta should be mindful of its heating qualities. The flour is a delicious gluten-free alternative for pancakes and is known as *sarrasin* in France. Buckwheat noodles (also known as

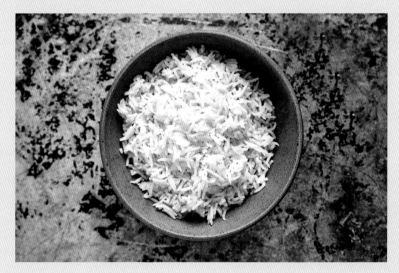

soba noodles in Japan) are naturally gluten-free, but check the ingredients list on packets as buckwheat flour is often mixed with wheat flour. Enjoy the nutty taste in soups, hot salads and as an alternative to spaghetti.

FATS

For a few generations now, many natural fats have been replaced with processed and refined oils as 'healthier' alternatives. Extra-virgin olive oil has thankfully remained at centre stage and recently butter has returned to its rightful place and been joined by coconut oil. Ghee is the fat favoured in Ayurveda – the deliciously sweet essence of butter, which is a very balancing ingredient.

HERBS AND SPICES

Behind the magic of Ayurvedic food, herbs and spices are respected medicinal foods, so unless prescribed by practitioners, enjoy them little and often. The main spices in my spice drawer are cinnamon, turmeric, fenugreek, fennel seeds, cumin, cardamom, curry leaves, turmeric, asofoetida, mustard seeds, coriander and ground ginger. Pink peppercorns and saffron are a bonus! Most of these spices are pungent and therefore heating, so Pitta types should keep these to a minimum.

MUSTARD SEEDS

Pungent and warming, mustard seeds are great for digestion, helping with gas and cramps, and can be used liberally to balance Kapha and Vata, but can be aggravating for Pitta. The black and brown seeds have a stronger flavour than yellow and white. When cooked in ghee they have a nutty rather than fiery flavour. Once they start popping, remove them from the heat, because you don't want to burn them, then stir and serve.

PINK PEPPERCORNS

These are not actually peppercorns but ripe berries that add a fruity flavour, along with a peppery bite. They are great for adding a touch of colour when used as a seasoning (lovely with fish) and add an unusual but delicious taste when incorporated into dressings, desserts and stews. Pink pepper has antiseptic, disinfectant and diuretic properties that can help with menstrual cramps and urinary infections, and can also be chewed as a simple remedy for coughs and colds. Be careful not to overdo it as it can be slightly toxic in large quantities. It belongs to the cashew family, and is not safe for those with tree-nut allergies.

GARAM MASALA

An aromatic spice mix, garam masala is used to add flavour and complexity to dishes like curries. You can either use shop-bought, or make it fresh (see pages 262–265).

GINGER

Wonderfully flavoursome, ginger is a signature healing ingredient in Ayurveda, being anti-inflammatory and antibacterial. It helps digestion and nausea and has an analgesic effect on joint pain. Add to a mug with hot water to clear congestion, awaken the taste buds, help saliva production and support the digestive process. It also stimulates the metabolism and is a great detox ingredient. If you buy organic, keep the skin on; if not, scrape it off with a teaspoon. Dry ginger is more heating than fresh, so Pitta types should use fresh and less of it.

CORIANDER

Both leaves and seeds are great for digestion and help with allergies, making them the perfect addition to spring cooking. The leaves are cooling and bitter, which is particularly beneficial for Pitta. Coriander kills meat-spoiling bacteria and fungi, which is why it's frequently used in meat dishes from India to Morocco. Coriander seeds can be used whole, but are usually used ground in dals or vegetable dishes. They are cooling, sweet, astringent and slightly warming.

CUMIN

This is the second most-used spice in the world. It adds a distinctive flavour to everything from curries to pickles. It's an amazing digestive aid, helping with gas, bloating, sluggish digestion and poor absorption of nutrients. It also has purifying properties, improves circulation and the metabolism. Its heating and drying qualities are ideal for spring, as it helps clear mucus. It's also great for menstruating women (helping with cramps) and new mothers (promoting the flow of breast milk). It's always best to buy the whole seed and grind it fresh when you need to use it.

CURRY LEAVES

These aromatic leaves are great for digestion and digestive disorders including stomach aches, cramps and loss of appetite. They are considered antimicrobial, anti-inflammatory and even anti-diabetic. Sub a small amount of fresh or dried curry leaves with a bay leaf – unlike the edible curry leaves, this will need removing after cooking.

ASAFOETIDA

Also known as hing, asafoetida is a pungent dried resin that is considered a super-power ingredient in Ayurveda, especially when cooking lentils or beans. It aids digestion, reduces gas, reduces Ama (see page 284), has anti-viral properties and helps with chest congestion (it was even used to treat the flu during World War I). It is an excellent flavour replacement for onion and garlic.

CARDAMOM

An aromatic spice that really throws its weight around, cardamom is especially good in desserts and is a must in biryanis and chais, too. If I'm cooking just for myself I'll bite into the pods to crush them before cooking; otherwise, shell them, remove the seeds and crush them in a pestle and mortar. Pre-ground isn't as easy to find and it loses freshness quickly. The amount of seeds per pod does vary, so be prepared to adjust the amount used every time you cook with this spice. Cardamom is a healing digestive tonic, helping to reduce bloating, nausea and gas. Its cleansing qualities also help dissolve mucus and detox the lymphatic system.

CINNAMON

This is the healing spice you probably already have in your cupboard. In Ayurveda, it is used to settle the stomach and balance digestion. Its warmth makes it perfect for those chilly days, on which all I crave is comfort. If you are Pitta, you should only have it in small doses. It acts as a circulation booster that will help warm your freezing toes and fingers, as well as keeping your lungs clear and joints lubricated. Cinnamon is great for adding natural sweetness without the blood-sugar spike, while also helping to metabolise fats and sugar. It freshens the breath, has antimicrobial properties and helps with nausea. When buying, make sure you get the best-quality cinnamon, especially if you use it frequently. You can substitute ground cinnamon for cinnamon sticks where appropriate – one 7.5cm (3in) stick is equal to ½ teaspoon ground cinnamon.

FENNEL SEEDS

A cooling spice, fennel has a hint of anise. It is the perfect go-to before and after a meal, since it stimulates the appetite before eating, while helping digestion and freshening the breath afterwards. Fennel seeds are a great digestive tonic, helping with gas, bloating, acid reflux, nausea and indigestion. Use whole or ground.

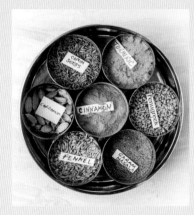

TURMERIC

Bright yellow in colour, turmeric is a spice that demands to be seen. A powerful anti-inflammatory and antioxidant, it is beneficial for liver cleansing, digestion improving and immunity boosting. Few spices offer turmeric's spectrum of benefits, which is why it has become a hero of the health world in all its forms. Unfortunately is is not easily absorbed by the body, so the best way to enjoy this spice is little and often, using good-quality roasted, dried and ground turmeric. In this form the root is heated again to activate it, then cooked with black pepper because the piperine (an active ingredient in black pepper) helps the body to absorb curcumin (the active ingredient in the turmeric) as well as fat. Raw turmeric is more heating, so dried is preferred – you'll be relieved to hear – so there is no fiddling around with fresh turmeric roots and staining your hands and kitchen surfaces yellow.

FENUGREEK SEEDS

While most bitter foods are cold in quality, fenugreek or methi is heating, so it is perfect for stoking the digestive fire. The seeds are often roasted to reduce bitterness and enhance flavour. Fenugreek combines well with fennel, cumin, coriander, turmeric and ginger. It is used in dosas to add viscosity and hold carbon dioxide as the batter ferments, to give you a lighter pancake.

SAFFRON

Saffron might seem more expensive than gold, but worry not, as you use barely any of it – it's that powerful. This luxurious spice is Tridoshic (see page 271) and is especially good for Pitta and Kapha. It helps flush out toxins, purifies blood, cleanses the skin, cools the mind, aids with urinary disorders and with the assimilation of nutrients. Use it for desserts, rice or vegetable and enjoy its regal colour tint in your food. When buying, make sure you are getting real saffron – there are lots of fake ones made from dyed safflower!

GARLIC

You won't find Ayurvedic cooking relying on this ingredient, or its usual pairing, onion, as much as many other cuisines. The right amount is stimulating, but too much will make you lethargic. Garlic has anti-viral, anti-fungal and anti-bacterial properties, and like the spices it is considered a medicine and should not be overdone. Fresh raw garlic is considered to have the most benefits. It's great for colds, coughs and the circulation. It also acts as a laxative and diuretic. Cooked garlic is more gentle on the system. Because garlic is considered to be Rajasic (stimulating to the nervous system and even considered a natural aphrodisiac), it is usually avoided by yogis. If you cut back on garlic for a while you'll really feel it when you do eat it and notice it in your sweat as well as your breath. The properties of onions are similar, which is why you'll find leeks are often given as an alternative in my recipes, and why the flavour of asafoetida is admired in Ayurvedic food, not least for its digestive powers.

SWEETENERS

Sweeteners are so ubitquitous in their refined form, with an addictive flavour and preservative properties. Kapha types in particular need to pay attention to how much they are eating, as the right amount is grounding, but more is highly stimulating (Rajasic), and too much will make you lethargic (Tamasic)! When it comes to sweet foods, less is more. Have a little often with meals (enjoy your dessert first or put a little in your chutneys, so you can enjoy all six Tastes with your meal rather than indulging all at once – see pages 285–287). The best option is to stick to natural sweeteners as much as possible – I use jaggery, which is the cheapest, raw honey and maple syrup. You can also use raisins and other dried fruit, such as dates. Dates and jaggery are good for sweetenening milk. Jaggery is better for Vata, honey for Kapha and maple syrup for Vata and Pitta.

JAGGERY

Made from raw, unrefined sugar cane juice (or palm tree sap), jaggery is available as crystals and molasses. You can find many types of jaggery sold very cheaply, from a pale golden shade (sold in 'cones', which you can find in large supermarkets) to a deep dark, almost black colour (available in Asian shops) – the dark one has more molasses and a stronger, caramel-like flavour. Your choice may affect the colours of certain baking recipes, so choose accordingly. Avoid granulated jaggery from health-food shops – not only is it much more expensive but it has also usually been treated to stop it clumping. It is also known as piloncillo in Hispanic supermarkets. It is different to demerara and other brown sugars in that the molasses is not stripped out and then reintroduced to the white sugar, meaning it has more nutrients. Jaggery is less heating than maple syrup and honey, and can be used in baking. You can either grate a block of jaggery and keep it in a jar, or just keep it on your chopping board with a bowl over it and chop some off when you need it.

RAW HONEY

Honey is a golden nectar, brimming with medicinal and nutritional properties. It is considered to be an all-purpose medicine because it is antiseptic, anti-fungal and anti-bacterial, and it also helps to stop bleeding both from skin wounds and stomach ulcers. It's considered by ancient Vedic civilisation as one of nature's gifts to mankind. It is very easily assimilated and used by the body, providing lots of energy. It stimulates the metabolism and can help with anaemia, lung health, skin issues, and also soothes coughs and helps keep your mouth, eyes and stomach healthy. It is very important that it is used raw, since cooked honey is considered a poison in Ayurveda. Do not use it in hot drinks; wait until they are at room temperature. Honey is particularly good for Kapha and is especially beneficial in spring. Support your local bee keepers, if possible, and buy direct from them – local honey can even be beneficial for allergies.

MORE FAVOURITES

CHICORY POWDER

This is my go-to when I fancy something bittersweet without the caffeine rollercoaster. It's made from the root of the chicory plant, which is dried and roasted, giving it a similar colour and smooth texture to coffee. In contrast to your regular cup of 'joe', chicory has lots of fibre, acts as a liver tonic and has sedative properties. It also helps keep your 'good' bacteria balanced.

BONITO FLAKES

Also known as katsuobushi, these flakes come from dried smoked bonito (a type of tuna). They take stocks to a whole new level, giving depth and a rich umami flavour to miso soup, hot pots and noodles. If you'd rather keep it vegan/vegetarian you can substitute them with kombu.

CHESTNUTS

The perfect winter food. According to Ayurveda, chestnuts help nourish kidneys and build Agni (see page 282). Their warming nature makes them a welcome addition in the cooler months – especially good for Vata. Although their astringent properties can help tone the bowels, they should not be eaten in excess to avoid Vata imbalances (such as constipation). Chestnut flour has a rich brown colour and is nutty, nourishing, gluten-free and naturally high in protein.

COCONUT

This ingredient seems to have taken the wellness world by storm: just visit a health-food shop to find coconut in all possible permutations. Fresh coconuts are best but are not widely available in the West. Instead, use good-quality unsweetened dried coconut or 'blocks' – sometimes called creamed coconut. Tinned foods are not encouraged but a dash of organic full-fat coconut milk can make all the difference to the flavour and appeal of a dish. It's cooling and sweet, making it ideal for hot days and for balancing Pitta, but can aggravate Kapha in excess. See page 257 for how to make coconut milk for drinking.

DASHI

Dashi is a simple Japanese stock that is easy to make at home and tastes of the sea. It can be made out of kombu (dried kelp), bonito flakes, sardines or a combination. The resulting clear broth adds umami to anything you mix it with. Use it for making a bowl of miso soup. If you want to keep your dashi vegan, use only kombu.

TAMARI

This Japanese soy sauce is traditionally a by-product of miso production; it's made from soy beans, sea salt and koji and is usually gluten-free. If you buy a good-quality brand it is more likely to have been made in the traditional way, which is much better for your health. Tamari has a stronger, richer taste and aroma than regular soy sauce. Most organic tamari sauces contain no preservatives or other additives – just make sure you check the ingredients.

TAMARIND

Sweet and tangy, tamarind is popular in Asian cuisine and adds an all-important sour note to dishes. It has potent laxative properties, which makes it good for Vata. It is usually available as a paste, but may contain additives, so make it at home if you can (see page 260).

COOKING EQUIPMENT

When cooking Ayurvedic recipes, old-fashioned pots on stoves or slowcookers are best. Because dried pulses need soaking and cooking time, pressure cookers are very popular. However, the Vaidyas (Ayurvedic practitioners) I have worked with note a difference: although both methods render soft and tender dishes, the pressure cooker is said to 'break down' the pulses rather than 'cook' them – and cooking is better for digestion. Where possible, use natural cooking utensils such as wooden spoons and spatulas, glassware rather than tupperware, cast-iron, stainless-steel and ceramic-lined saucepans and frying pans. Avoid having aluminium foil and cling film touching foods.

THE RECIPES

Morning milks

Most of us can testify that a hot drink is the best way to start the day. I recommend gently waking up the body with a mug of hot water, sipped slowly to help get your system moving. These Morning Milks are delicious to follow – they make excellent breakfasts, or at least breakfast starters if you're feeling particularly hungry or lunch is a long way off!

Other than the Matcha Latte and Masala Chai, which contain caffeine, these recipes also work as an evening wind-down, especially if you've got in late and need something nourishing to fill you up without overworking your body before bed.

Dairy and almond milk (see recipe on page 256) are classic Ayurvedic milks but you could also try coconut milk if you have a tree-nut allergy or just want to change things up (see drinking coconut milk recipe on page 257). Cow's milk is the most nutritious, although goat's milk is lighter and another good option. To make dairy easier to digest, it's best to choose the natural stuff: unhomogenised, organic, whole (full-fat) and raw where possible, and avoid eating around the same time as anything salty or sour (which will make the milk curdle in your stomach). Ayurveda also insists on cooking the milk first by adding water and simmering gently for 10–15 minutes to break down the lactose and make it lighter. Because of the longer simmering time, you'll need to start with a little more water than with the nut milks to allow for evaporation.

If you're feeling Kapha, you might find that one of these milks is all you need for breakfast, while if you're feeling Vata, you may need a bigger portion or something else to follow. On a more regular basis, Kapha types should use rice milk (see recipe page 257) or dilute dairy milk with even more water to better suit their digestion.

Dairy milk is deliciously sweet but if you are feeling Vata, or you are a newbie to spiced milk, you could add a little sweetener and even some ghee to make it more unctuous. Avoid sweetening with honey or maple syrup – neither are very compatible with dairy milk and honey shouldn't be heated. Instead choose jaggery or dates.

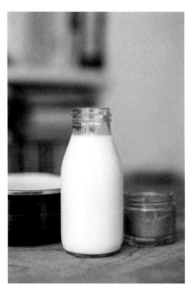

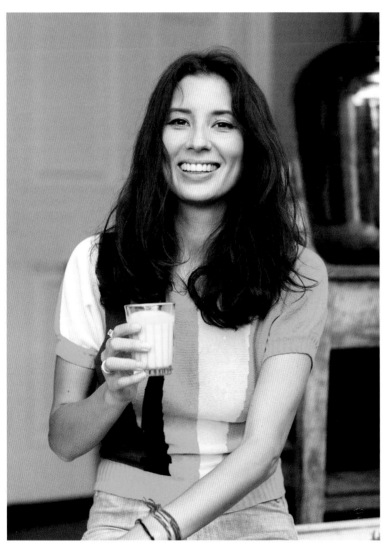

Gorgeously bright, rich and caffeine-free, Golden Milk is the ultimate Ayurvedic recipe and can help improve digestion and circulation. Versions of the drink, known as turmeric latte, have hit the hip cafes, meaning that non-coffee drinkers can enjoy something different from herbal tea!

Serves 1

Turmeric is a joy to drink when you mix it with a little sweetness and spices and it is a lovely way to start and end the day. I choose this if wake up early and want something small and warming. It is also calming for the mind and healing to the body, so helps me wind down – if I've had a huge lunch, been snacking or get home late then this becomes my dinner. If I get to bed late and suddenly become peckish, this is my go-to recipe.

It is more beneficial to cook turmeric with black pepper, and as dairy milk is simmered for a while to make it more digestible it's the perfect time to get everything cooking together. The spices still need the simmering time even if you use almond milk, so add a little water to allow for evaporation.

Golden Milk

175ml (¾ cup) whole milk or 250ml (1 cup) almond milk
water, for simmering
3 cardamom pods, cracked
½ tsp ground turmeric

2.5cm (1in) piece of fresh ginger, grated (around ½ tsp), or
1 tsp ground ginger
½ tsp ground cinnamon
¼ tsp freshly ground black pepper
½ tbsp jaggery

1   Place the milk in a small pot or milk pan. If you are using dairy milk, add 120ml (½ cup) of water. If you are using almond milk, add 60ml (¼ cup) of water. Add the remaining ingredients, apart from the jaggery, and gently simmer for 10–15 minutes.

2   Add a splash more hot water if needed. Stir through the jaggery to taste, strain and serve.

FEELING VATA

This is very calming, especially in autumn and winter. Try increasing the spices, and break up your routine by enjoying this a few days on and then one day off.

FEELING PITTA

For an extra boost in the summer, add a tiny pinch of saffron – this is beneficial to all Doshas, but especially cooling to Pitta types, who can also use it instead of ginger.

FEELING KAPHA

Go for a light almond milk or rice milk (see pages 256–257). Ground ginger is even better than fresh as it's more heating. Up the spices if you like and avoid adding the jaggery.

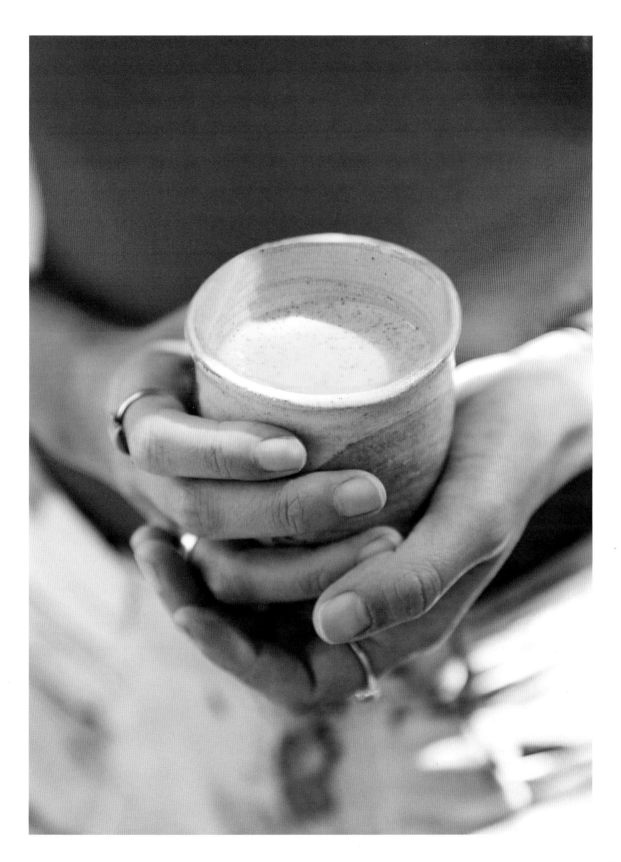

This delicious pink concoction is a pretty way to introduce spices and the earthy sweetness of beetroot to new taste buds. I asked several Vaidyas (Ayurvedic practitioners) about the combination of milk with beetroot and although none had come across it before, they said it seemed A-OK. The easiest way to make this recipe is with beetroot powder, which is one of my favourite non-essentials in the cupboard – it's great for decorating cakes in a hurry! Otherwise blend in about 50g of cooked or raw beetroot (save a wedge when cooking beetroot for another dish). I find this recipe sweet enough, but add a little jaggery if you like.

Serves 1

Beetroot latte

175ml (¾ cup) whole milk plus 120ml (½ cup) water, or 250ml (1 cup) almond milk
¼ tsp ground cinnamon
1 tsp vanilla extract
1cm (½ in) piece of fresh ginger, grated, or ¼ tsp ground ginger

¼ tsp freshly ground black pepper (optional)
pinch of ground cardamom (optional)
1 tsp beetroot powder, to serve

1   If using dairy milk, place the milk and water in a small saucepan over a medium heat. Bring to the boil and then gently simmer for 10–15 minutes – this stage makes dairy milk easier to digest. For almond milk, gently heat until piping hot.

2   Add the remaining ingredients, and simmer for a few minutes. Stir through the beetroot powder and serve.

. . . .

Enjoy this drink in the morning for a gentle caffeine buzz rather than an instant high – avoid boiling the matcha to keep its antioxidant goodness. If you like this, you might want to invest in a special matcha whisk, which the Japanese use to get this nice and smooth.

Serves 1

Matcha latte

175ml (¾ cup) whole milk plus 120ml (½ cup) water, or 250ml (1 cup) almond milk

1 tsp matcha tea powder
¼ tsp vanilla extract
tiniest pinch of sea salt
½–1 tsp jaggery

1   If using dairy milk, place the milk and water in a small saucepan over a medium heat. Bring to the boil and then gently simmer for 10–15 minutes – this stage makes dairy milk easier to digest. For almond milk, gently heat until piping hot.

2   Whisk the matcha, vanilla, salt and jaggery in a mug to form a thick paste. Add a dash of hot milk to loosen the mixture, then whisk in the remaining hot milk and serve.

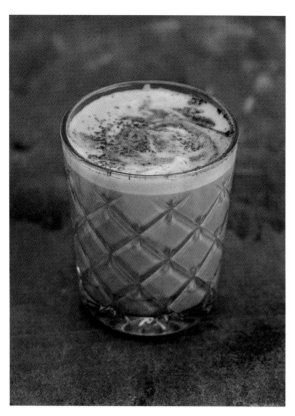

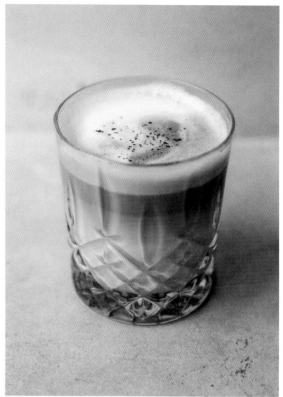

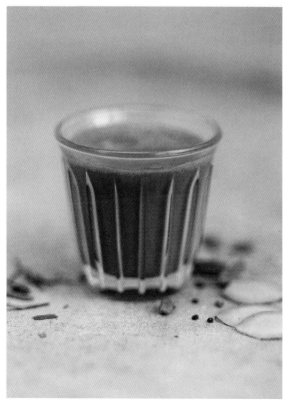

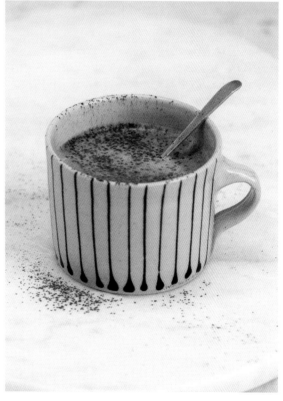

Coffee and I have had a long-distance relationship for many years now, as it makes my Vata crazy! But we're okay with it. What helps is good old Indian chai. Sometimes we can feel a bit short-changed when it comes to having a herbal tea at home or in a coffee shop. Not that the provenance and preparation of tea leaves are any less important than for coffee beans, or the act of making tea any less 'wow' than a barista with his or her coffee, but in this tea-loving country we tend to overlook the perfect way to make our brew. A real chai tea is rich and bitter and sweet, and filling and totally satisfying. If you've only ever had a chai tea bag in a mug with a splash of milk then you really need to try this again.

This recipe is inspired by the Ravva family in Hyderabad, India, who invited my partner Nick and me to breakfast one day. This tea was just the start of it. The bronze pot was part of the mother of the house's inheritance, and is apparently important for the flavour. I'm happy to make this in my little milk pan at home – but then again I'm no chai wallah! Of course, every family has their own chai recipe – to make some delicious variations try adding ½ star anise, ½ teaspoon of coriander seeds or a pinch of nutmeg or allspice when you're simmering. And if you're caffeine-sensitive, try a Rooibos Chai – a lovely one for the evening. PICTURED ON PAGE 37.

○◐●

Serves 2

Masala chai

175ml (¾ cup) whole milk or 250ml (1 cup) almond milk
water, for simmering
1½ tsp fine-grind black tea powder or contents of 1 black or rooibos tea bag
2 cardamom pods, cracked
good grind of black pepper
5cm (2in) piece of fresh ginger, sliced
½ tsp ground cinnamon
½–1 tsp jaggery

1   Place the milk in a small bronze pot or milk pan. If you are using dairy milk, add 120ml (½ cup) of water. If you are using almond milk, add 60ml (¼ cup) of water.

2   Add the remaining ingredients, apart from the ginger, cinnamon and jaggery, and gently simmer for up to 15 minutes. Add the ginger, cinnamon and jaggery and simmer for another 2–5 minutes, depending on your preferred strength of ginger. Strain and serve.

TIP
·
If you can't find black tea powder, you could break open a tea bag of any black tea blend.

This is the perfect hot drink for kids. Enjoy it French-style for breakfast or American-style in the evenings. The beauty of this recipe is that it has the nourishing spices and the nutritious milk but none of the stimulating caffeine from cocoa. Just a little chicory powder gives you the depth of flavour and the cinnamon, vanilla and milk do the rest. Sweeten with just a touch of maple syrup or jaggery (dairy milk needs less sweetener than homemade almond milk) or when it's more than cool enough to drink, add a little raw honey instead. PICTURED ON PAGE 37.

Serves 2

Ayurvedic caffeine-free hot chocolate

175ml (¾ cup) whole milk
    or 250ml (1 cup)
    almond milk
water, for simmering
pinch of freshly ground
    black pepper (optional)
½–1 tsp jaggery

½–1 tsp ground chicory
½ tsp ground cinnamon
½ tsp vanilla extract
cocoa powder or extra
    chicory, for dusting
    (optional)

1   Place the milk in a small saucepan. If you are using dairy milk, add 120ml (½ cup) of water. If you are using almond milk, add 60ml (¼ cup) of water.

2   Add the remaining ingredients, apart from the jaggery, and cook over a medium heat. Bring to the boil and then gently simmer for 10–15 minutes. Add the jaggery to taste and serve.

TIP
.

To froth your milk, place a milk frother on the top of the liquid in the pan and turn on the power, allowing the milk to froth and foam until it reaches your desired texture. Alternatively, reserve a little of the hot milk and froth it separately in a cup, then gently pour into the mug, barista-style. Serve, or transfer to an insulated flask.

FEELING
KAPHA

Throw in some
black pepper for an extra
flavour dimension.

This drink is nourishing, filling, refreshing and great for all Doshas. Traditionally consumed during Lent or fasting days in Ethiopia, Suff makes a great snack for in-between meals on hungry days. For a special meal with friends this drink goes beautifully with my Lamb and Vegetable Biryani on page 154. Traditionally, the sunflower seeds are toasted – making them more digestible as well as all the more tasty – but you can skip this stage if you find raw foods easy to digest. The rose water is a new addition and takes it up to the next level, giving it a Middle Eastern or Indian feel. It's also essential for those skipping the toasting stage as it adds flavour. A powerful blender gets this really smooth but otherwise be prepared for 'bits', which are brilliant for stopping you from gulping too quickly – savour that smoothie!

Serves 2

Suff – Ethiopian sunflower seed smoothie with rose water

80g (½ cup) sunflower seeds, soaked overnight, or quickly soaked in boiling water

2.5cm (1in) piece of fresh ginger, or 1 tsp ground ginger

2 cups (500ml) water

1 tbsp raw honey

½ tsp rose water (or to taste – I use Nielsen-Massey as it's strong)

dried rose petals, to serve (optional)

FEELING PITTA

Swap the ginger for fresh mint, cardamom or cinnamon to taste. Use maple syrup or jaggery instead of raw honey.

1   Rinse and drain the sunflower seeds. Toast them in a dry pan, over a medium heat, for 10–20 minutes, or until they turn a deep golden brown, taste nutty and smell fragrant. After toasting, transfer them to a blender or food processor with the ginger and a little of the water and blend until very smooth.

2   Add the rest of the water, raw honey and rose water. Blend again and serve in a drinking vessel or as a smoothie bowl, decorated with rose petals, if using.

TIP
·

If you have digestive issues with raw food, then be sure to soak the seeds overnight and toast them well.

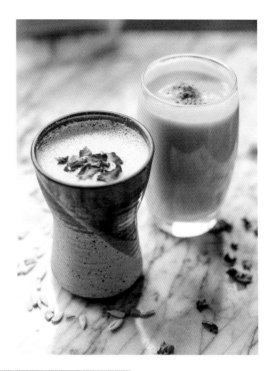

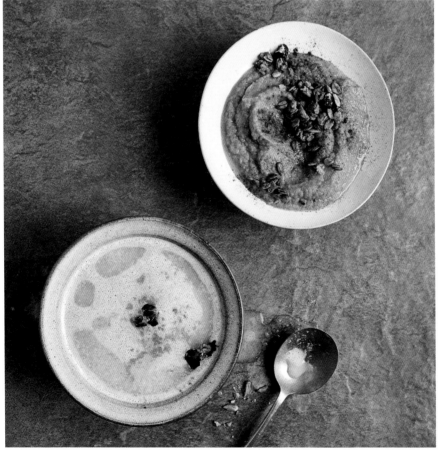

Ayurveda loves a hot meal, so here's a warming, cooked variation on the usual smoothie. Perfect for breakfast all year round, think of this as a sweet soup or a hot-house smoothie. The carrots are simmered until tender, which not only makes them easy to digest, but also makes the smoothie deliciously smooth, even if you don't have a power blender.

For variety, swap in butternut squash or sweet potato – just like the porridge opposite. Try different nuts and seeds, but avoid cashews and peanuts as they are very heating and heavy. Top with your favourite granola, if you fancy, for a gorgeous smoothie bowl.

If you want to thin this into a drink, follow the instructions below, adding another 250ml (1 cup) of water to the blender. PICTURED ON PAGE 41.

Serves 2

Hot carrot cake and walnut smoothie bowl

2 large carrots, chopped (about 400g)
2 large pitted dates
250ml (1 cup) water
40g (scant ½ cup) walnut halves, soaked overnight (and toasted if you have issues with digestion)
1 tbsp raw honey
¼ tsp ground cinnamon, plus more to decorate

2.5cm (1in) piece of fresh ginger, finely chopped
seeds of 2 cardamom pods, ground
¼–½ tsp vanilla extract
pinch of sea salt (optional – to bring out flavours and help rehydrate after a workout)
2 tbsp granola, to serve (optional)

1 Simmer the carrots and dates in the water until tender.

2 Add to a blender with the rest of the ingredients. Blend until smooth. Dust with cinnamon, top with granola, if using, and serve.

TIP
.

In the summer, enjoy this as a refreshing drink using raw carrot and fresh mint instead of spices. Served at room temperature, it's good for calming Pitta. Simply grate the carrots and add to a powerful blender with the rest of the ingredients. Use 250–500ml (1–2 cups) of water, according to how thick you want it.

FEELING
VATA

Add more spices and some ghee if you like.

FEELING
PITTA

Reduce the ginger, black pepper and cardamom slightly to keep your cool, and swap the honey for maple syrup or jaggery.

FEELING
KAPHA

If you're having this regularly, halve the amount of walnuts and up the pungent spices.

This is an excellent winter dish that's also great on a cool summer's day. It's a simple vegetable porridge that's very Kapha-friendly; unlike the usual comfort dishes containing dairy, potatoes and pasta, sweet potatoes are very pacifying and light for heavy digestive systems and provide an easy-to-digest sweetness. They can satisfy the appetite for long stretches, making this an excellent breakfast, snack or addition to your lunch.

Serves 2

The volatile oils of the orange zest are used across many traditions for low Agni (see page 278), nausea and indigestion, and can help to clear congestion. They are also a natural appetite-suppressant for Kapha types, who might want to eat a lot of this! Orange zest and cinnamon bring out the natural sweetness of this dish, without needing any sweeteners. Adding a dollop of fat with ghee, butter or almond butter makes it satisfying and creamy. PICTURED ON PAGE 44.

Sweet potato and orange porridge

1 large sweet potato, cut into chunks (about 640g)
500ml (2 cups) water
½–1 tsp orange extract
pinch of sea salt

1–2 tbsp ghee, butter or almond butter, melted
ground cinnamon and orange zest, to serve

1 Simmer the sweet potato with the water for about 15–20 minutes, or until completely tender.

2 Add to a blender with the orange extract and salt and blend until smooth, adding more water if you like. Top with the ghee, butter or almond butter, and serve with orange zest and cinnamon.

FEELING VATA

Sweet potatoes are a diuretic and can provoke dryness, so it's best to use carrots or orange yams instead. Top with more ghee or butter.

FEELING PITTA

Top with lime zest or ground cardamom and coconut.

FEELING KAPHA

Use only 1 tablespoon of ghee, or try 1 tablespoon of pumpkin seed butter.

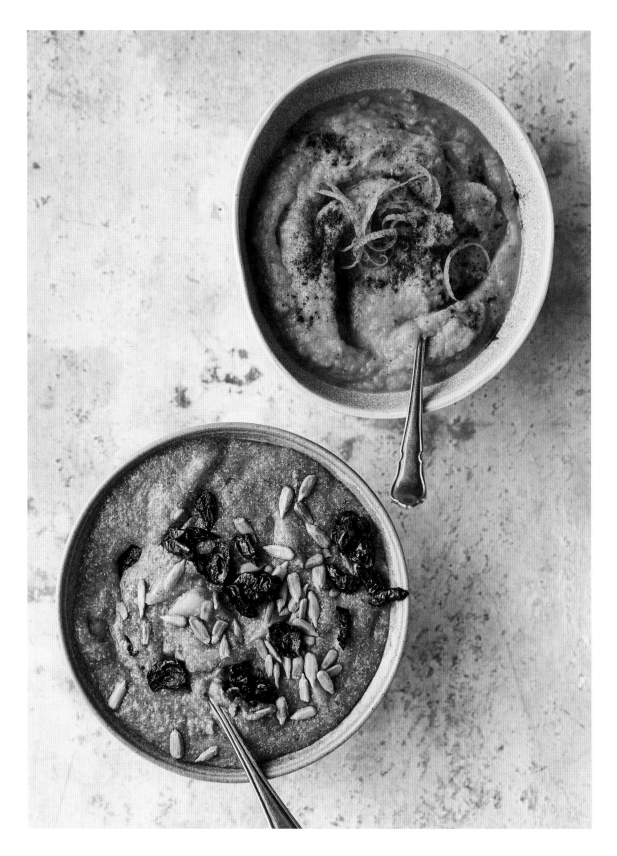

I love amaranth seeds but they can be a bit tricky for digestion – the little seeds are so tiny that unless you chew them really thoroughly they can pass straight through you, making them an expensive waste of goodness that can also upset your gut! Amaranth flakes totally solve the problem and are also quicker to cook. Much like a rolled oat, the flakes have been broken down and flattened, thereby killing off some of the antinutrients and allowing the amaranth to be digested more easily. If you can't get hold of the flakes, you can always blitz soaked whole seeds in a powerful blender before or after cooking.

Soft cooked pear breaks up the texture and the sunflower seeds add crunch. This dish is very filling so you only need a small bowl, unless you want to add more water to make it soupy.

○◑●

Serves 5–6

Amaranth porridge with pear and cinnamon-spiced sunflower seeds

125g (1 cup) amaranth flakes (or whole amaranth seeds, soaked overnight, rinsed and drained)
250ml (1 cup) full-fat coconut milk
370ml (1½ cups) water
½ tsp ground nutmeg
½ tsp ground turmeric
2 cardamom pods, cracked
1.5cm (¾in) piece of fresh ginger, grated, or 1½ tsp ground ginger
1½ tbsp maple syrup or jaggery
pinch of sea salt and freshly ground black pepper
2 medium pears, peeled and chopped into 2.5cm (1in) chunks (about 150g/1½ cups)

1 tsp vanilla extract
1 tsp ground cinnamon, plus extra for dusting

TO SERVE
4 tbsp sunflower seeds
1 tbsp ghee, butter or coconut oil
handful of dried cranberries or sour cherries (optional)

1 Simmer all of the ingredients, apart from the pears, vanilla and cinnamon, lid on, for about 5 minutes, or up to 20 minutes if using whole amaranth seeds.

2 Add the pears and continue to simmer for 5–10 minutes, stirring frequently. Add more water if necessary during cooking to reach your desired consistency.

3 Stir through the vanilla and ground cinnamon. To serve, lightly toast the sunflower seeds in a dry frying pan, add the ghee and sprinkle with cinnamon. Spoon the porridge into bowls and garnish with the toasted seeds and dried cranberries, if using.

TIP
·

To make this in a slowcooker, add all of the ingredients, apart from the vanilla and cinnamon, to the slowcooker and cook on high overnight, or for at least 8 hours. Stir through the vanilla and cinnamon, add the toppings and serve.

This sweet and comforting porridge is packed with protein and filling enough in small amounts. When I was a personal health-food chef, I found that at least 1 in 10 people couldn't bring themselves to eat anything savoury first thing, so I created this to encourage us all to eat dal for breakfast. Mung beans contain protein that's easy to digest if prepared properly. In Asia, beans and lentils are used in sweet dishes more often than not, and in India you can also eat a variation of this as a rich pudding. This is a more subtle breakfast version that can be pimped up or watered down to suit your needs, whether you want a breakfast to hike on or a breakfast to fast on!

The good news is that you don't need to soak mung dal the night before – so this is a great porridge to get on with at the last minute. I also like to pop this in a slowcooker just before bed so it's ready when I wake up. Toasting the mung dal gives it a nuttier flavour, but if you're feeling lazy you can also skip that step.

Beware – if you use mung dal (which are tiny little split yellow mung beans) you'll get sunshine in a bowl, but if you use whole mung beans with their green jackets you may end up with something one of my clients calls 'Dung Dal', ha!

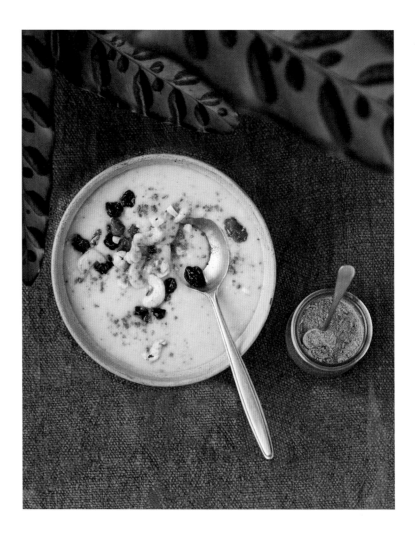

○◑●

Serves 1–2

Sunshine yellow porridge

100g (½ cup) mung dal
(or whole mung beans,
soaked for 4–6 hours
or overnight)
500ml (2 cups) water
½ tsp ground turmeric
½ tsp coriander seeds
250ml (1 cup) full-fat
coconut milk or
whole milk
3 tbsp jaggery, maple
syrup or coconut sugar
seeds of 1–2 cardamom
pods, ground
1.5cm (¾ in) piece of fresh
ginger, grated, or
1½ tsp ground ginger

TO SERVE
1 tbsp ghee
2 tbsp cashews,
chopped
2 tbsp raisins
1 tsp Dosha Churna
Spice Mix (see
page 247, no salt)

1 Toast the mung dal in a dry frying pan until fragrant
   and lightly toasted. Simmer with the water, turmeric
   and coriander seeds, lid on, for about 15 minutes or
   until very soft.

2 Mash the mixture well with the back of a spoon or
   blitz with a powerful blender, depending on your
   preferred texture.

3 Stir in the milk, along with the jaggery, cardamom
   seeds and fresh ginger, and bring to the boil, then
   reduce the heat and simmer, lid on, for 10–15 minutes.

4 Melt the ghee in a small saucepan and toast the
   cashews, then stir in the raisins and cook for a
   few seconds until soft and puffy. Stir into the
   porridge and serve.

FEELING
VATA

When you make the
Dosha Churna Spice Mix,
leave out the sea salt and
asafoetida otherwise it will
taste too pungent – and
milk does not combine
well with salt.

FEELING
KAPHA

Dry-toast the cashews and
raisins rather than using
ghee. Cook the dal in
the water, then add rice
milk or 1 tbsp creamed
coconut or just a splash
of coconut milk.

TIP
.

To make this in a slowcooker,
toast the mung dal as above and
then add all of the ingredients and
cook on high overnight, or for
at least 8 hours. Then add
the toppings.

Move over green smoothies and smashed avocado – this is the new green brekkie! I first discovered this creamy rice and herb soup at Cape Welligama – a beautiful resort in Sri Lanka where the chefs were proud to make me a traditional breakfast. A steaming bowl of comfort might not be the first breakfast you consider in a hot country, but it totally hit the spot after a morning's surfing, and even my beloved breakfast papaya made room for this dish.

The name comes from chief ingredient gotu kola, which is a nutritious wonder herb that grows in Southeast Asia. I've had to adapt it to what's available here, and watercress fits the bill – the bitterness of this superfood works with the sweet creamy coconut. In April, make the most of asparagus's short season. Traditionally made with broken, mushy red rice, Kola Kanda is served steaming hot with a piece of jaggery that you nibble between mouthfuls – this is particularly beneficial for Vata and Pitta types, to control the bitterness of the watercress.

Serves 1

Kola Kanda – watercress, coconut and rice herbal porridge

50g (scant ¼ cup) red rice or brown basmati rice, soaked overnight, or white basmati rice
water, for cooking rice
pinch of asafoetida or 1 garlic clove, crushed (optional)
50g (1 cup) watercress, or other green leaves, such as mustard leaves

50ml (scant ¼ cup) full-fat coconut or almond milk, shaken well
sea salt and freshly ground black pepper, to taste
piece of jaggery, to taste

1   Rinse and drain the rice and transfer it to a saucepan. If you're using red or brown rice, pour 200ml water over the top. If you're using white basmati rice, pour 150ml (⅔ cup) water over the top. Add the asafoetida or garlic, if using, then bring to the boil and simmer until slightly overcooked. Remove from the heat.

2   Meanwhile, wash the watercress thoroughly. Mix it with 100ml water and the milk and blend until it's as chunky or smooth as you like.

3   Add the watercress smoothie to the rice and bring to a rolling simmer. Taste and season with sea salt and black pepper. Add more water for a thinner texture and serve immediately with jaggery, if desired.

FEELING
PITTA

In summer, enjoy fresh coriander leaves instead of watercress.

FEELING
KAPHA

Try this with rice milk, or use a little less coconut milk and a little more water.

TIP
.

This is great for using up leftover rice – swap in 100g of cooked rice and heat through thoroughly. Also delicious for dinner (but avoid if you are feeling Vata).

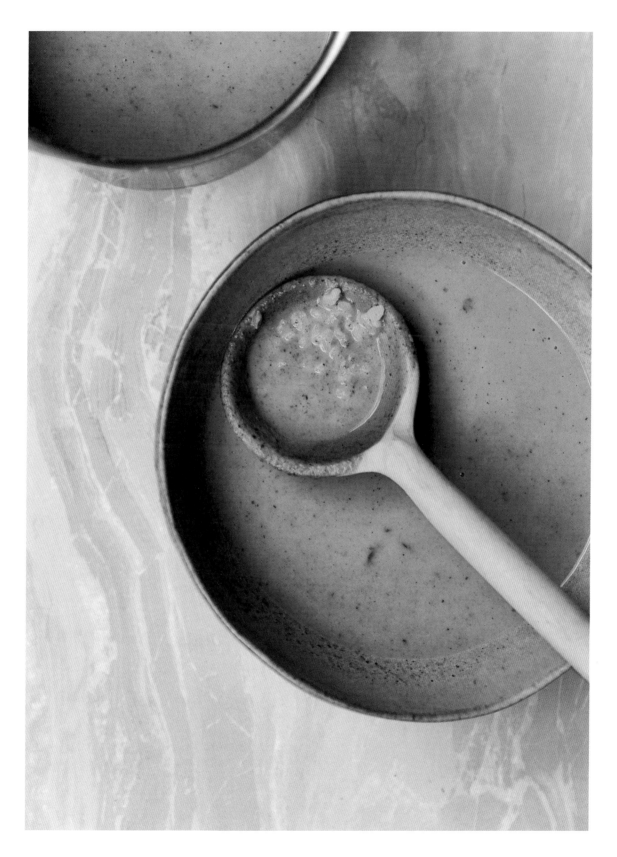

Based on the Chinese 'breakfast for longevity', this congee is the perfect way to wake up your digestion and ease into the day. It's incredibly light and easy to digest and perfect for a detox day.

I first enjoyed congee on a trip to Hong Kong 15 years ago – it's a thin rice gruel (thinner than porridge) with garlic, ginger, shiitake mushrooms and spring onions. As a breakfast dish it may take some getting used to, so here's a sweet version.

This is my go-to overnight breakfast. All of the ingredients come straight from the cupboard – I just pop them into my slowcooker the night before and turn it on. You can also cook this on the stove, but allow at least 2 hours because the longer the congee cooks, the more medicinal it becomes. This breakfast is a great way to enjoy brown rice, because the long cooking process breaks it down while keeping some texture – but remember to soak it the night before you cook it.

Serves 3

Fig, cinnamon and cardamom slowcooker congee

55g (¼ cup) white basmati rice, rinsed
55g (¼ cup) brown basmati rice, soaked overnight, rinsed and drained
3 cups (750ml) water
3 cardamom pods, cracked
3 dried figs, halved
2.5cm (1in) piece of fresh ginger, cut in half, or 1 tsp ground ginger
tiny pinch of sea salt
½ tsp ground coriander

TO SERVE
fresh figs or pear slices sautéed in ghee, butter or coconut oil
drizzle of maple syrup
½ tsp ground cinnamon
2 tbsp coconut cream, cream or almond milk (optional)

1 Add the ingredients to a slowcooker (putting them in a small ovenproof bowl if your slowcooker is a large one) and cook on low for 8 hours.

2 Alternatively, use a medium saucepan with a tight-fitting lid – it's important that the lid fits tightly or the water may steam away. Add the ingredients to the saucepan, bring to a boil, and then place the lid on. Reduce the heat to the lowest setting and cook for 2–6 hours, checking every now and then and adding a little water if necessary.

3 To serve, remove the ginger and figs (they may have lost their flavour, but eat them if you like!) and cardamom pods. Add enough boiling water to reach your desired consistency, then stir and ladle into bowls. Top with cooked fruit, maple syrup, cinnamon and a swirl of coconut cream, if you like.

TIP
.
Change it up by topping with a handful of raisins, dried apricots or chopped apple.

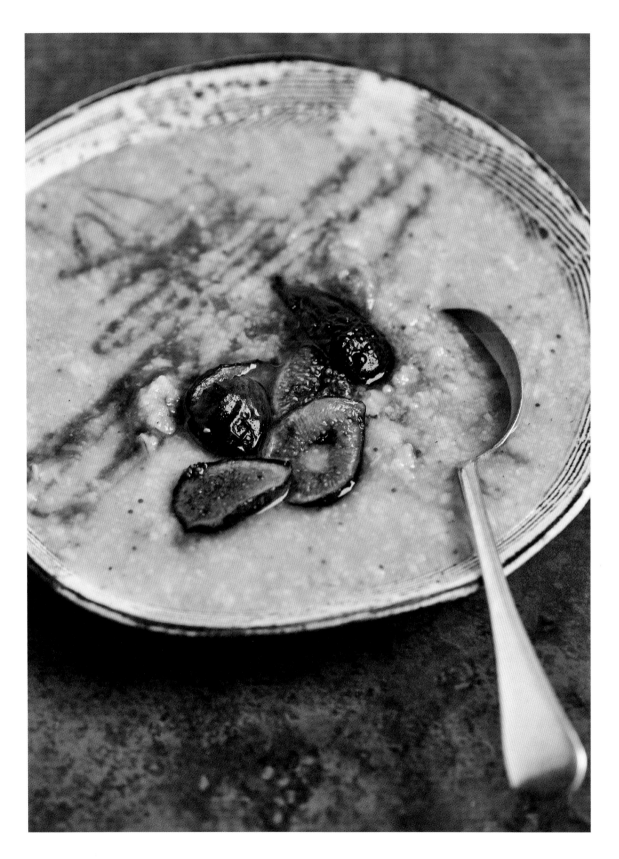

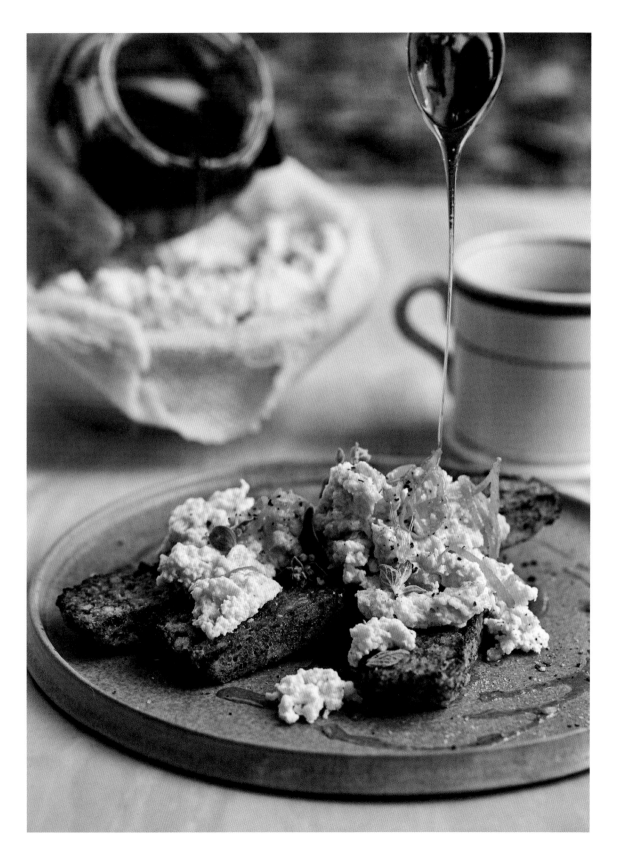

This recipe has a Mediterranean or Persian flavour to it, with its creamy, sweet ricotta, honey, fresh herbs, zest, and a good glug of olive oil. I usually bake a loaf of mung bean bread every other week and save a slice or two for this. The ricotta only takes 30 minutes to make and it's also delicious with the Buckwheat Banana Bread (see page 60), Ragi Roti (see page 62), Teff Waffles (see page 78) or sourdough. If you've got the ingredients ready then this dish can be assembled quickly and easily for a beautiful brunch with friends. Ayurveda advises against mixing fresh fruit with dairy for optimum digestion, but fresh orange zest helps to bring a fruity flavour.

Serves 4

Olive oil toast with ricotta, honey and orange zest

250g (½ quantity) homemade whole-milk ricotta (see page 254)
8 slices of homemade Rosemary Mung Bean Bread (see page 232)
1 tbsp extra-virgin olive oil, for drizzling
2 tsp raw honey, for drizzling

flaky sea salt and freshly ground black pepper, to taste
zest of ½ orange
few sprigs of oregano or rosemary, to decorate

1 Around 30 minutes before you wish to serve, make your ricotta, following the recipe on page 254.

2 Toast the bread and drizzle it with olive oil (you can also rub the herbs on the toast at this point to infuse with some of their aroma).

3 Divide the ricotta between the pieces of toast. Serve drizzled with olive oil and honey and seasoned with sea salt, black pepper, orange zest and herbs.

FEELING
PITTA

Skip the black pepper, reduce the olive oil and swap the honey for maple syrup.

FEELING
KAPHA

Enjoy only occasionally as cheese can be heavy for your system – otherwise, spread the ricotta thickly like butter on your toast and top with plenty of black pepper and a little chilli instead of honey.

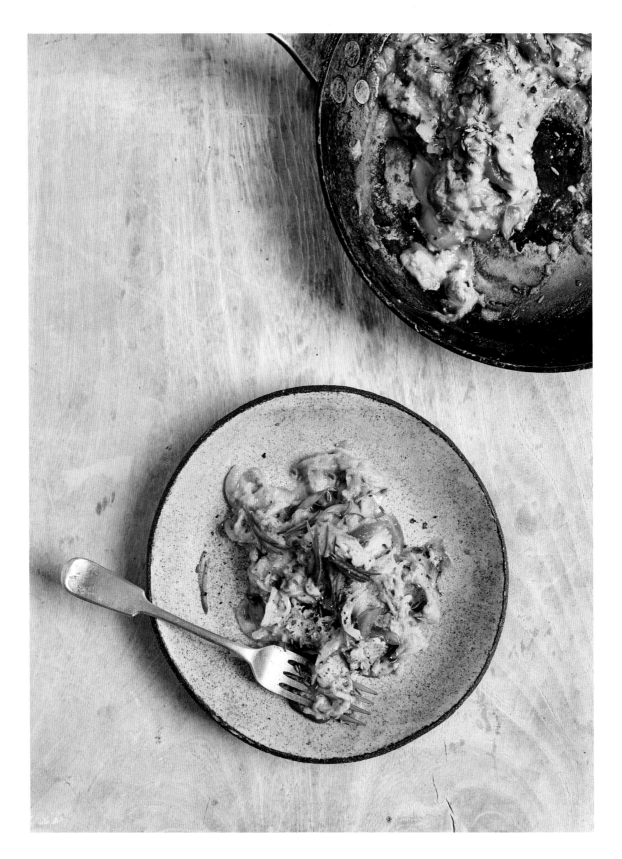

This is a classic Indian breakfast – think scrambled eggs, Spanish-style, with onion and tomatoes, made even more tasty with a selection of spices. This is a proper East meets West start to the day and a delicious way to introduce spices, for a savoury breakfast as opposed to the usual English fry-up. As your taste buds become accustomed, you can start to make it more of a Sattvic dish (see page 14) by swapping the tomatoes for a squeeze of lime, halving the onion and garnishing with plenty of fresh coriander.

Serves 2,
or 3 with a side dish

Akuri
scrambled eggs

1 tsp ghee, butter or
    coconut oil
1 onion, sliced
1 tomato, skinned and
    deseeded (see
    page 260), and
    roughly chopped
2.5cm (1in) piece of fresh
    ginger, grated
pinch of asafoetida
½ tsp ground turmeric
½ tsp ground coriander
½ tsp ground cumin
4 medium eggs
sea salt, to taste
1 green chilli, finely
    chopped (optional)

TO SERVE
2 tbsp fresh coriander
    leaves, chopped
½ tsp ground cumin,
    to garnish

1   Melt the ghee in a saucepan over a medium heat and sauté the onion until pinkish brown. Add the tomato, cook until tender and then add the ginger and asafoetida and cook for a few minutes.

2   Add all of the ground spices and sauté for a few minutes, then reduce the heat to the lowest possible.

3   Break the eggs into a clean bowl and beat with a fork until frothy. Add the beaten eggs to the pan and stir continuously until you get your perfect consistency. Season with salt and stir through the chopped chilli, if using. Serve with coriander and ground cumin.

FEELING
VATA

FEELING
PITTA

FEELING
KAPHA

Enjoy with your choice
of bread or some
savoury porridge.

Skip the chilli, reduce the
spices and enjoy with your
choice of sides, including
salad if you like.

Serve with sautéed greens
and enjoy the chilli.

This recipe was born of a Saturday with my mum a few years ago when neither of us could decide what to eat for breakfast. I was hungry but had just come back from the first book tour, where I'd been lucky enough to enjoy many delicious dishes but was suffering from a massive bout of jetlag. I knew I wanted eggs and my body knew it wanted veggies. My genius mum made this, and I added the cumin to create a match made in heaven. Quick and simple, this recipe is great for a weekday breakfast – it can feed a family with minimal fuss, but watch out for sticky fingers!

Serves 2

Soft-boiled eggs with cumin courgette and broccoli dippers

½ head of broccoli and 1 courgette
dash of extra-virgin olive oil, plus extra for serving
4 medium eggs
sea salt, to taste
pinch of toasted ground cumin (see cooking with spices, page 265)

FEELING
VATA

Stick to courgettes, rather than a mix of broccoli and courgette.

FEELING
KAPHA

Eggs are already grounding, so lighten with just one egg and loads of veggies.

1 Cut the broccoli into thin florets and the courgette into soldiers – try to make them all roughly the same size so they cook at the same rate.

2 In a steamer set over boiling water, lightly steam the vegetables until they have slightly softened but still retain their bite. Alternatively, put them in a saucepan with 3 tablespoons of water, cover with a tightly fitting lid, and steam for 1–2 minutes for the courgette and 4 minutes for the broccoli. Keep checking to make sure that the water doesn't steam away.

3 While the broccoli and courgette are steaming, put the eggs in a medium pan, cover with cold water and place over a high heat. Bring to the boil, then reduce the heat to low and simmer for about 3 minutes for runny eggs.

4 When the vegetables are cooked, either toss them with the olive oil or place them on a plate and drizzle with olive oil. Sprinkle over some salt and cumin.

5 Using a slotted spoon, carefully remove the eggs and place them in egg cups. Remove the tops of each egg by tapping the shell with a teaspoon or using a knife to slice the top off. Serve with the plate of veggies and extra salt, oil and cumin on the side – and dip away!

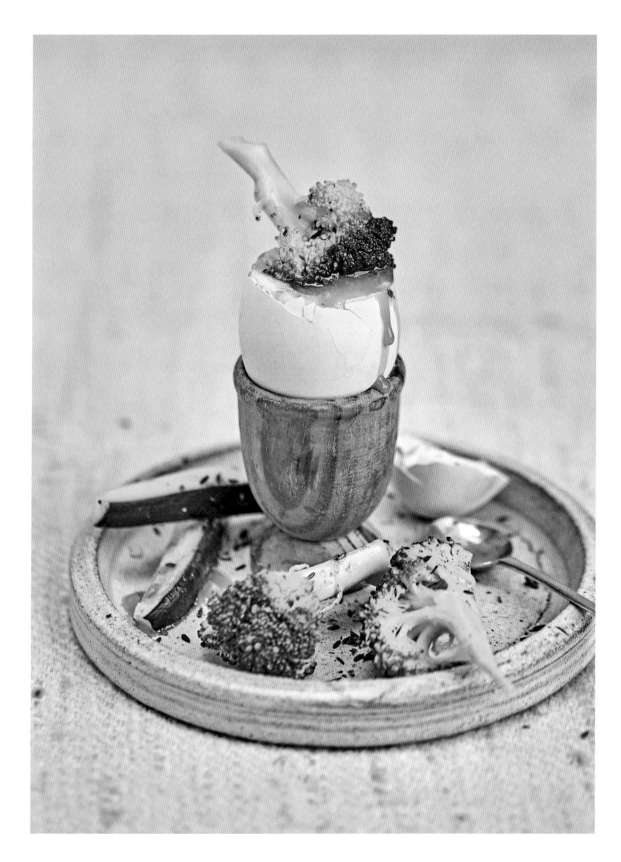

One of the most popular breakfast dishes at my pop-up cafe, those in the know even asked us to rustle it up for lunch! In Ayurveda, eggs should not be eaten with meat, fish or dairy, so this is my answer to the British fry-up.

There's a lot going on in this recipe and it's quite heavy, so if your digestion is feeling off, remove one of the elements to simplify it and make sure that the egg whites are well cooked and the yolks are just runny, because this makes them easier to digest. You can prepare the chutney and flax crunch in advance, then cool and store in the fridge.

Serves 2

Sunny-side-up eggs with flax crunch and tomato chutney

1 tbsp ghee, butter
   or coconut oil
4 medium eggs
pinch of sea salt
1 avocado

FOR THE
FLAX CRUNCH
65g (½ cup) golden or
   brown whole flaxseeds
½ tsp sea salt
10g dulse, cut into small
   pieces with scissors

FOR THE
TOMATO CHUTNEY
1 tbsp sunflower oil
500g tomatoes, skinned
   and deseeded (see
   page 260), chopped
2 tsp ground cumin
½ tsp sea salt
1 tsp jaggery
1 tbsp apple cider vinegar
8 fresh or dried curry
   leaves, chopped
3 garlic cloves, chopped

FEELING
VATA

Swap the flax crunch
for dulse flakes or
sunflower seeds.

FEELING
PITTA

Avoid eating too many egg
yolks in one week.

FEELING
KAPHA

Enjoy occasionally –
with cooked greens
instead of avocado.

1 To make the flax crunch, heat a frying pan and very lightly dry-toast the flaxseeds with the salt until they have a light aroma. Remove from the heat, toss through the dulse and set aside.

2 To make the tomato chutney, heat the sunflower oil in a pan. Add all of the remaining chutney ingredients to the pan. Stir to mix well and cook for 15 minutes until the tomatoes have broken down to a mush, then take the lid off and simmer off the excess liquid until you get quite a dry chutney.

3 Melt the ghee in a frying pan, crack in the eggs and season with a pinch of sea salt. Cook until the egg whites are cooked through but the yolk is still runny (if you tend to overcook the underside and undercook the top, try cooking the eggs with a lid on after the first minute or so).

4 Meanwhile, slice the avocado in half and de-stone. Scoop out the avocado and slice lengthways. When the eggs are ready, transfer them onto the plates. Arrange the avocado slices on top, sprinkle over the crunch and serve with a dollop of the chutney.

5 Once it has cooled, you can store the flax crunch in an airtight container in the fridge for a couple of weeks – it adds texture, crunch and seaweed goodness to almost any meal. Store leftover chutney in the fridge for up to a week.

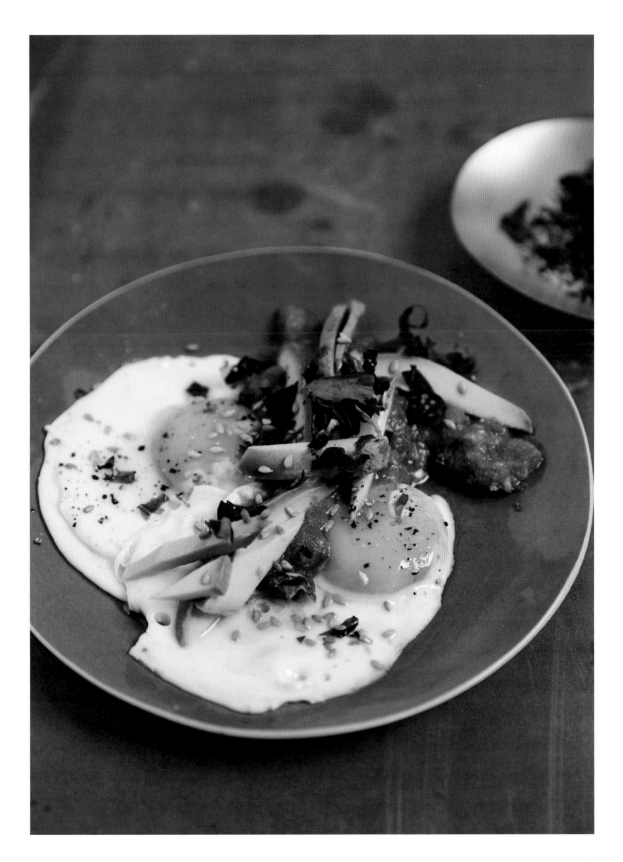

I've been baking this bread and variations of it for years, and now many of my friends make it on a regular basis. Banana bread is everyone's favourite and this malty, not-too-sweet version toasts beautifully and was a stand-out hit at the cafe. Bananas not only flavour the bread in this recipe but also work with the buckwheat to make the dough – that's right, no eggs or gluten needed.

I've thrown in cinnamon and raisins to sweeten and walnuts for crunch. It's made all the more glorious with some salty butter. For something fancy, whip up the butter to make it fluffy and sprinkle with black or flaky salt – or serve with olive oil and ricotta (see page 52).

Makes 1 large loaf

Buckwheat banana bread with salty butter

290g (2⅓ cups)
    buckwheat flour
2 tsp baking powder
1 tsp baking soda
½ tbsp ground cinnamon
¼ tsp sea salt
4 ripe bananas (about
    400g), mashed, plus
    1 ripe banana, sliced
    (about 90g)

120ml (½ cup) water
1 tsp vanilla extract
60g (½ cup) raisins
30g (¼ cup) walnuts
lightly salted butter,
    to serve

1 Preheat the oven to 180ºC (fan 160ºC/gas mark 4). Mix the buckwheat flour, baking powder, baking soda, cinnamon and sea salt together in a large bowl.

2 Mix the mashed bananas, water and vanilla together, then add to the bowl. Mix in the raisins, walnuts and remaining banana slices.

3 Transfer the mixture to a 750g (1½ lb) loaf tin lined with baking parchment. Bake for 25 minutes, then turn the tin around and bake for another 15 minutes until the bread is firm-ish to the touch. Allow to cool before slicing, then serve with butter.

FEELING
VATA

Try using half rice flour and half buckwheat flour, or exchange the buckwheat for spelt flour and serve with plenty of butter or ghee.

FEELING
KAPHA

Enjoy infrequently.
Skip the butter.

TIP
.

Use sprouted buckwheat flour if you can find it!

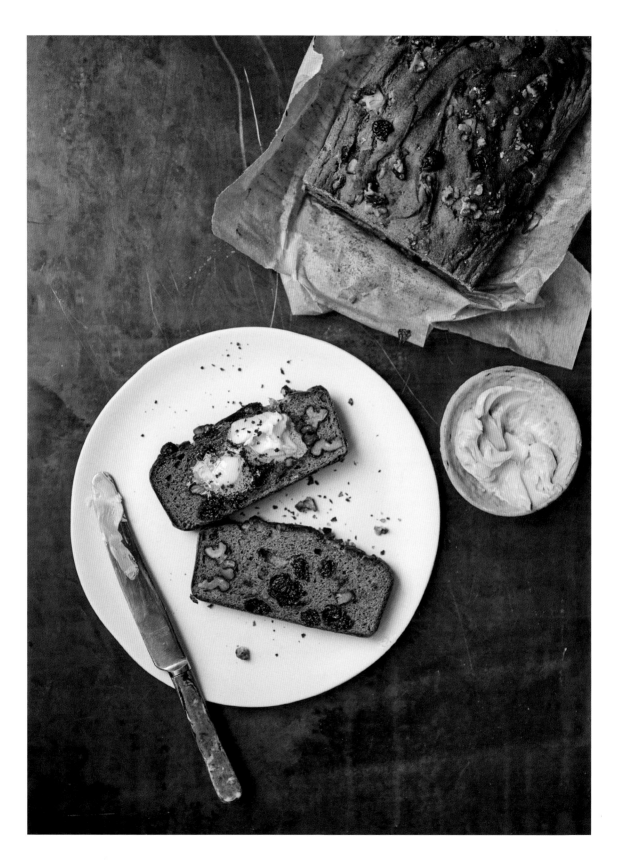

These freshly cooked rotis, smeared with creamy, savoury avocado and miso butter have become my go-to breakfast, snack or lunch. Making rotis might sound like hard work but this recipe is so easy you'll be impressing guests with your hot-off-the-press flatbreads in no time.

I love the nutty flavour of ragi – a small brown finger millet from Africa and Asia. It can be quite dense by itself in recipes, so I like to mix it 50:50 with either rice or gram flour. You can also mix it with flour from an older variety of wheat, such as spelt or einkorn, for a roti that puffs up slightly – these varieties are easier to digest than modern wheat and naturally lower in gluten. Naturally gluten-free flours tend to be dry, so that is why I've used yoghurt and ghee to bind it together. My mum grew up using mashed avocado like butter, picking them straight from the tree in her garden. Despite that little story, I didn't eat the 'green mush' until I was 12 and my auntie told me how good it was for my skin. Vanity won and now it's a favourite. Adding the salty umami miso makes this savoury butter taste a bit like creamy Marmite (says my Marmite-loving other half). You can also serve the rotis with your favourite stews, soups or pakti bowls.

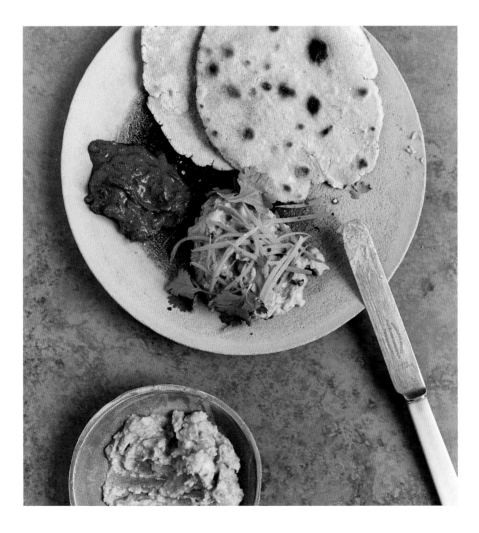

○ ◐ ●

Serves 2

Ragi roti with miso and avocado butter

38g (¼ cup) ragi flour
38g (¼ cup) rice flour
   or gram flour
¼ tsp sea salt
½ tbsp ghee, at room
   temperature
¼ tsp nigella seeds
1 tbsp homemade yoghurt
   (see page 259)
2 tbsp water

FOR THE 'BUTTER'
1 large ripe avocado,
   de-stoned
1 tbsp dark or sweet miso
splash of lemon or lime
   juice (optional)

TO SERVE
freshly ground black
   pepper
1 tbsp parsley, or your
   favourite herb
½ carrot, grated (optional)

1 Sift both flours together and mix well. Add the salt, ghee, nigella seeds and yoghurt. Starting with 1 tablespoon, add the water a little at time and mix together with your fingers until you get a soft elastic dough. Divide into eight balls about the size of a large walnut.

2 Cover a chopping board with baking parchment and roll out each ball into a roti using a rolling pin. If the dough is very sticky, I use another piece of parchment on top to stop it sticking to the rolling pin – better than adding more flour, which can make it too dry.

3 Cook each roti on a hot griddle pan for 2 minutes or so until lightly toasted. Turn the roti over and cook for 1 minute on the other side. You can also start them in a pan and then finish them in a toaster!

4 While the rotis are cooking, make the butter: mash the avocado and miso together and add a tiny splash of water to loosen, if needed. Taste and adjust the seasoning. If you're making this in advance, add a splash of lemon or lime juice to keep the colour.

5 The rotis are best served immediately while hot, so simply spread a generous amount of the butter and finish with lots of black pepper, herbs and grated carrot, if using.

WORKS WITH

PIZZA PUDAS
page 204

BRAISED GEM
LETTUCE WEDGES
WITH FENNEL AND
SESAME GOMASHIO
page 218

BEETROOT RAITA
page 226

FEELING
KAPHA

Replace the avocado
with 200g of cooked
kale and blend.

TIP
.

This also works with buckwheat
flour instead of ragi flour, or
50:50 gram and rice flour.

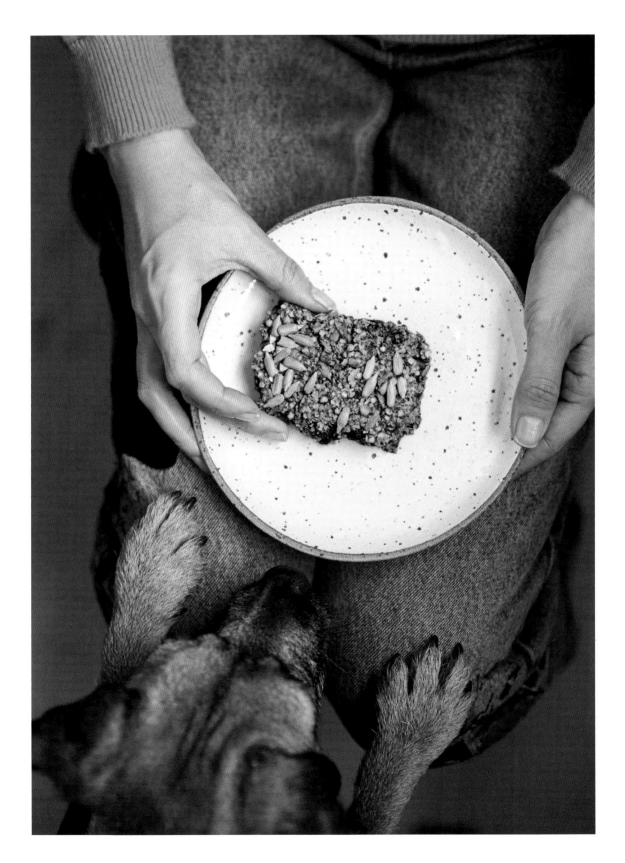

This is my kind of flapjack – savoury, sweet, crumbly and perfect with a cup of tea. Nice and portable, it doesn't go mushy and isn't full of sugar. It's an excellent recipe for practising your chewing and tuning in to the subtle flavours of the coriander seeds and cardamom. In taste tests, this is a recipe that people fall in love with ... on second bite! Oats and sunflower seeds are great for Vata and Pitta. Quinoa is Tridoshic (see page 271), and this recipe has many dry qualities so this makes a really lovely breakfast or snack for Kapha types. If you like, you can also make these sweeter and cut them smaller as little desserts.

Makes 8

Quinoa and coriander seed flapjack

5 tbsp ground flax
175ml (¾ cup) water
100g (1 cup) quinoa flakes
70g (½ cup) sunflower seeds
4 tbsp ghee, butter or coconut oil
1½ tsp coriander seeds, crushed
seeds of 15 cardamom pods, ground, or ½ tsp ground cardamom
2 tbsp maple syrup
½ cup (65g) raisins
½ tsp baking powder
¼ tsp flaky sea salt
110g (1 cup) fine oats

FEELING
VATA

Add more fat to make it unctuous, or cook the grains into a thick porridge first to get a squidgy bar (see tip).

TIP
·

For a softer bar, place the untoasted quinoa flakes and oats in a medium saucepan with 925ml water and cook over a medium-high heat for 15 minutes, stirring continuously until you have a cooked porridge. Continue with the rest of the recipe, adding 2 tablespoons more butter, ghee or coconut oil, and leaving out the water. Bake it for an extra 15 minutes.

1 Preheat the oven to 200ºC (180ºC fan/gas mark 6) and line a 20cm (8in) square tin with baking parchment. To make the flax eggs, mix the ground flax with 120ml (½ cup) of the water and set aside.

2 Spread the quinoa flakes in a 5mm-thick layer on a baking tray, and repeat the process with the sunflower seeds on another baking tray. Bake both for 10 minutes until toasty and fragrant, stirring halfway through.

3 Remove from the oven and allow to cool. Reduce the oven temperature to 180ºC (160ºC fan/gas mark 4).

4 Melt the ghee in a small pan and fry the coriander and cardamom for 2 minutes over a medium-high heat, until fragrant. Remove from the heat.

5 In a medium bowl, stir together the rest of the water, the maple syrup, flax egg and raisins and then stir in the baking powder, oats, quinoa and two-thirds of the sunflower seeds, reserving the rest for the top.

6 Spread out the mixture in the prepared tin, pressing down firmly. Scatter over the remaining seeds and press again, using the back of a spoon. Bake in the oven for 25 minutes or until firm.

7 Allow the flapjack to cool in the tin before slicing into 8 rectangles. The flapjacks store well in the fridge, or will keep for a few days at room temperature.

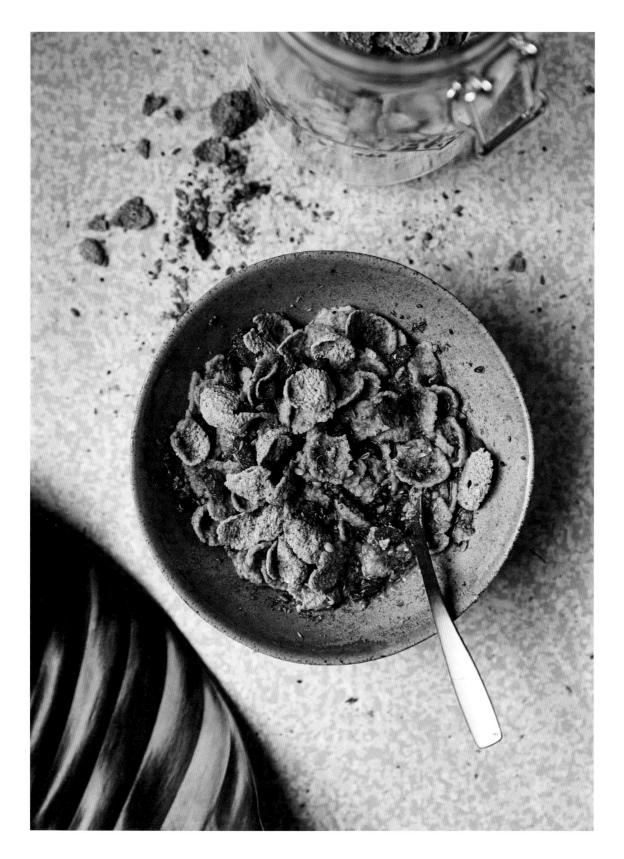

Eating well while travelling can be either a match made in heaven or a nightmare, depending on where you're going and how you're getting there! This is my little travel mix, inspired by my stay at Vana Ayurvedic Retreat when I combined dried fruits and cinnamon with ragi flakes (a type of dark millet found in Asia) in a jar for my flight home. For the absolute lightest meal I added hot water, allowed it to sit and enjoyed the malty simplicity and all-important dose of spices.

Ragi flakes are not easy to source in the UK but you can usually find regular millet flakes in health-food shops and online – either in crunchy breakfast cereal form or the even more cost-effective rolled millet flakes (think porridge-oats style). Be sure to toast the raw, rolled millet flakes first so that they are easier to digest.

This is a great mix to make ahead, ready for a quick breakfast or your travels. It lasts without the need for a fridge, and if you make it using roasted rolled millet flakes it's pretty compact. It might seem strange eating cereal without milk, but once the hot water has softened the flakes, you'll end up with a sweetly spiced porridge.

○◑●

Serves 4–5

Millet flake travel mix

120g crunchy millet flakes (or rolled millet flakes)
1 tbsp fennel seeds
4 tbsp ghee or coconut oil
50g goji berries, raisins or other dried berries
30g desiccated coconut
seeds of 5 cardamom pods, ground
1 tbsp ground ginger (omit if you're feeling Pitta)

2 tbsp ground coriander
2 tbsp ground cinnamon
3 heaped tbsp chia seeds
3 heaped tbsp whole flaxseeds
1 tbsp jaggery, chopped

1   If you're using rolled millet flakes, toast them. Preheat the oven to 170ºC (fan 150ºC/gas mark 3). Spread the flakes on a baking tray, in a 5mm-thick layer. Toast for 5 minutes. Alternatively, toast in a dry frying pan over a low-medium heat, stirring continuously for 1–2 minutes until golden. Add the ghee, stir to coat and allow to cool. Forgo this step if the millet flakes are crunchy, and simply melt the ghee.

2   Toast the fennel seeds in a dry frying pan until fragrant and set aside. Leave to cool and then grind in a pestle and mortar. Transfer to a mixing bowl with the millet flakes and ghee.

3   Add the rest of the ingredients and mix together well. Transfer to a glass jar or stainless-steel container with a tightly fitting lid and store somewhere cool. To serve, shake the mix and pour 25g (1 cup) into a bowl or large mug. Pour over 120ml (½ cup) of boiling water, cover and leave for a few minutes, then enjoy.

FEELING
VATA

Be sure to add some ghee and jaggery – if you're eating it at home you can add at the table.

FEELING
KAPHA

Skip the ghee. There's no need to wait for the cereal to soften – enjoy it crunchy and chewy!

TIP
.

Also try rolled oats or crunchy millet, rice and oat flakes from health-food shops. These may be sweetened, though, so watch the jaggery.

Nothing says summer like the abundance of local fruit. Ripe seasonal fruit is the easiest to digest, and it's even better to choose fruit that suits your Dosha. Tridoshic fruits include melons, blueberries, apricots and raspberries, but you can also follow the individual Dosha suggestions below. It's tempting to eat a fruit salad medley, but it's best to stick to one or two types of fruit in one sitting and leave a 30-minute gap before you eat other foods. Make sure that fruit is at room temperature, or even griddled or roasted, and that melon is eaten without any other fruit to optimise digestion. Enjoy with the spiced dip for a fresh breakfast or a 4pm snack.

Serves 2

Fresh fruit with spicy dip

¼ tsp arrowroot

60ml (¼ cup) water

1 tsp ground cinnamon

seeds of 30 cardamom
   pods, ground, or 1 tsp
   ground cardamom

¼ tsp ground nutmeg

5mm (¼ in) piece of fresh
   ginger, grated

½ tbsp ghee

1 tbsp maple syrup
   or jaggery

⅛ tsp sea salt

fruit of your choice
   (see below)

1   In a cup or small bowl, dissolve the arrowroot in 1 tablespoon of the water and then whisk in the rest of the water until smooth.

2   To prepare the spice mix, sauté all of the ground spices and the ginger in the ghee over a medium-high heat for about 2 minutes, or until the aromas are released. Add the maple syrup or jaggery, salt and the arrowroot water. Simmer for about 2 minutes until reduced, then pour into a dipping bowl.

3   Prepare your choice of fruit, making sure it is ripe and at room temperature. Dip the pieces of fruit into the sauce and chew thoroughly.

TIP
.
The sauce begins to thicken as it cools. Add 1–2 teaspoons of hot water to return it to the desired consistency.

**FEELING
VATA**

Choose from apricots, bananas, mango, papaya, peaches, strawberries, grapes and cherries.

**FEELING
PITTA**

Choose from sweet apples, pears, berries, plums and pomegranates.

**FEELING
KAPHA**

Choose from apples, pears, strawberries, mango, peaches and cherries. Add chilli.

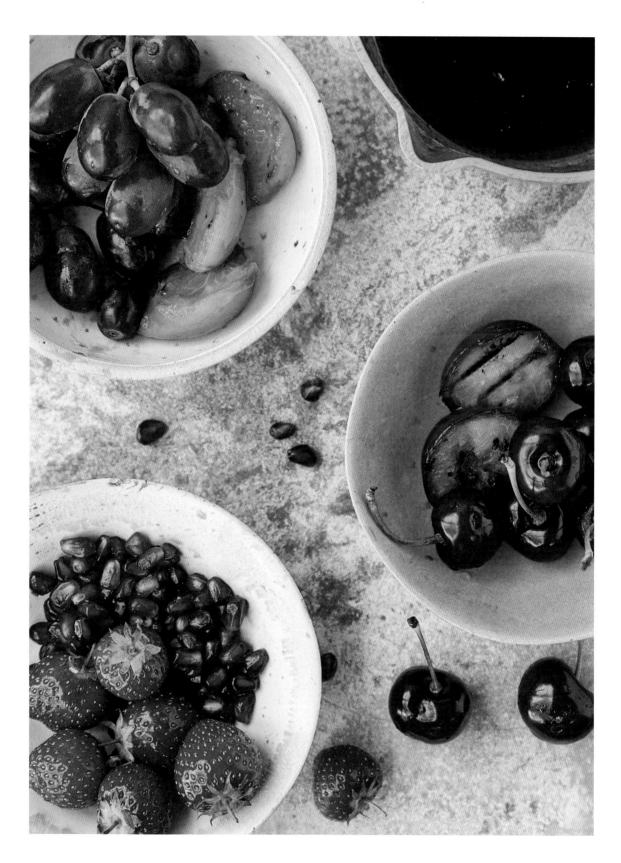

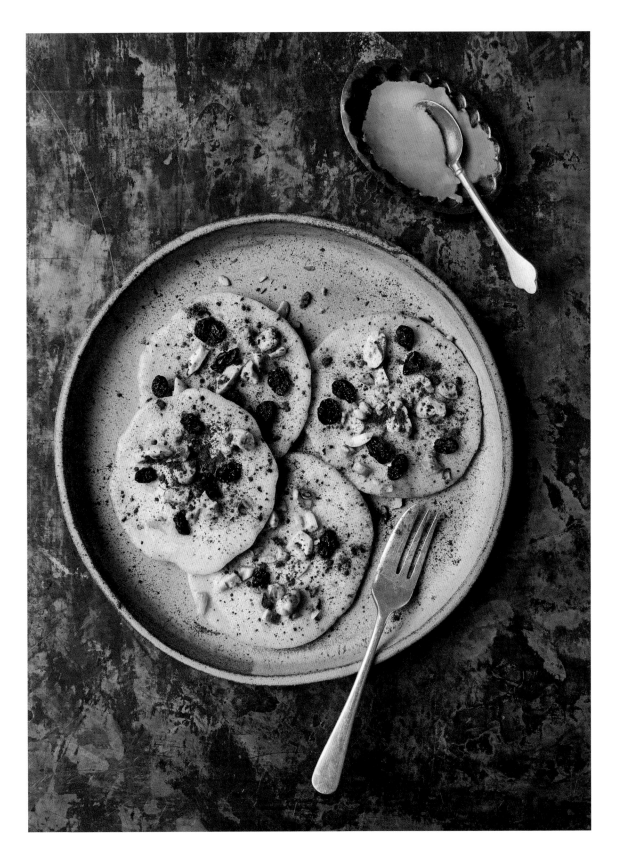

I'm pretty proud of this recipe, which is inspired by the original savoury uttapams I discovered during my first trip to India – I say discovered, but they are everywhere and hard to miss! Originating from the south of India, traditional uttapams are thick mini pancakes served with onion, tomatoes, spices and herbs and are made of the same fermented rice and dal batter as the Breakfast Dosas (see page 80), although ratios can vary slightly. After ordering masala uttapams accompanied with the usual breakfast chutneys and sambar every day for nearly a week, I fancied a sweet version, so I suggested some changes to the chef: raisins, vanilla and cashews with a sprinkling of cinnamon. He thought I was mad, but we both loved the results!

Serves 3

Sweet cashew, raisin and cinnamon uttapams

½ quantity of Dosa batter
(see page 80)
60ml (¼ cup) water
1 tbsp maple syrup or
jaggery
1 tsp vanilla extract
1 tsp ground cinnamon,
plus extra for
sprinkling
18 cashews, crushed or
roughly chopped

20g raisins
1 tsp ghee or coconut oil,
plus more if necessary

1   Make half the dosa batter from the Breakfast Dosas on page 80. This makes enough for about twelve pancakes. Mix in the water, maple syrup, vanilla extract and cinnamon.

2   Melt the ghee in a 25cm (10in) ceramic-lined or seasoned cast-iron frying pan on a medium-high heat.

3   Pour 2 tablespoons of the batter into the hot pan, which should spread out to make a 9cm (3½ in) thick pancake. Working quickly, stud the pancake with five or so raisins, a few crushed cashews and a tiny pinch of cinnamon. Repeat, working your way around the pan (you should be able to fit four pancakes).

4   Fry on low heat until small bubbles appear on the surface. Flip over and cook for a few seconds to toast the cashews, being careful not to burn the toppings. Remove and repeat until all the batter is used up, adding a little more oil or ghee if needed.

FEELING
VATA

Skip the cashews and
dot with ghee.

FEELING
KAPHA

Go traditional and make
these with spices and
vegetables.

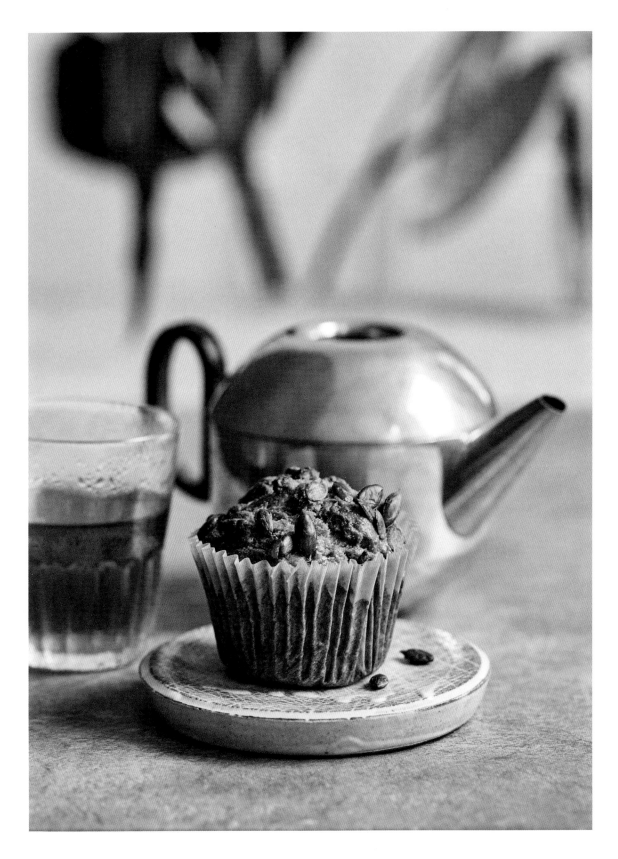

A recipe challenge is guaranteed to make me tick, and this proved to be just that! I'm all about adding carrots to baking where possible, and I've also been working with chestnut flour, sweetened with a little maple syrup, for years. However, it turns out that combining these three sweet ingredients is a big ask for digestion. My Ayurvedic doctor put a question mark by this recipe when I showed it to him, so I went back to the drawing board! I knew I didn't want an overly sweet muffin – something just sweet enough for breakfast, or as a snack if I know a meal is going to be delayed – so I took out the maple syrup and worked on the spices to make it a delicious little bran-style muffin.

These keep well in an airtight container for a day or two or longer in the fridge, but allow them to come to room temperature before you eat them.

○◑●

Makes 6

Chestnut, carrot and ginger muffins with pumpkin seeds

115g (1 cup) chestnut flour
1 tsp baking powder
1 tsp ground cinnamon
2 large pinches of sea salt
5 medium eggs or 5 flax eggs (see page 256)
2cm (¾in) piece of fresh ginger, grated

5 tbsp butter, melted
2 medium carrots, coarsely grated (about 125g)
handful of pumpkin seeds, to garnish

1   Preheat the oven to 220ºC (fan 200ºC/gas mark 7).

2   Mix together the flour, baking powder, cinnamon and salt in a large bowl. In a separate bowl, mix together the eggs, ginger, butter and carrots. Pour the wet ingredients into the dry mixture, stirring gently.

3   Divide the mixture between six muffin cases, top with pumpkin seeds and bake the muffins for 20 minutes until they turn a deep golden colour. Allow to cool before serving.

FEELING
VATA

The eggs and chestnut flour makes this suited to winter and Vata nature. Enjoy with ginger tea.

FEELING
PITTA

Enjoy with fennel tea and use flax eggs. You could try 50:50 chestnut flour and rice flour.

FEELING
KAPHA

Enjoy with black tea and use flax eggs. You could try 50:50 chestnut flour and buckwheat flour.

These buttery crêpes go really well with the tartness of plum compote. The batter works best with 30 minutes rest, which is the perfect amount of time to stew the plums with the spices. Play around with the spice combination by adding some cloves, allspice or cayenne pepper. This also makes a delicious jam: if you have a sweet tooth or the plums are not as ripe as you'd like, simply up the jaggery and cook for longer.

Makes around
12 crêpes

Chestnut crêpes with vanilla chai plum compote

FOR THE CRÊPES

115g (1 cup) chestnut flour

3 large eggs, at room temperature

120ml (½ cup) water or buttermilk

⅛ tsp sea salt

melted ghee or coconut oil, to cook

FOR THE PLUMS

around 12 ripe plums (900g)

60g (¼ cup) jaggery

1 star anise

1 vanilla pod or 2 tsp vanilla extract

1 cinnamon stick or ½ tsp ground cinnamon

1 tsp freshly ground black pepper, or more to taste

FEELING
PITTA

Use rice flour instead of chestnut flour, and try apricots as an alternative to plums.

FEELING
KAPHA

Use buckwheat or millet flour, and try apricots as an alternative to plums.

1 To make the batter, place the flour in a large bowl and make a well in the middle. Beat in the eggs, one at a time. Add the water a little at a time, whisking continuously until you have a smooth batter. Stir in the salt and set the batter aside to rest for 30 minutes.

2 Quarter the plums, removing the stones. Put the fruit into a heavy-based pan with the jaggery, star anise, vanilla pod, cinnamon stick and black pepper.

3 Cook gently on a medium heat, lid on, then reduce the heat and simmer for 15 minutes, or until the plums are just tender or completely falling apart, depending on your preference. Remember to fish out the whole spices – star anise, vanilla pod and cinnamon stick.

4 Once the compote is cooked, heat a ceramic-lined or seasoned cast-iron frying pan on a medium heat and brush with melted ghee. Whisk the batter again, then add 2–3 tablespoons to the pan. Tilt the pan to thinly but evenly coat the bottom with batter. Cook for 1 minute or so until the pancake lifts easily from the pan and is golden brown on the underside. Turn (or flip!) the pancake to cook the other side – don't overcook, to keep them chewy rather than crisp.

5 Repeat with the remaining batter, stacking pancakes on top of each other to keep them warm. Serve each pancake with a helping of the compote. Store the remaining compote in the fridge for up to 1 month.

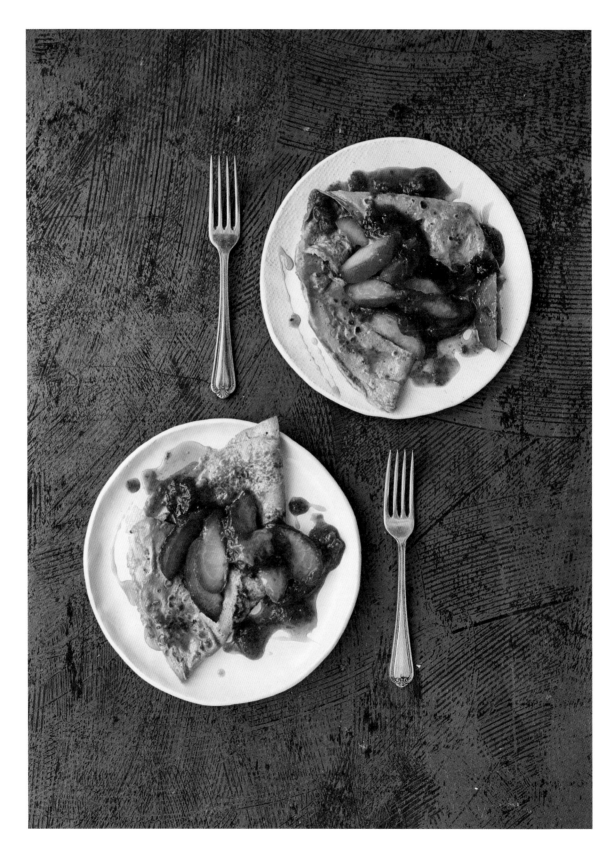

Stewed apple is an Ayurvedic classic. From the first time I tried this simple recipe, I loved it – it smells reassuringly nostalgic and sets the tone for the whole day. Light to digest, warming and deliciously spiced, this is so easy to make and all the ingredients are readily available.

Serves 1

Apples are a great source of vitamin A and potassium, cinnamon is medicinal and anti-inflammatory, and cloves are metabolism-activating and great for oral health – so in combination, this little dish forms part of the perfect morning ritual. Best enjoyed as early as possible in the morning, it suits all Dosha types and can stimulate your system, build an appetite for lunch and increase vitality and alertness.

This makes enough for one, but it is easy to double or triple the recipe to feed more. If I'm making this for more than one then I usually pop it all into my slowcooker the night before and let it cook gently overnight on low, or in the morning on high for an hour. Fill the slowcooker with 5cm (2in) of water to prevent it from burning, or use the ovenproof bowl method on page 50.

For a heartier breakfast, follow this with some sweet cooked cereal such as Fig, Cinnamon and Cardamom Congee (see page 50), Milk Rice (see page 82) or Amaranth Porridge (see page 45). For easier digestion, peel the apples – you can simmer the peel with the apples to get the benefits and then discard. Please note: if you've got blood-sugar issues it's best to avoid this recipe.

Stewed apple with star anise and cinnamon

1 apple, cored
(and peeled if skin
is thick)
5 whole cloves
around 60ml
(¼ cup) water,
depending on the
size of your pan

1 star anise
pinch of ground
cinnamon

1 Cut the apple into quarters or chunks. Add it to a very small pan with the cloves, water and star anise and bring to the boil. Lower the heat to a simmer, then cover and cook for about 5 minutes until tender.

2 Add the cinnamon, then remove from the heat and allow to sit for another 10 minutes. Serve.

TIP
.

It's important to use a very small pan with a tight-fitting lid for this recipe. If you use a bigger pan you may need to increase the volume of water.

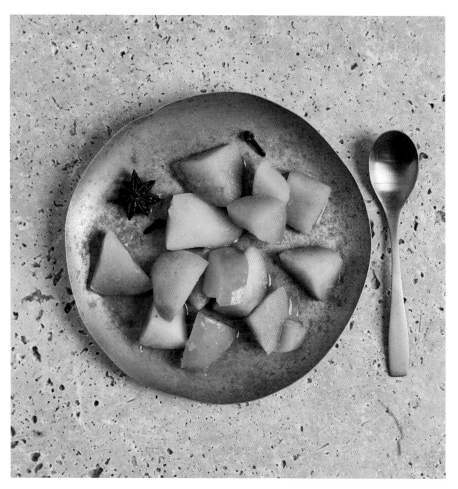

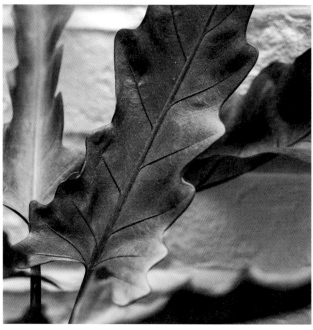

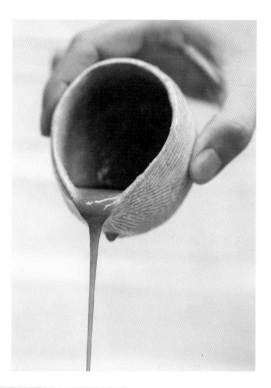

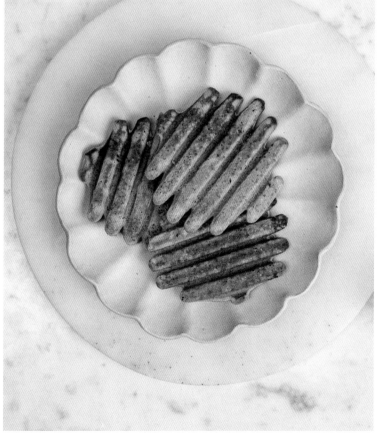

The inspiration for this recipe came from one of my besties, Taylor, who's living in New York and works above a cafe selling teff waffles drizzled with ghee. I set to work making them myself and they've since become a firm breakfast favourite – especially when entertaining. The addition of molasses is optional since it's not a common ingredient around these parts and I don't use it in this book again. The turmeric and honey drizzle is a must, or serve with Goldenspoon (see page 91) if you've got a batch of that ready. For the turmeric and honey drizzle it's important to get the ratio of ghee to turmeric right, according to your Dosha. The golden (!) rule is not to use equal weights: for Kapha, use more honey than ghee, and for Vata and Pitta, use more ghee than honey.

I'd love a waffle maker but don't need another piece of equipment in my kitchen, so on the weekends I pull out the griddle pan and make thick pancakes with grooves on them, close my eyes and pretend! This makes four thick, scotch-style pancakes, but feel free to double the recipe if you're feeding a crowd.

◌◑●

Makes 4

Teff waffles with turmeric and honey drizzle

125g (¾ cup) teff flour
1½ tsp baking powder
¾ tsp ground cinnamon
pinch of sea salt
1 tbsp maple syrup
120ml (½ cup) whole milk, nut milk or water
1 medium egg, beaten, or 1 flax egg (see page 256)

1½ tbsp melted ghee, butter or coconut oil, plus extra for greasing
2½ tsp molasses (optional)

FOR THE TURMERIC AND HONEY DRIZZLE
1 tbsp raw honey
1 tbsp melted ghee
½ tsp ground turmeric

1   Mix the teff flour, baking powder, cinnamon and salt in a medium bowl. Whisk together the wet ingredients and add them to the dry. Stir well to combine.

2   Heat a large, ceramic-lined or seasoned cast-iron griddle pan over a medium heat. Grease with ghee. When hot add a quarter of the batter and lightly smooth with the back of a spoon, until you get a flat pancake that's around 1cm (½ in) thick and 7–8cm (2¾–3in) across.

3   Cook for 3–4 minutes on one side then flip it over with a spatula and cook for 3–4 minutes on the other side. Repeat with the remaining batter until you get four thick pancakes.

4   For the drizzle, combine the honey, ghee and turmeric in a small bowl or jug. Drizzle over the pancakes and serve.

TIP
·
If you're using a waffle iron, preheat it according to the manufacturer's instructions. Add 60ml (¼ cup) extra water to the batter, and drop onto the preheated waffle iron.

If you've been to India then you are probably already a fan of these light and crisp southern Indian crêpes made from a fermented batter of rice and dal. Traditionally served for breakfast with a tangy sambhar and a chutney, these are also delicious with any manner of toppings you might have in the fridge. Be warned – some of these toppings may be considered sacrilegious by purists!

Serves 4

The batter is simple but requires prepping two nights in advance if you want them for breakfast, or start it in the evening if you want them for dinner the next day. Like all the best things in life, it needs a little time to do its thing.

You'll need a fairly strong blender or grinder for this, as well as a seasoned cast-iron or ceramic-lined pan. Once the batter is prepped it will last for 2 days in the fridge, and is the same batter used to make the uttapams on page 71. Make sure it is at room temperature before using and proceed as if making thin pancakes or crêpes – with good humour until you get it right!

Breakfast dosas

160g (1 cup) basmati rice
80g (⅓ cup) urad dal
¼ tsp fenugreek seeds
250ml (1 cup) filtered
    water (see tip), plus
    extra if necessary
½ tsp salt
melted ghee, for cooking

1 At least 24 hours before you wish to serve, rinse the basmati rice and urad dal and place in a bowl with the fenugreek. Pour over enough water to reach 5cm (2in) above the surface of the ingredients. Cover with a lid and leave to soak for 5–6 hours.

2 Drain and blend in a strong blender with the water and the salt until you get a fine but grainy consistency.

3 Transfer to a bowl (or leave in the blender) and cover loosely. Leave in a warm place like an airing cupboard or in an oven with the light on for 8 hours or more until the batter is lightly fermented, doubled in volume and has bubbles and a slightly sour aroma.

TIP
·

Blend the batter with filtered water at the fermenting stage, as the chlorine in tap water will kill the friendly bacteria.

4 Stir the batter lightly, adding a little water if necessary to reach a pouring consistency.

5 Heat a seasoned cast-iron or ceramic-lined pan over a medium-high heat. Smear lightly with ghee as if making a pancake. Do not use too much, otherwise you won't be able to spread the dosa batter properly.

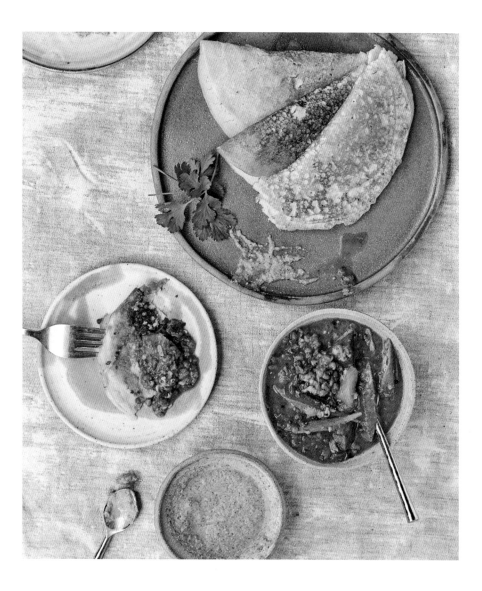

WORKS WITH

SRI LANKAN
CELEBRATION PICKLE
page 237

APRICOT TAHINI AND
CARDAMOM CREAM
page 96

VANILLA CHAI PLUM
COMPOTE
page 74

LEMON, TURMERIC
AND BLACK PEPPER
SALMON
page 125

GOLDENSPOON
page 91

6   Take a small ladleful of the batter and spoon into the centre. Gently spread using the back of the ladle in a circular movement from the centre outwards.

7   Drizzle a little ghee over the top and sides of the dosa and allow to cook until the base is nicely golden and crisp and lifts off the pan easily. If the dosa is thin, fold and serve hot with the South Indian Moong Sambhar (see page 183) and Green Chutney (from the Dhokla recipe, see page 229). Otherwise flip and cook for a minute or so, then continue with the rest of the batter.

Rice pudding can divide a room. However, this Ayurvedic version, contributed by my friend and meditation teacher Jess Cook, has certainly ignited a renewed passion for rice pudding in anyone who has tried it! When I first ate this, one summer morning on a retreat, a warm feeling washed over me and I never forgot it.

Serves 2

This balancing and calming dish is dedicated to our Ayurvedic family friends, the Rajus. The recipe contains the most Sattvic Ayurvedic foods – basmati rice, milk, ghee, dates and almonds – making it perfect for a breakfast or evening meal, especially for Vata types. I also recommend it for ladies on their moon cycle to really make the most of this cleansing time. As this recipe includes milk, avoid eating around the same time as sour and salty foods.

Milk rice

60g (generous ¼ cup) white basmati rice
300ml whole milk
100ml water
½ tsp ghee
1 tbsp pitted medjool dates, chopped
10g currants or raisins
10g blanched almonds or cashews, chopped and soaked for 1 hour
5 cardamom pods (you can add these whole, or just use the seeds)

large pinch of ground turmeric
2.5cm (1in) piece of fresh ginger, finely chopped

FOR THE TOPPING (OPTIONAL)
½ tsp coconut oil
1 tsp coconut flakes
½ tsp jaggery

1   Rinse the rice in a sieve with cold water, then drain and add it to a saucepan. Add the milk, water, ghee and other ingredients.

2   Bring the mixture slowly to the boil, stirring occasionally. Allow it to simmer for about 20 minutes, until the rice is soft and the consistency is thick and creamy.

3   For the optional topping, add the coconut oil, coconut slices and jaggery to a small saucepan over a medium heat. Cook for 1–2 minutes, stirring constantly, until lightly golden and crisp.

4   Divide the milk rice between two bowls and add the topping, if using.

TIP
.
You might find that you feel hot during and after eating this, and expel some gas as Vata is released – these are both good signs!

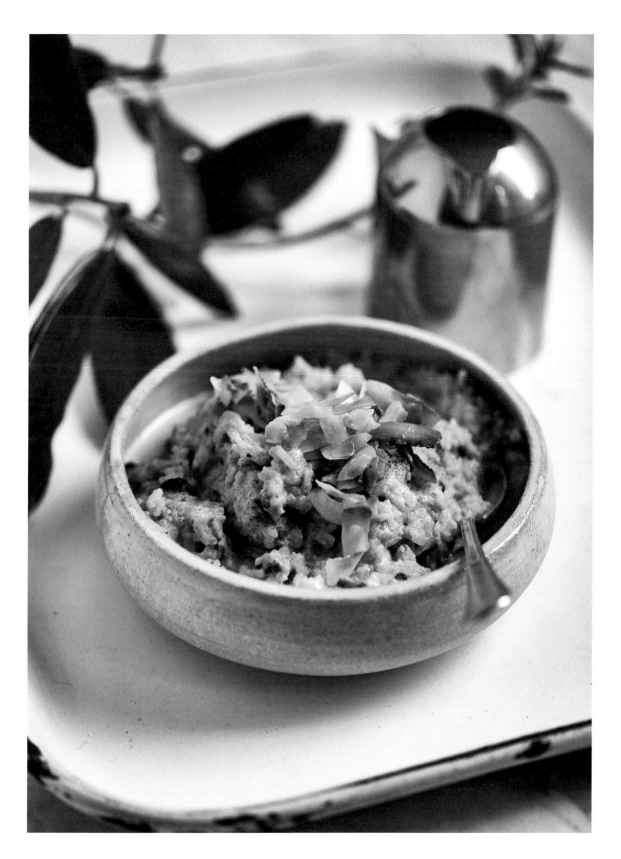

The original bliss ball or 'energy ball', an Indian ladoo is a ball-shaped sweet that's usually made of nuts and dried fruit. The traditional name in Ayurveda is 'modak', which means a preparation that makes the inner body happy. Pilgrims were traditionally given ladoos on arrival at the holy sites, to boost energy and strengthen the spirit during meditation and prayer. The process of turning the quick mixture into even-sized balls is like a little meditation in itself! And a fun one to involve the kids. In Ayurveda, ladoos are seen to promote Agni (see page 278) and so make the perfect starter for lunch.

Makes 24 balls

Coconut, lime and mint ladoo

200g (1¾ cups) ground
    almonds
140g (1¾ cup) desiccated
    coconut
3 tbsp maple syrup
zest of 2 limes
½ tsp vanilla extract
1 tsp peppermint extract
100g (½ cup) coconut oil
pinch of sea salt

1 Blitz the ground almonds, 60g (¾ cup) of the desiccated coconut, the maple syrup, zest, vanilla extract, peppermint extract, coconut oil and sea salt in a food processor, until chunky but evenly mixed.

2 Taste the mixture and add a drop more of the peppermint extract if needed, then blitz again.

3 Take small pieces from the bowl and roll them into twenty-four bite-sized balls with the palms of your hands. Refrigerate for around 20 minutes, until firm.

4 Spread out the remaining desiccated coconut and roll each ladoo in it until completely covered. Store somewhere cool or in the fridge for up to a week.

FEELING
VATA

Enjoy in
warm weather.

FEELING
PITTA

Make the most of the
cooling effects of the lime,
coconut and mint by
serving straight from
the fridge. Be sure to
savour slowly.

FEELING
KAPHA

Enjoy very
occasionally in
warm weather.

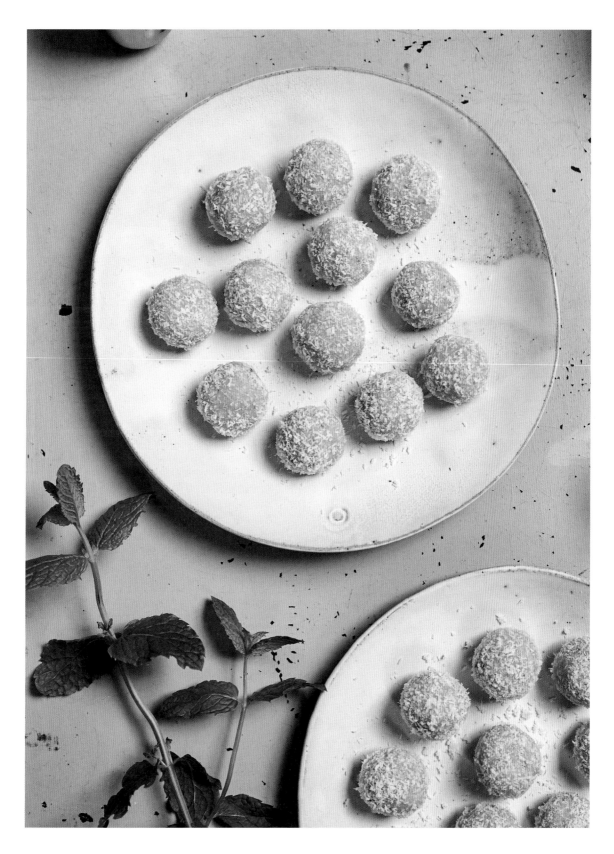

To ladoo or not to ladoo, that is the question! Perhaps only a question when it comes to digesting peanuts. A staple in many parts of the world, peanuts can be a bit tricky to digest, especially if wolfed down without chewing. Peanut butter is much better for digestion, especially when savoured slowly and eaten occasionally in small amounts.

These easy ladoos, paired with fresh ginger to help things along and eaten before lunch as part of the Surya Agni (see page 11), keep well in the freezer, ready for a peanut fix in perfect measure. Tune in to your body and see how well you digest peanuts and other nuts – we're told they are very healthy but if our digestion says otherwise we need to listen to that first. Look for good-quality, organic peanut butter as peanuts are prone to mould. You could also use almond butter if you prefer.

Makes about
30 balls

Sesame, peanut, ginger and honey ladoo

130g (¾ cup) peanut
    butter, mixed well
85g (¼ cup) raw honey
⅛ tsp sea salt
3–4 tbsp coconut flour
2.5cm (1in) piece of fresh
    ginger, grated (avoiding
    stringy bits) or 1 tsp
    ground ginger
35–75g (¼–½ cup)
    sesame seeds

1   Place all the ingredients, apart from the sesame seeds, into a mixing bowl and stir until well combined.

2   Take small pieces from the bowl and roll them into bite-sized balls with the palms of your hands. If the mixture is difficult to work with, chill it for 10 minutes before rolling.

3   Place the sesame seeds in another bowl. Roll the peanut butter balls in the sesame seeds until they are completely covered. Refrigerate for around 15 minutes, until firm. Store in the fridge for up to 5 days or in the freezer for up to a month. If you've opted for dried ginger they will keep for a month in a cool, dark place.

FEELING
PITTA

FEELING
KAPHA

Swap the honey for
jaggery and stick to fresh
ginger or swap for
cinnamon or fennel seeds.

Roll these balls very small
– they are so nourishing,
but can be too much of
a good thing.

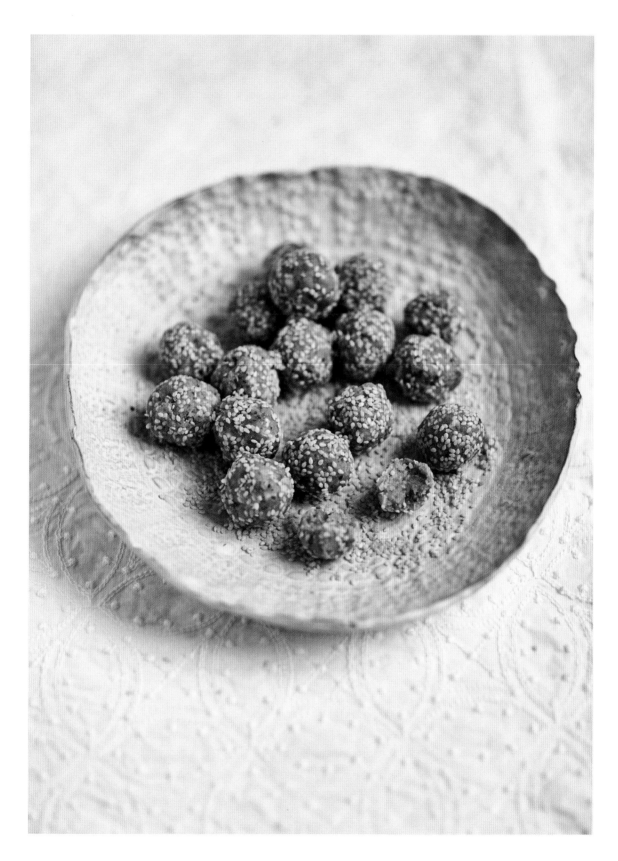

This little recipe was developed at home in my kitchen just before opening the cafe – it's a super-simple whipped dessert using up the dried mango that one of my aunties had brought back from the Philippines. Fresh fruit and yoghurt are usually a digestive 'no-no', but using dried mango changes the properties of the fruit and makes it more compatible – as does blending it, which is a bit like cooking and helps the two different ingredients come together. Rather than making a rich mousse, this one is light and creamy – especially if you have a powerful blender. If using a food processor, use the smallest bowl possible to ensure the smoothest mousse, or make more than one portion.

Mango is considered the king of fruits in Ayurveda because of its many medicinal uses. Unluckily for us, we rarely get to try a truly ripe, sublime one – if you do, save it to enjoy on its own.

Serves 1

Mango lassi mousse

35g dried mango pieces
100ml water
125g (½ cup) homemade yoghurt (see page 259)
¼ tsp finely grated lemon zest (optional)

¼ tsp ground turmeric (optional)
pinch of sumac and mint leaves, to garnish

1 Soak the mango pieces in the water until soft. Remove the pieces from the water and reserve 50ml of the soaking water.

2 Blend the reserved water and mango with the yoghurt for 5 seconds until smooth and whipped, then mix through the lemon zest and turmeric, if using. Top with the sumac and mint leaves and serve at room temperature.

FEELING
KAPHA

Enjoy very infrequently, due to the mucilaginous properties of both mango and yoghurt.

TIP
.
Save the leftover soaking water to add a little sweetness to dals and stews.

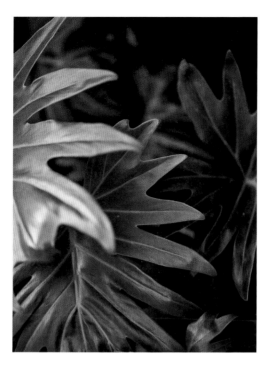

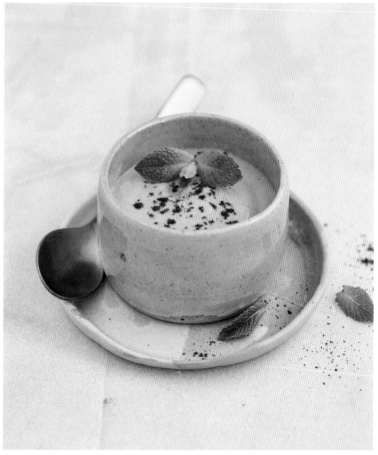

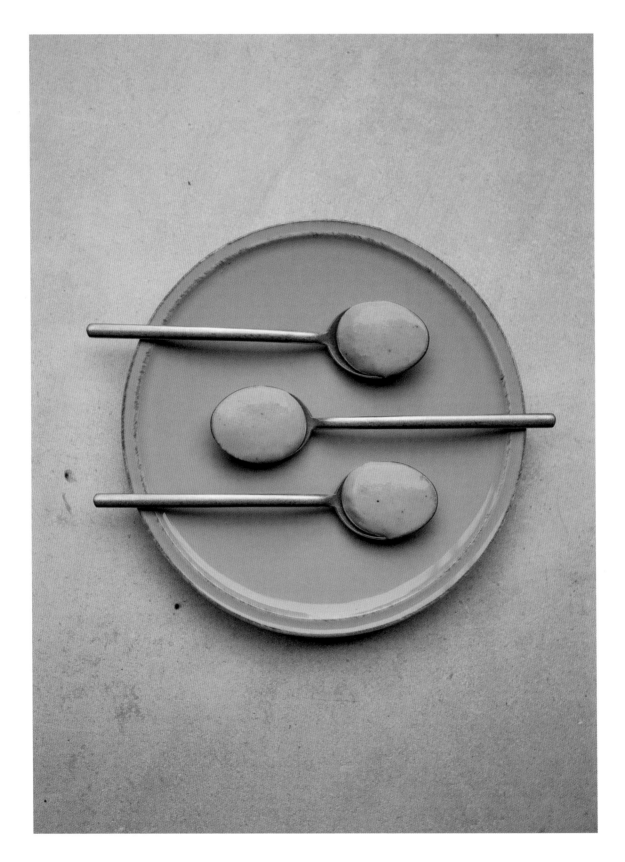

Welcome to the Goldenspoon! This immune-boosting elixir served on a spoon was my signature recipe at the pop-up cafe. The eye-catching and oh-so-delicious paste was ordered by everyone in the know – and everyone who just had to know, as little dishes of Goldenspoon circulated and people demanded it by the jar. Not only do ground turmeric and black pepper have excellent antioxidant benefits, but also black pepper contains the active ingredient piperine, which enhances the bioavailability of curcumin – the active ingredient in turmeric.

Coconut oil also helps the body to absorb the benefits of fat-soluble turmeric and makes for a smooth and creamy paste that you can also use as a spread. Since coconut oil is cooling, in winter I switch to avocado oil, which also thickens in the fridge, although it becomes more syrup-like than a paste.

Goldenspoon needs to be kept in the fridge, so be sure to enjoy it slowly, savouring the flavour and warming it up before it hits your belly and your digestive fire! You can also enjoy this paste in warm water or almond milk, but make sure it is not too hot and avoid using dairy milk – in Ayurveda, combining honey and dairy milk is a 'no-no'. Always allow the mixture to cool down before adding the honey, because it's also important not to heat honey.

Makes 320g

Goldenspoon

120ml (½ cup) water
35g (¼ cup) ground
   turmeric
1½ tsp freshly ground
   black pepper
75g coconut oil,
   melted and at room
   temperature (or
   avocado oil)
100g (scant ⅓ cup)
   raw honey

1   Mix the water with the ground turmeric and black pepper in a small saucepan over a medium heat. Slowly simmer for up to 10 minutes, stirring until it becomes a thick paste. Set aside to cool for 5 minutes.

2   Gradually add the coconut oil, and continue stirring until all the ingredients are completely mixed together. When cool enough to touch, gradually add the honey, stirring continuously.

3   Pour the paste into a clean, sterilised jar and leave to cool for 1 hour. Then seal the jar and place in the fridge for 6 hours, mixing at 2-hour intervals until it solidifies.

4   Store in the fridge for up to a month.

The traditional Indian recipe for almond barfi calls for blanched or soaked almonds, peeled, then ground to a paste that's cooked in condensed milk or sugar syrup. I've swapped the condensed milk and sugar syrup for ghee and jaggery, of course, and in addition to saffron I've included pistachios and rose extract to flavour – both expensive but that's what makes this sweet an absolute delicacy! Remember nuts should be eaten in small amounts, so just one piece is enough.

I've also included a cheat's version using ground almonds (see the tip, opposite): it's slightly more expensive but it saves an extra step. Make sure the packet is in date and fresh as possible – don't grab the stuff lurking at the back of your cupboard, as the delicate nut oils become rancid easily. If you have digestive issues, skip the pistachios, so you are only digesting one type of nut, and add some fresh ginger while cooking.

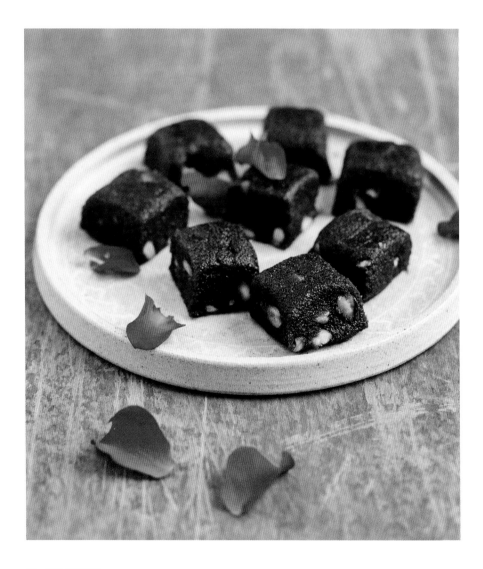

Saffron and almond barfi with pistachios and rose

180g (1⅓ cups) whole
   almonds, soaked
   overnight, or ground
   almonds (see below)
250ml (1 cup)
   boiling water
175ml (¾ cup) cold water
40g (¼ cup) pistachios
65g (⅓ cup) jaggery,
   finely chopped

pinch of saffron strands,
   soaked in 2 tbsp
   warm water
4 tbsp ghee
¼ tsp rose extract,
   or to taste

1   Line a 900g (2lb) loaf tin with baking parchment. Soak the almonds in the boiling water. Cover and leave to blanch for 30 seconds.

2   Drain the almonds and then press each one out of its skin. Add them all to a blender with 120ml (½ cup) of the soaking water and pulse the almonds to get a fine texture, but not too fine.

3   Place the ground almonds with the pistachios and the 175ml (¾ cup) cold water in a heavy-bottomed, medium saucepan. Heat the pan over a medium-high heat, stirring continuously for 2–3 minutes until the almonds are fragrant. Reduce the heat to medium.

4   Add the jaggery and stir well until it starts to melt. Keep on stirring for 7–10 minutes, or until the mixture thickens and starts to come together.

5   Stir in the soaked saffron solution and add the ghee. Cook until the ghee is absorbed and the mixture is thick and begins to clump together – avoid cooking too much to retain a chewy texture. This process should take around 15–20 minutes. When it has reached the correct consistency, you will see that all the liquid has been completely absorbed, that it comes away from the pan easily and has become very smooth.

6   Add the rose extract and transfer the mixture into the loaf tin, spreading it out to about 2.5cm (1in) thick. Serve warm or at room temperature. The barfi stays fresh for 3–4 days at room temperature or you can refrigerate it for longer.

TIP
·

If you're using ground almonds, skip the first stage and place the ground almonds with the pistachios and 120ml (½ cup) water in the heavy-bottomed, medium pan at step 3. Continue with the recipe.

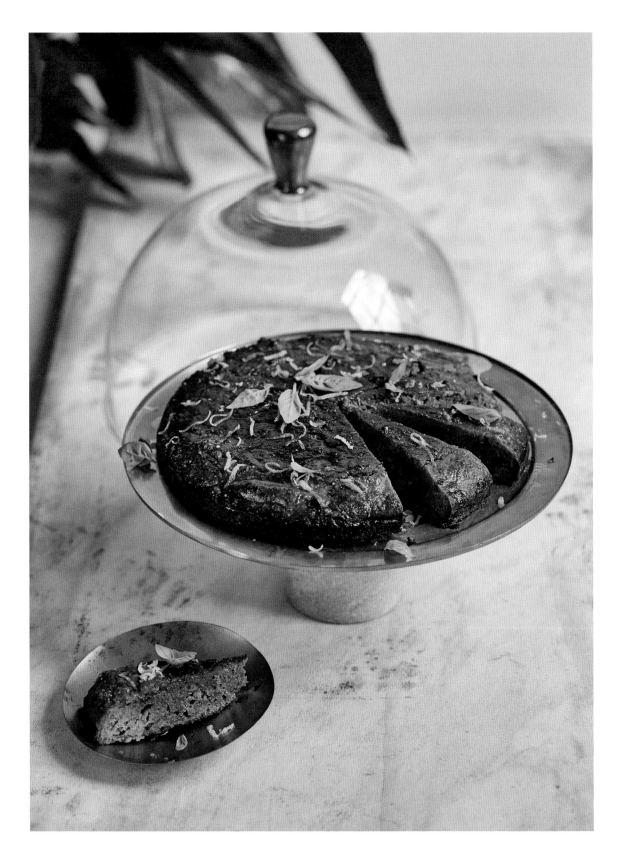

I love cakes that are flavoured with herbs, such as rosemary and fennel. The light aniseed flavour of basil gives a new dimension to a lemon cake. My other half loves lemon tarts and cakes, but I usually find them too sharp, so I've created this – an olive oil, almond sponge, made lighter with tapioca and given a herby aroma with the fresh basil. For any cake connoisseurs who want to make this even lighter, feel free to whip up the whites and all that jazz. I usually put the ingredients straight into the food processor and whizz away before stirring in the basil by hand. Bake as mini cakes or cupcakes, if you like – they'll need less time in the oven. This is also delicious with limes, which are more cooling and less harsh than lemons.

Serves 12

Lemon basil almond drizzle cake

75ml (⅓ cup) extra-virgin
   olive oil, plus extra
   for greasing
280g (2½ cups)
   ground almonds
95g (¾ cup) tapioca
½ tsp baking powder
¼ tsp sea salt
20g (½ cup) fresh basil,
   torn, plus extra to
   decorate (optional)
150g (¾ cup) jaggery
   or maple syrup
60ml (¼ cup) lemon juice
1 tsp vanilla extract
3 medium eggs
finely grated zest of
   1 large lemon

FOR THE GLAZE
3 tbsp lemon juice
85g (¼ cup) raw honey
pinch of sea salt
zest of 1 large lemon
   (plus extra to decorate,
   optional)

1   Preheat the oven to 180ºC (fan 160ºC/gas mark 4), and grease a 23cm (9in) round springform tin with olive oil.

2   Mix together the ground almonds, tapioca, baking powder and salt in a large bowl. Whisk together all the remaining ingredients in a separate bowl. Then add the wet mixture into the dry mixture and stir until well combined.

3   Pour the mixture into the prepared tin, smooth with a wet spatula and bake for 30 minutes or more, until the middle is set and a toothpick comes out almost clean.

4   Allow to cool completely in the tin. Meanwhile, make the glaze by whisking the ingredients together in a glass jug. Pour the glaze over the cake. Allow to stand for another 30 minutes.

5   Carefully run a thin knife around the edges of the cake to loosen it, then transfer onto a plate to serve.

FEELING
PITTA

Use lime juice and zest
instead of lemon and
replace the egg yolks with
extra egg whites. Use
maple syrup instead of
honey in the glaze.

TIP
·

I managed to get enough juice and zest
for this recipe from 2 large lemons, but
I'd recommend having a third lemon on
hand just in case, especially if you are
decorating with extra zest.

These nourishing teff pancakes filled with an easy tahini and and apricot sauce are my take on the peanut butter and jam sandwiches that I used to tuck into after school. So you don't eat too many of them, we've rolled them up and sliced them to make pinwheels – perfect for little fingers, too! Apricots are great for all the Doshas but they're not the easiest fruit to find nice and ripe as they have a short season; this dried apricot cream is brilliant and lasts for up to a month in the fridge.

Serves 4

Teff pinwheels with apricot tahini and cardamom cream

125g (¾ cup) teff flour
1½ tsp baking powder
¾ tsp ground cinnamon
pinch of sea salt
1 tbsp maple syrup
120ml (½ cup) whole milk, nut milk or water
2 medium eggs, beaten, or 3 flax eggs (see page 256)
1½ tbsp melted ghee, butter or coconut oil, plus extra for greasing
75ml (⅓ cup) water
zest of 1½–2 lemons

FOR THE CREAM
450g unsulphured dried apricots
250ml (1 cup) boiling water
seeds of 20 cardamom pods, ground
60g (⅓ cup) tahini or more

FEELING
KAPHA

Swap the tahini for pumpkin or sunflower seed butter – or leave it out altogether and stick to plain apricot spread, sprinkled with toasted sesame seeds for flavour.

1 To make the cream, soak the apricots in the boiling water for 30 minutes or until soft. Blend with the soaking water, cardamom and tahini, adding a little more tahini if needed to reach your desired consistency. To increase the cream's shelf-life, transfer to a small, heavy-based pan and cook it through for 5 minutes, stirring frequently.

2 Mix the teff flour, baking powder, cinnamon and salt together in a medium bowl. Whisk together the wet ingredients, apart from the ghee. Add them to the bowl and stir well to combine.

3 Heat a large ceramic-lined or seasoned cast-iron frying pan over a medium heat and grease with ghee. When hot add a ladleful of the batter, then immediately swirl the pan around and lightly smooth with the back of a spoon to create a thin pancake. Cook for1½ minutes on one side, then using a spatula flip over and cook the other side for about a minute. The mixture makes enough for six thin pancakes.

4 Spread each pancake with 2 tablespoons of the cream, then roll up the pancakes to create a long cigar. Cut the cigar into 2.5cm (1in) slices and serve as little pinwheel bites, garnished with lemon zest.

5 Store leftover cream in a clean, sterilised glass jar in the fridge for up to a month.

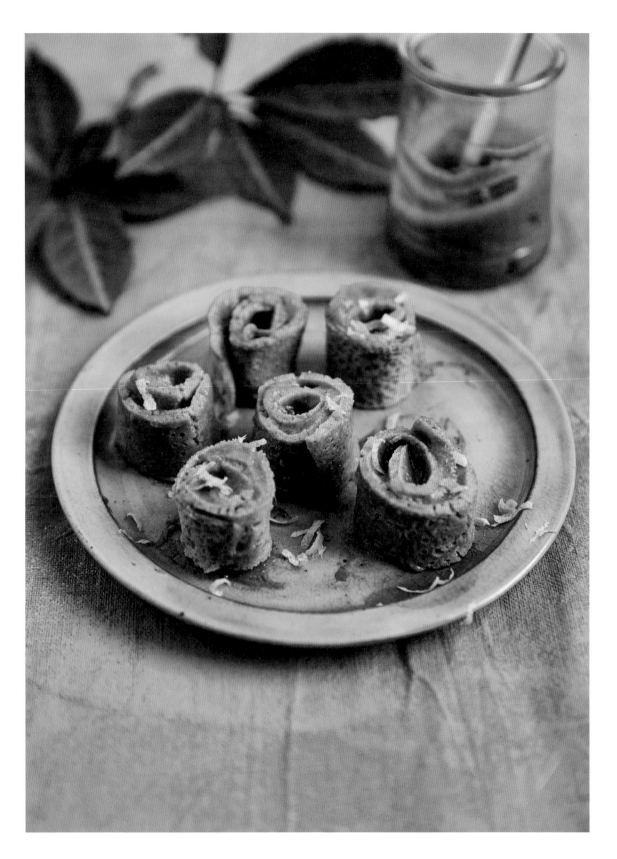

I was inspired to make these chocolate Dosha walnut balls (or 'chocolate brains', if you like) for my friend Toni, who was pregnant and in need of snacks. I went through the cupboards in her kitchen, mixed up some maple syrup and ghee into a paste, spread it between two walnut halves and presented her with a little walnut whip sandwich – without the whip! She loved it and sent me back to make a few more. The next time I made them I took it up a level by dipping them in chocolate to transform them into delicious sweets that are also worthy of a gift.

Although it's often presented as a low-sugar, antioxidant-rich treat, good-quality dark chocolate is often rich in caffeine due to its high cocoa content. This makes it very stimulating and therefore best enjoyed in very small amounts and earlier in the day. By lightly coating in chocolate you keep the caffeine on the down-low while still enjoying the flavour of real chocolate, along with a satisfying creaminess and crunch. Vata types don't do so well with caffeine but are good with creamy and sweet – so it's white chocolate for you. Nearly all nuts aggravate Kapha because they are rich and very nourishing, but walnuts are definitely the best option.

○◑●

Makes 10 balls

Chocolate Dosha walnut balls

FOR VATA

20 walnut halves
    (around 30g/¼ cup)
2 tbsp ghee
1 tsp jaggery
1 tbsp fennel seeds,
    toasted and ground
    (see page 265)
pinch of sea salt
100g white chocolate

FOR PITTA

20 walnut halves
    (around 30g/¼ cup)
2 tbsp ghee
1–2 tsp coriander seeds,
    toasted and ground
    (see page 265), plus
    extra to decorate
1 tsp jaggery
¼ tsp peppermint extract
pinch of sea salt
100g dark chocolate

FOR KAPHA

20 walnut halves
    (around 30g/¼ cup)
2 tbsp ghee, at room
    temperature
2 tsp maple syrup
¼ tsp or more chilli flakes,
    plus extra to decorate
½ tsp ground cinnamon
pinch of sea salt
100g dark chocolate

1 Preheat the oven to 170ºC (fan 150ºC/gas mark 3) and toast the walnuts on a baking tray for 5 minutes. Alternatively, toast them in a dry frying pan over a low-medium heat until fragrant and golden all over. Continuously stir and watch closely – they'll take around 1–2 minutes to toast. Allow to cool.

2 Mix together the rest of the ingredients, apart from the chocolate, in a small bowl. Place the bowl in the freezer and chill until firm (around 1 hour).

3 Run a ½ teaspoon measuring spoon along the chilled mixture until full, then sandwich the ball of mixture between two walnut halves. Continue until you have ten sandwiches. Place in the fridge or freezer to chill.

4 Meanwhile, gently melt two-thirds of the chocolate over a bain-marie until just melted. Immediately remove from the heat and stir in the remaining chocolate until melted. Working quickly, dip each ball into the chocolate using two forks and then place on a plate or board lined with baking parchment. Decorate according to your Dosha.

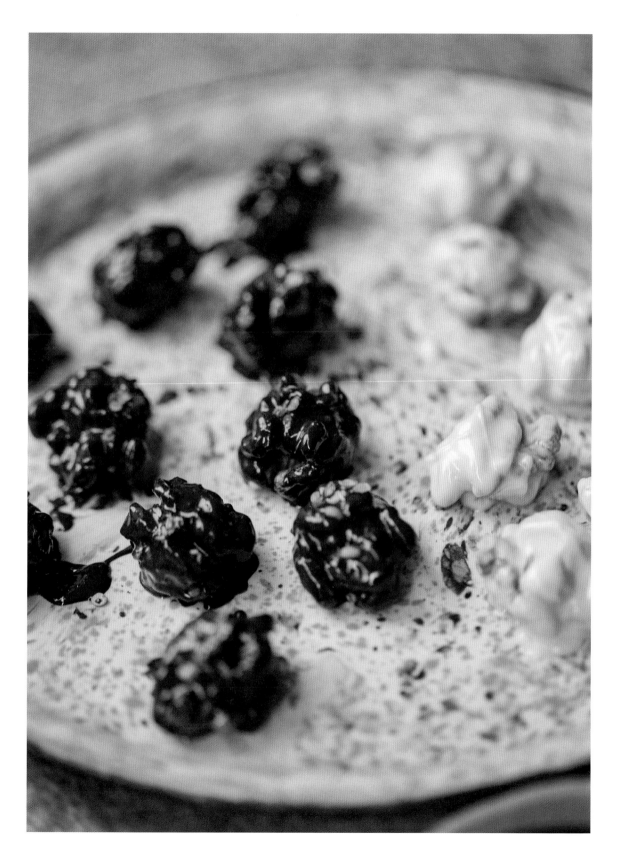

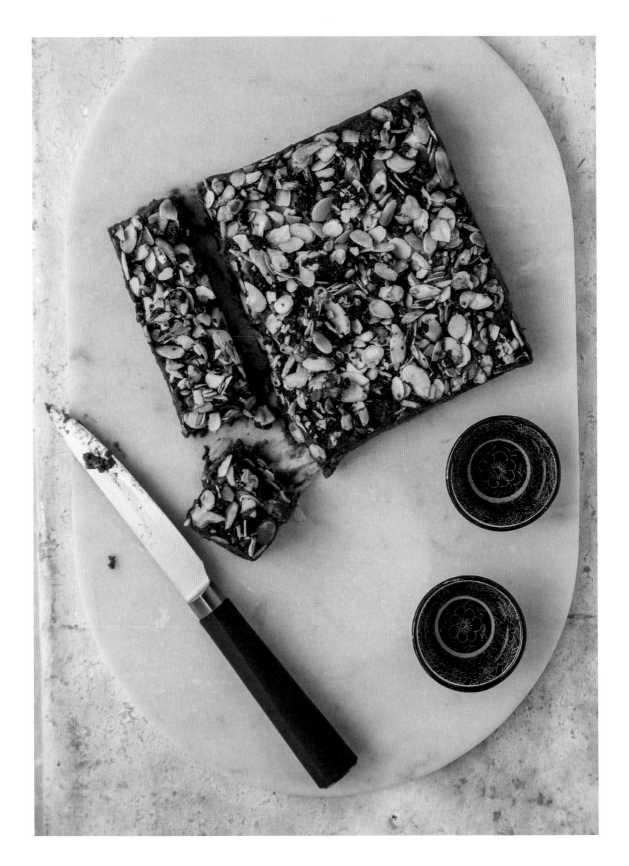

Growing up, I loved Hoppia – little pastry buns from the Philippines that originated in China – stuffed with a stodgy sweet red bean paste. In Asia, beans such as these adzuki beans (also known as aduki beans) or mung beans are very commonly served in dessert form. I remember trying to convince my Thai friend to eat mung dal and he wasn't having any of it! This fudge is very easy to make, creamy and caramel-like. Simply boil up the beans until soft and mashable, then cook with the rest of the ingredients to make a thick paste that will set in the fridge. You can also bake or steam this to make little cakes, using the same technique as for Dhokla (see page 229) but this one-pan version is so easy. If you want a nice dark colour, use dark jaggery, which will also give it even more of a caramel flavour. Feel free to halve this recipe.

Serves 16

Bean and jaggery fudge with toasted almonds

255g (1½ cups) adzuki beans, soaked overnight
3 tbsp rice flour
1.5 litres (6 cups) water
100g (½ cup) dark jaggery (for better colour), finely chopped
50g (¼ cup) butter
pinch of sea salt

FOR THE TOPPING
50g (½ cup) flaked or slivered almonds
50g (¼ cup) jaggery, finely chopped

TIP
·
Add a little cocoa powder to the mix at step 4 for chocolate fudge.

FEELING
VATA

Enjoy only very occasionally.

FEELING
PITTA

Use as little jaggery as you can for flavour, and enjoy occasionally.

1   Rinse and drain the adzuki beans. Place the beans in a saucepan with the water. Bring to the boil and then simmer, lid on, for about 30-40 minutes or until completely soft.

2   Drain any remaining water. Mash using a potato masher or the back of a spoon to your liking – I like it quite chunky. Or blitz in a food processor if you want it smooth.

3   Return to the pan and mix in the rice flour, jaggery, butter and pinch of salt. Cook for around 10 minutes until it becomes a really thick mash. Line an 18cm (7in) shallow square dish with baking parchment and push the bean paste into the dish, smoothing the top as neatly as possible using a piece of baking parchment. Place in the fridge to set for 1 hour.

4   Half an hour before serving, remove the fudge from the fridge and allow it to come to room temperature. When you're ready to serve, lightly toast the almonds in a dry frying pan until golden, add the jaggery and a pinch of salt, toast for a little longer, then spread evenly over the fudge and press down firmly.

5   Remove the fudge from the tray using the parchment to help lift it out and transfer to a wooden board. Slice the fudge into squares and serve.

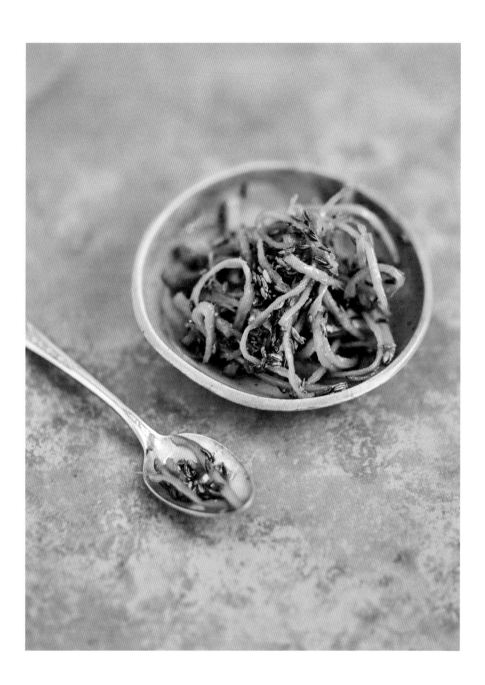

Both ginger and fennel seeds stimulate digestion, so if my digestive fire is feeling low, I eat two or three of these matchsticks to get the fire going! To make the mild version of this recipe, separate the ginger cooking water, which you could enjoy as a tea. Otherwise, see the tip below for a slightly easier method that gives you a kick up the backside and gets your nose running if you're feeling congested! The jaggery or maple syrup helps to tame the fiery flavour of the ginger with sticky sweetness, so I've included this in the sweet treats section because it's a great way to start your meal with that all-important sweet taste while stimulating digestion without filling you up. If you feel you've overdone it with eating (easily done during festive times!) then a couple of these chews work well to end a meal.

A word of caution: no matter how more-ish they are, avoid snacking on these willy-nilly or you will keep your digestion forever on edge.

Makes 200g

Ginger anise chews

1 tbsp fennel seeds or
   1½ tsp ground fennel
   seeds
200g fresh ginger
120ml (½ cup) water
100g (½ cup) jaggery
   or maple syrup (less if
   you're feeling Kapha)
pinch of flaky sea salt
   (optional)

FEELING
PITTA

This isn't good for you on a regular basis, because you don't usually need help to feel fiery!

TIP
·

If you're hardcore like me and love the ginger burn, you don't have to strain away the cooking water at step 3. Instead, simmer the ginger in 60ml (¼ cup) water, lid on, until tender. Add the jaggery or maple syrup, then simmer, lid off, until the liquid evaporates. Continue with the recipe.

1 Lightly toast the fennel seeds in a dry frying pan until fragrant. Set aside to cool.

2 Peel the ginger using the back of a teaspoon, then slice into matchsticks or grate using the coarse side of a grater. Place the strips of ginger in a small saucepan with the water, cover and bring to the boil. Lower to a simmer and cook for 30−45 minutes, lid on, until tender. Keep an eye on it and add water if needed.

3 Drain the ginger cooking water into a jug and set aside. You can enjoy this hot or chilled as ginger tea or tonic − dilute with more water as needed.

4 Add the jaggery and salt to the pan with the ginger. Simmer, uncovered, over a low heat for another 30 minutes, stirring occasionally to make sure it doesn't burn, until the ginger has turned darker in colour, is slightly translucent and the water has completely evaporated. Remove from the heat and stir in the fennel seeds.

5 Spoon the mixture onto a baking tray lined with parchment paper. Sprinkle with a little flaky sea salt, if desired, and leave to cool. If it still feels wet, you can transfer to the oven next time it's on and let it dry on a low heat. Transfer to an airtight jar and enjoy to stimulate appetite before a meal or to aid digestion afterwards.

I've been dreaming about making the perfect wholefood millionaires shortbread for years – many recipes skip the white-sugar-based caramel and the white flour in favour of an almond biscuit base but this ends up being too crumbly or too crisp, and the whole thing is usually too sweet. This is a millionaire recipe that makes you pay attention – from the medley of flavours to the sublime texture, with a hit of cardamom to add pungency and aid digestion. The deep, nutty and slightly bitter flavour is thanks to the toasted gram flour (also known as besan or chickpea flour), which creates the perfect biscuit-y base, contrasting beautifully with the sweet date layer and rich dark chocolate. Serve these cool, or at room temperature for melt-in-the-mouth chocolate. These are super-rich and sweet, so you can cut down on the jaggery and dates a little if you like. The gram shortbread base is also delicious by itself or as a base for the Saffron Cardamom Cheesecake (see page 212). Yum!

Makes 16

Cardamom millionaires with gram shortbread

150g dark chocolate, 70–80% cocoa content
1 tbsp ghee

FOR THE CARAMEL LAYER
18 soft pitted dates or 18 dried, pitted dates (290g), soaked in just enough hot water to cover for 30 minutes
4 tbsp ghee
½ tsp vanilla extract
3 tbsp of water (use the soaking water if using dried dates)

FOR THE GRAM SHORTBREAD
150g (1¼ cup) gram flour
seeds of 6 cardamom pods, ground
100g (½ cup) jaggery, chopped finely, or coconut sugar
100g (½ cup) ghee or butter
pinch of sea salt

1   Line an 18cm (7in) square tin with baking parchment. To make the gram shortbread, toast the gram flour for 15 minutes in a dry heavy-bottomed frying pan over a medium heat, stirring frequently to ensure even toasting and to keep the flour from burning. At the end of this process the flour should be fragrant and a few shades darker.

2   Stir in the cardamom, jaggery, ghee and salt, stirring constantly to ensure that the ghee and jaggery melt and the mixture is as lump-free as possible. It will be liquid-like at first, but keep cooking for 3–4 minutes, until the mixture is thick and smooth. Ghee is absorbed quickly and jaggery doesn't melt as easily, so you won't get a thick, smooth mixture, but this is fine as long as it's well combined.

3   Spread the mixture into the lined tin, pressing flat and evenly into all four corners with the back of a metal spoon. Transfer to the fridge and allow the mixture to chill for about an hour.

4   Meanwhile, blend the pitted dates with the ghee, vanilla and the water, until as smooth as possible, stopping to scrape down the sides a few times. Spread on top of the chilled base and put back into the fridge to set for a further hour.

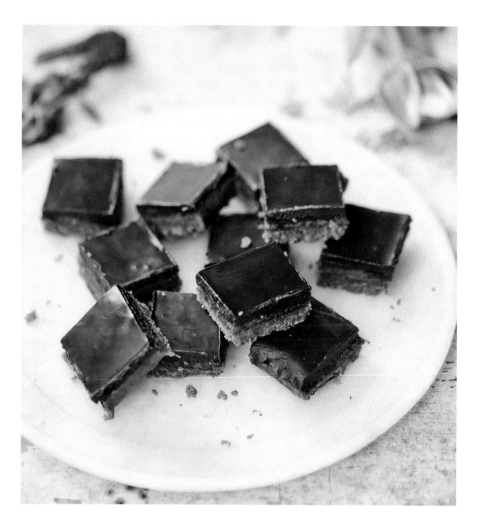

.

If you are using very soft, plump dates, which are easily blendable, do not soak them or add water to the blender at step 4 or your caramel layer might be too runny. You can always add 1 tablespoon of hot water to get the blender going.

5   Melt two-thirds of the chocolate slowly in a bain-marie, stirring frequently until fully melted. Remove from the heat and stir in the final third of the chocolate and allow to melt in the residual heat (this is a way of tempering chocolate without a thermometer, to avoid the 'white bloom' that can appear). Stir in the ghee and pour the melted chocolate over the date layer.

6   Place the tin in the fridge and allow to set for 20–30 minutes. Once set, lift out using the baking parchment to help, then place on a cutting board. Using a large sharp knife, slice into sixteen squares. (You can wipe the knife between each cut with paper towel to avoid getting crumbs on the squares).

7   Store in a container in the fridge for up to 3 days, but bring back to room temperature before eating.

Combining milk and banana is an Ayurveda digestive 'no-no', so banana milkshakes are out – but, thank goodness, banana cookies are still in. These little cookies, with their nostalgic banana flavour, remind me of being a kid. Mixing banana with dates and desiccated coconut makes an easy dough, which is then baked into cookie shapes – filling the kitchen with a delicious aroma. Watch the children and adults alike descend on you! One of these cookie bites is the perfect way to begin your lunch.

Makes 18

Banana and date cookie-dough bites

2 ripe medium
    bananas (each
    around 150g, peeled)
2 tbsp butter
    or coconut oil, at
    room temperature

125g (1½ cups)
    desiccated coconut
1 tsp baking powder
pinch of sea salt
675g (scant ½ cup) pitted
    dates, chopped

1 Preheat the oven to 180ºC (fan 160ºC/gas mark 4).

2 Place everything in a food processor except the dates. Pulse until well blended. Then add the dates and pulse again until evenly distributed.

3 Divide the mixture into eighteen balls. Place them on a lined baking sheet and flatten so they are around 1cm thick and 4cm wide.

4 Bake for 15 minutes, then turn them over and bake for another 10 minutes or until golden brown all over. They will still feel a bit soft, but they get crunchier as they cool. Leave on a wire rack until completely cool and enjoy!

FEELING
KAPHA

Replace the desiccated
coconut with rice flour or
buckwheat flour, making
sure to roll them thinner
so they cook well.

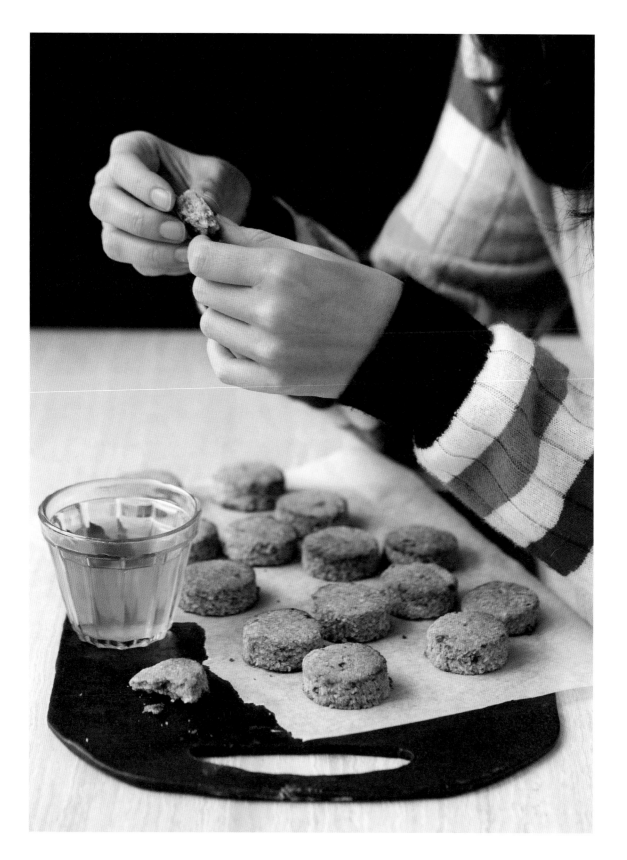

The smell of pear, thyme and buckwheat makes me feel very French, because I imagine it's the kind of thing you'd find in Provence (not that I've ever been there!). The French use buckwheat flour (*sarrasin*) to make their famous galettes. I found out after creating this recipe that buckwheat is also used to make something similar to this, called butter cake, which is enjoyed as a snack because it's dense and less sweet than most pâtisserie.

Instead of using egg yolks to bind it together as the French do, I've used yoghurt, which I also soak the buckwheat in overnight or for at least a few hours – this helps make it all the more digestible while slightly mellowing the buckwheat flour flavour. In go the delicious fragrant digestive spices of cinnamon and cardamom, then the cake is studded with pears and thyme before being baked. Faintly sweet and nicely filling, this is perfect for breakfast with a cup of tea. For another type of buckwheat cake, try the Buckwheat Banana Bread on page 60.

Serves 4–6

Pear and thyme buckwheat cake

70g (½ cup) buckwheat flour

60g (¼ cup) homemade yoghurt (see page 259)

60ml (¼ cup) water

1 tsp baking powder

pinch of fine sea salt

3 tbsp jaggery or maple syrup

1 tsp vanilla extract

1½ tsp ground cinnamon

seeds of 3–4 cardamom pods, ground

2 medium, ripe but firm, pears (peeled if the skin is tough), cut into 2cm (¾ in) cubes

butter, for greasing

1 tsp fresh thyme, leaves picked

1   The day before you wish to serve, combine the flour with the yoghurt and water, mix, then cover and leave the batter overnight at room temperature.

2   When you are ready to bake, preheat the oven to 200ºC (180ºC fan/gas mark 6) and line an 18cm (7in) square tin with baking parchment. Lightly grease the baking parchment.

3   Add the baking powder, salt, jaggery, vanilla, cinnamon and cardamom to the batter. Mix well, then spread out in the lined baking tin.

4   Distribute the pears evenly across the batter, pressing them down lightly so they are just showing. Bake for 25 minutes, or until golden and firm to the touch.

5   Decorate with small thyme leaves, pushed in gently. Eat hot or leave to cool and cut into squares or rectangles.

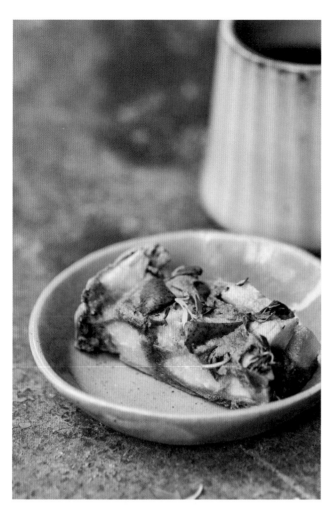

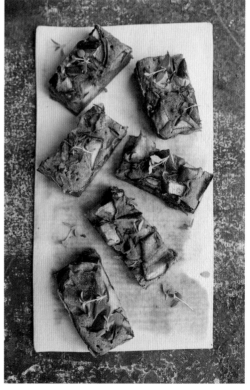

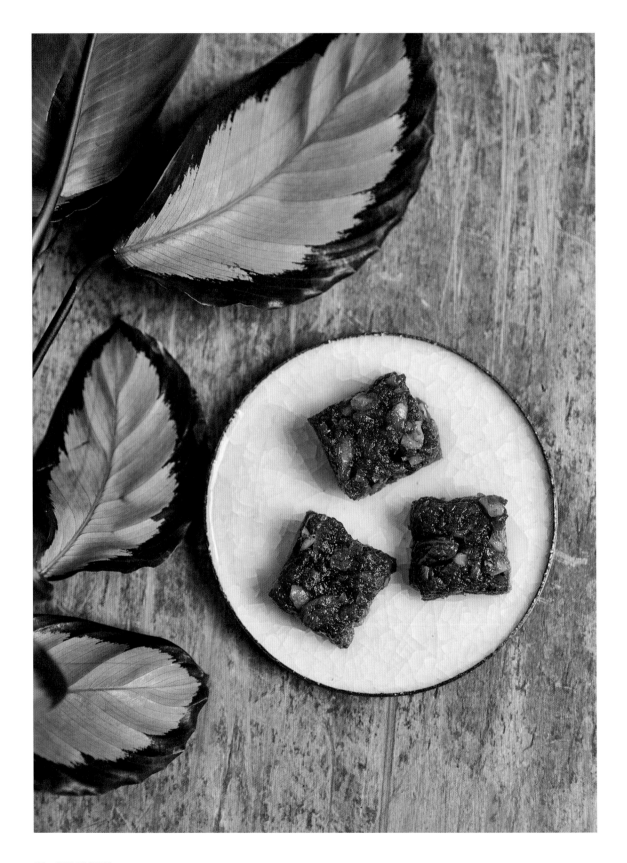

Halwa is delicious strands of grated carrot, slowly cooked in milk and ghee until deliciously creamy. I first came across the recipe after wondering about new ways to use carrot in sweet treats. I still remember I had my head in the freezer doing a clear out when I thought of this – I imagined it with butter and toasted nuts. I wasn't far off the gajwar halwa or carrot halwa: a famous Indian confection, steeped in tradition. Halwa comes in many forms, including grain- and nut-based versions, and has Arab origins, from where it travelled both East and West in various recipes using gourd, mung beans, semolina and rich nuts or gelatinous sweets (think of Turkish delight). It also has the same roots as the popular Mediterranean, Balkan and Middle Eastern halva, which is usually made from crushed sesame seeds and honey. For something similar, try the Chinese or Filipino take on this: Bean and Jaggery Fudge with Toasted Almonds (see page 101).

This recipe requires the same patience and attention as a risotto. The sugar content of halwa varies wildly – especially as it invariably appears at special occasions like weddings, where everyone gets high on an abundance of sugar in every form. Some recipes also use a lot of ghee – now I love ghee (can't you tell?) but I like to use less here to keep the delicate texture and stop it from becoming too rich. I have used cashews and golden raisins, but it's just as lovely with regular raisins. You could also use other nuts, such as almonds or pistachios.

○◑●

Makes 6 squares

Carrot Halwa

2 tbsp ghee or unrefined
   sesame oil
75g (½ cup) golden raisins
80g (½ cup) cashews,
   blanched almonds or
   pistachios, chopped
450g carrots,
   coarsely grated
750ml (3 cups) whole milk
   or almond milk, or
   250ml (1 cup) full-fat
   coconut milk and
   500ml (2 cups) water

3 tbsp jaggery
   or maple syrup
seeds of 5 cardamom
   pods, ground, or ¼ tsp
   ground cardamom
1½ teaspoons ground
   cinnamon

1 In a heavy-bottomed pan, heat 1 tablespoon of the ghee, then stir in the raisins. When they puff, remove them from the pan and set aside. In the same pan, fry the cashews until golden brown and set aside.

2 Melt the remaining ghee and sauté the grated carrots for 2–3 minutes. Pour in the milk and cook on a medium heat, stirring frequently to prevent the carrots from sticking to the bottom of the pan. Continue cooking for about 25 minutes.

3 Stir in the jaggery, cardamom, cinnamon, raisins and nuts and continue cooking on medium-low, stirring occasionally, for about 25 minutes, or until all the liquid is absorbed. Take care that the halwa doesn't stick to the pan as it dries out.

4 You can serve this in little bowls while it is hot, or at room temperature. Otherwise, cook until almost dry and allow to cool in a baking-parchment-lined container (about 12cm/4½ in square). Chill in the fridge before cutting into squares.

TIP
·
To make this vegan, use unrefined sunflower oil instead of ghee and almond milk instead of dairy milk.

This steamed pudding is very reminiscent of the Filipino-style desserts I grew up with. I find this recipe quite filling, and perfect for sharing between two – but if you're a cake lover you might disagree!

No need to turn on the oven or use the microwave, simply steam the batter in a ramekin in a good old-fashioned saucepan with a lid, or make multiple 'cupcakes' in a big saucepan for friends! If you don't have a ramekin, you can use a mug or small bowl, making sure you have a saucepan deep enough for it.

I've given a weight measurement for the coconut flour, because it is different to other flours in that it can expand to up to three times its volume – how tightly or loosely you pack that spoon makes all the difference! And you can also play with the texture, using 1 tablespoon of coconut flour for a flan-like pudding, or 1½ tablespoons for a lighter cake. Use coconut oil for a strong coconut flavour, or ghee or butter for something more subtle.

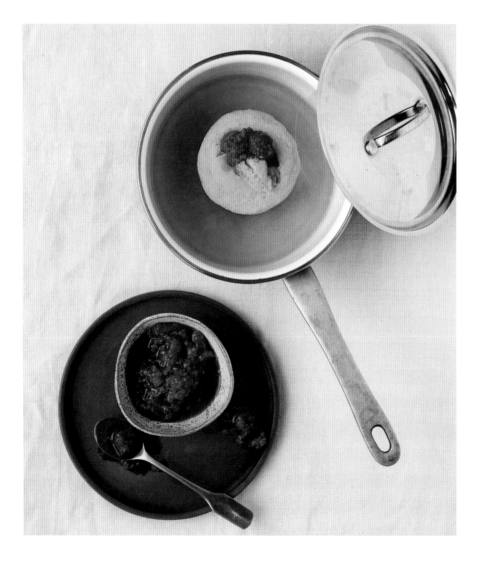

Steamed coconut pudding with raspberry sauce

1–1½ tbsp (10–15g)
  coconut flour
¼ tsp baking powder
pinch of sea salt
1 tbsp coconut oil
  or ghee, melted
2 tsp maple syrup
  or jaggery (plus 1 tsp
  extra for stewing the
  raspberries, optional)

1 tbsp water
½ tsp vanilla extract
1 medium egg, beaten
75g (about ½ pack)
  raspberries

1　Add the coconut flour, baking powder and sea salt to a mug or small mixing bowl and combine with a fork. Mix in the coconut oil, maple syrup, water, vanilla extract and egg until the mixture is completely smooth.

2　Grease a ramekin (8cm wide and 4cm deep). Pour in the batter and place it in a small saucepan with a tight-fitting lid. Pour 3cm (1½ in) of boiling water into the pan and bring it to the boil. Once the water starts to boil, lower to a gentle simmer, cover with the lid and steam for 15 minutes.

3　Meanwhile, stew the raspberries. Place them in a small pan over a low heat, and place a lid on top. Allow to cook down in their own juices, adding 1 teaspoon of maple syrup if desired.

4　When the pudding is ready, enjoy hot from the ramekin, or let it cool a little and ease it out with a knife, then allow to cool completely. Serve with the stewed raspberries.

WORKS WITH

GOLDENSPOON
(at room temperature)
page 91

BLACK PEPPER, PRUNE
AND SESAME SEED
CHUTNEY
(thinned with water)
page 236

VANILLA CHAI PLUM
COMPOTE
page 74

APRICOT TAHINI AND
CARDAMOM CREAM
page 96

FEELING
KAPHA

Enjoy
infrequently.

TIP
·

This is delicious with chopped dried fruits, or pop a square of chocolate into the middle before steaming. You can flavour with the usual suspects – cardamom, cinnamon and star anise, or give some of my other topping ideas a try.

This little dessert was created at the last minute for my friend Sjaniel's baby shower. I was in charge of the afternoon tea with cakes, sandwiches and pots of tea, and she requested something cool and creamy to serve in her beautiful little vintage sherry glasses from a car-boot sale (we're both car-boot crazy). With just four ingredients from the cupboard, these mini cooling coconut creams came together.

Serves 2–3

If you can get good gelatine you can also use that instead of the agar flakes, which give it a loose pannacotta-like consistency. Make use of the Vanilla Chai Plum Compote from my Chestnut Crêpes recipe (see page 74).

Coconut creams with vanilla chai plum compote

1 x 400ml tin of full-fat coconut milk, or 400ml rice milk (see page 257)
100g (½ tbsp) jaggery (plus extra for garnish, optional)
tiny pinch of sea salt
¼ tsp ground cinnamon

2 tsp agar flakes
1 quantity of Vanilla Chai Plum Compote, to serve (see page 74)
1 tbsp brazil nuts, finely sliced, to serve (optional)

1   Shake the tin of coconut milk (if it's cold, give it a really good shake), then pour into a small saucepan. Stir in the jaggery, salt and cinnamon and give it a stir.

2   Sprinkle over the agar flakes and heat gently without stirring for a minute or two, then bring to a gentle simmer, stirring occasionally, for 5 minutes.

3   Allow to cool slightly (if using delicate glassware) and then divide between two or three glasses or ramekins. Allow to set in the fridge. Top with the compote and finely sliced brazil nuts, if using, and serve.

FEELING
VATA

Enjoy at room temperature.

FEELING
KAPHA

This is a bit heavy, so enjoy only occasionally at room temperature, and use rice milk every now and then.

TIP
·

In the summer, serve the coconut creams with the compote at room temperature, and in the winter try warming up the compote over a low heat.

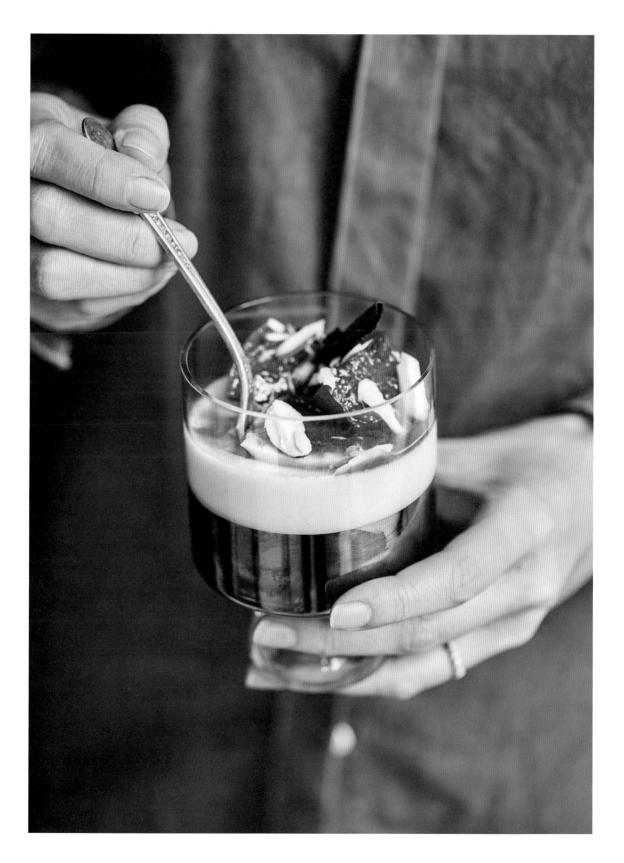

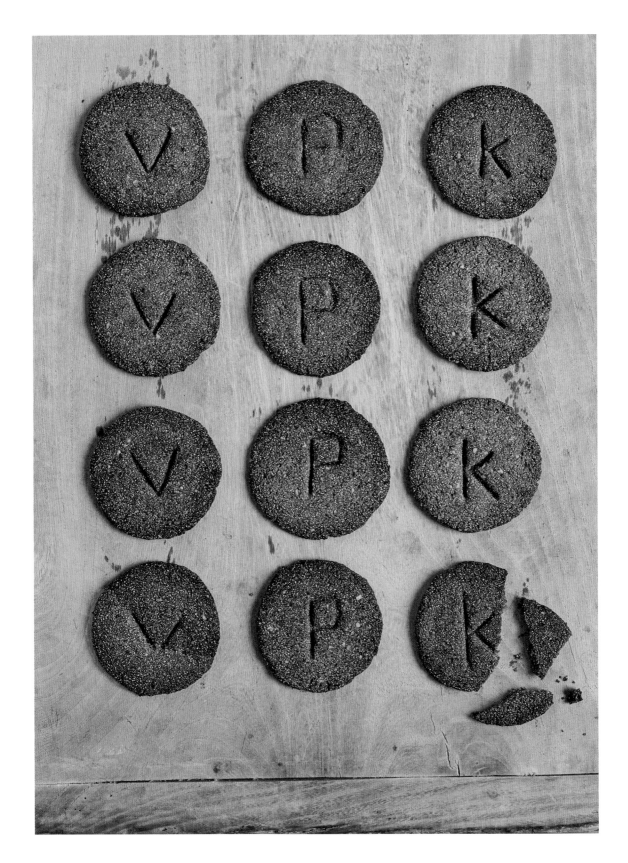

I loved digestive biscuits growing up – for me they are the perfect mix of sweet and salty, with a malty flavour. In Ayurveda, the main focus is always digestion and one day, while in the kitchen with my friend Jeanine rustling up digestive spice mixes, she said 'We should make our own digestive biscuits!'. Below is the result of her cute idea for celebrating the spices that help bring balance to the different Doshas. The biscuit base is a mix of ground amaranth and almonds, bound with coconut oil and ground flax, resulting in a crisp biscuit that crumbles beautifully.

Amaranth flour can be pricey – for a fraction of the price you can grind your own from whole amaranth or flaked amaranth, if you have a powerful blender. Or try oat flour (again you can make it in a blender from oat flakes). You can also swap the ground almonds for ground sunflower seeds (again made in the blender).

Makes 15

Dosha digestive biscuits

140g (1 cup)
   amaranth flour
90g (scant ½ cup) jaggery,
   broken into pieces,
   or coconut sugar
6 tbsp coconut oil
   (or ghee for Vata
   and Kapha)
60g (½ cup)
   ground almonds

3 tsp Dosha Churna
   Spice Mix (see
   page 247)
1 tsp baking powder
2 tbsp ground flax
2 pinches of sea salt
50ml (scant ¼ cup) water

FEELING
VATA

Make the Dosha Churna
Spice Mix without the salt
and asafoetida, which will
make this too savoury.
These biscuits can be
a bit drying, but you
could spread a little
butter on top.

1 Preheat the oven to 170ºC (fan 150ºC/gas mark 3) and line a baking tray with baking parchment.

2 Toast the amaranth flour in a dry saucepan until fragrant. Add the jaggery and the coconut oil.

3 Remove the pan from the heat and add the ground almonds, spice mix, baking powder, flax and salt and mix well.

4 Add the water and mix until it makes a dough. If it's still hot then leave to come to room temperature.

5 Take 1 tablespoon of the mixture and roll it into a ball, then flatten it with your palms on the baking tray until it is just under 1cm high. Repeat with the rest of the mixture. You can also try the technique of rolling the dough in a sheet of baking parchment to create a sausage and then slicing it into biscuits.

6 Make a pattern on the top, if you like, using the end of a chopstick. Bake for 20–25 minutes or until browned at the edges – the biscuits will be delicate while hot but harden as they cool.

7 When completely cool, store the biscuits in an airtight container – they will keep their crunch for a couple of days.

Light lassis

In Ayurveda, lassis are known as Takras: super-light, drinkable digestive aids made from a little yoghurt or buttermilk whipped with water and spices to help increase Agni (see page 282). Said to be beneficial in cases of irritable bowel syndrome, Crohn's disease, haemorrhoids and obesity, these lighter lassis are typically served after lunch to counter the symptoms of digestive disorders by increasing assimilation of nutrients and reducing post-meal discomfort. You can also enjoy one of these refreshing, nourishing and easy-to-digest Dosha-specific drinks as a mid-morning snack if needed.

Perfect for pacifying the Vata Dosha, thanks to the heavy, sweet qualities of yoghurt, the effect is further enhanced with pungent spices and a touch of sea salt. Since lassis are Agni-increasing, if you're feeling Pitta, add cooling ingredients such as rose water and jaggery. If you're feeling Kapha, dilute the lassi with more water and add extra digestive spices such as black pepper. It is essential to whisk the yoghurt with water to help remove the natural fat of the yoghurt and transform the heavy, heating properties of the yoghurt into the light digestive qualities of a Takra – so don't skip it!

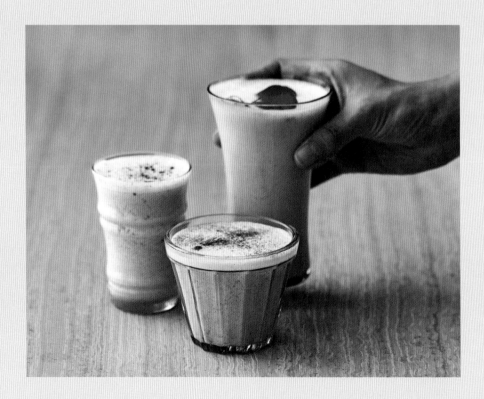

VATA

Serves 1

Warm cinnamon lassi

125g (½ cup) homemade
   yoghurt (see page 259)
250ml (1 cup) warm water
¼ tsp ground cumin or
   toasted cumin seeds
½ tsp ground cinnamon,
   plus extra for dusting
   (optional)
¼ tsp ground ginger
⅛ tsp sea salt

1   Place all of the ingredients in a blender and blend
    for 30 seconds until light and foamy. Alternatively,
    whisk by hand for a few minutes.

2   Skim off any fat that rises to the top and sprinkle
    with cinnamon to serve.

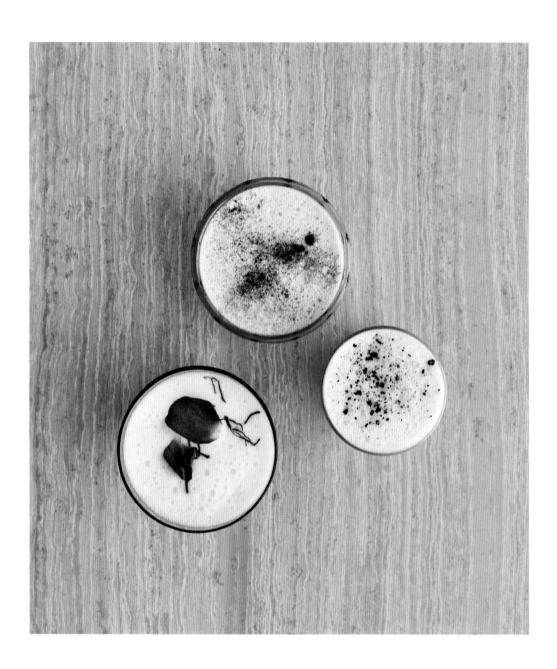

○◐●

PITTA

Serves 1

Cumin and rose lassi

125g (½ cup) homemade yoghurt (see page 259) or yoghurt made from coconut

250ml (1 cup) water

½ tsp ground cumin

¼ tsp ground ginger

1–2 drops of rose water or ⅛ tsp rose extract

½ tbsp jaggery

1–2 strands of saffron (optional)

rose petals (optional)

1 Place all of the ingredients, apart from the saffron and rose petals, if using, into a blender and blend for 30 seconds until light and foamy. Alternatively, whisk by hand for a few minutes.

2 Skim off any fat that rises to the top and sprinkle with saffron or rose petals, if using.

TIP
.

Coconut is cooling for Pitta but doesn't combine very well with dairy, so try using yoghurt made from coconut instead.

. . . .

○◐●

KAPHA

Serves 1

Ginger and coriander lassi

60g (¼ cup) homemade yoghurt (see page 259)

250ml (1 cup) water

½ tsp ground ginger

seeds of 1 cardamom pod, ground, or ⅛ tsp ground cardamom

3 strands of saffron (optional)

½ tsp freshly ground black pepper, plus extra for dusting (optional)

½ tsp ground coriander or 5–6 fresh coriander leaves

1 tsp raw honey (optional)

1 Place all of the ingredients into a blender and blend for 30 seconds until light and foamy or whisk by hand for a few minutes.

2 Skim off any fat that rises to the top and sprinkle with black pepper to serve, if desired.

This all-year-round favourite is one of the first recipes I created for the pop-up cafe. It has Middle Eastern flavours, proving that Indian food is not the only outcome when you combine lentils with Ayurveda! For dinner parties, I like to raise the flavour profile by slightly caramelising the celeriac to make it even more sweet and nutty, but as an everyday dish it's delicious as it is.

Serves 4

If you're serving this in winter, make it more warming by braising the gem lettuce before setting it aside and gently sautéing the red cabbage until tender. If you have strong digestion – Pitta types take note! – then you can enjoy the veggies raw, but remember to chew thoroughly. You can serve this dish as either a salad or a stew, depending on whether the lentils are cooked until crunchy or soft.

Celeriac and Puy lentils with hazelnuts, red cabbage and mint

60g (scant ½ cup) hazelnuts, cut in half

200g (1 cup) Puy lentils, preferably soaked for 8 hours or overnight

750ml (3 cups) water

2 bay leaves

4 sprigs of thyme

1 small celeriac (650g), peeled and cut into 1cm (½ in) wedges

4 tbsp extra-virgin olive oil

3 tbsp hazelnut oil

3 tbsp apple cider vinegar

sea salt and freshly ground black pepper, to taste

¼ red cabbage, very finely sliced

4 tbsp fresh mint, chopped

2 gem lettuces, outer leaves removed and hearts quartered

1 Preheat the oven to 140ºC (fan 120ºC/gas mark 1) and scatter the hazelnuts on a small baking tray. Toast in the oven for 10–15 minutes. Alternatively, toast them in a dry frying pan over a low–medium heat until they smell fragrant and are golden all over. Continuously stir and watch closely – they'll take about 1–2 minutes to toast. Set aside to cool.

2 Combine the lentils, water, bay leaves and thyme in a small saucepan. Bring to the boil, then simmer for 15–20 minutes, or until tender. Drain in a sieve.

3 Meanwhile, place the celeriac in another saucepan and gently cook in just enough salted water to cover for 8–12 minutes, or until just tender. Drain.

4 In a large bowl, mix the still-warm lentils (if they have cooled down they won't soak up all the flavours) with the olive oil, 2 tablespoons of the hazelnut oil, the vinegar, black pepper and plenty of salt. Add the celeriac and stir well. Taste and adjust the seasoning.

5 To serve, stir in the red cabbage, half the mint and half the hazelnuts. Pile onto a serving dish with the gem lettuce. Drizzle the remaining hazelnut oil on top. Garnish with the rest of the mint and hazelnuts.

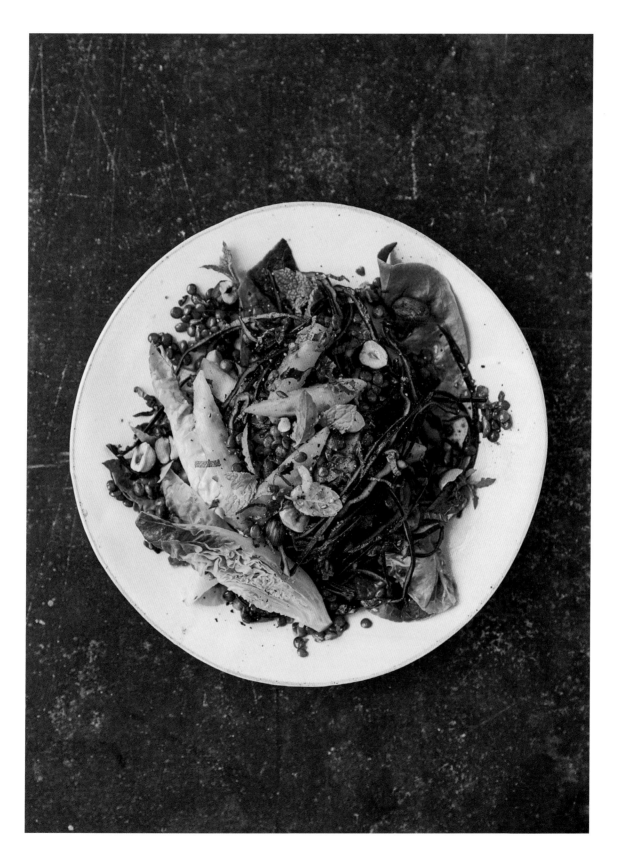

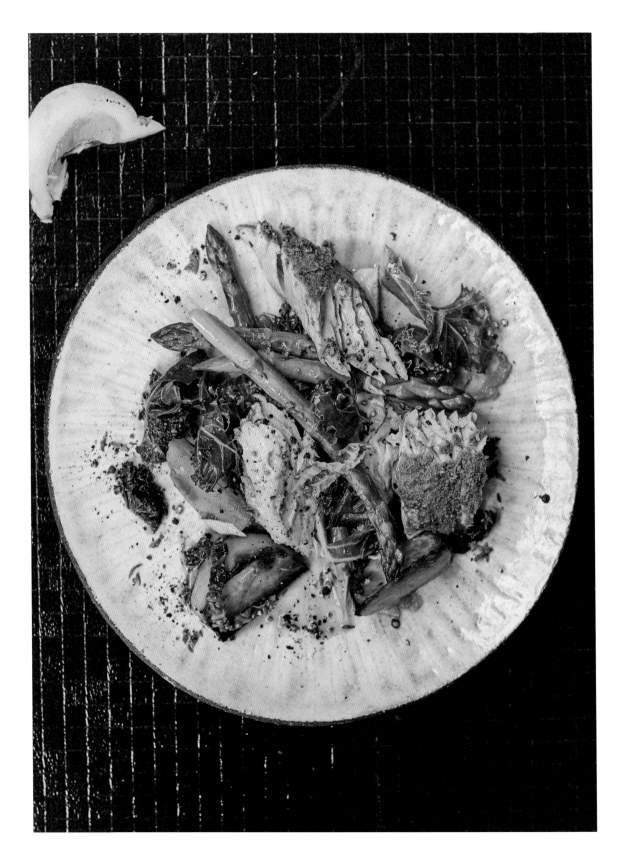

Melt-in-the-mouth chunks of delicately spiced salmon started off as an addition to any dish on the menu at my pop-up cafe. It was so popular that it soon made a weekly appearance. This recipe is a delicious way to show off the subtle flavours of turmeric without making a curry (or Golden Milk!). I always team black pepper and turmeric where I can, to improve the bioavailability of turmeric's nutrients. Here, the sharp pungency of the pepper cuts through the rich fatty sweetness of the salmon. This dish is a great one for feeding a crowd – the salmon looks impressive, yet all you need to do is dust it with some spices, pop it in the oven and serve over some sautéed seasonal veg. Yum.

Serves 6

Lemon, turmeric and black-pepper salmon with spring greens

850g side of salmon
or 6 salmon fillets
zest of 3 lemons
1 tbsp coarsely ground
black pepper
2 tbsp ground turmeric
1 tsp sea salt

FOR THE VEGETABLES
1½ tbsp ghee
3 garlic cloves, chopped
200g (2 cups) spring
greens, chopped
½ Savoy cabbage,
finely sliced
3 bay leaves
3 tbsp apple cider vinegar
250g asparagus
sea salt and freshly
ground black
pepper, to taste

1 The day before you wish to serve, line a large baking sheet with baking parchment. Place the salmon on it, skin-side down. Mix together the lemon zest, black pepper and turmeric. Spread it all over the fish and leave to marinate overnight in the fridge.

2 Preheat the oven to 200ºC (fan 180ºC/gas mark 6). Season the marinated salmon with sea salt and then bake for 22 minutes. If you're using fillets, reduce the cooking time slightly.

3 About 7 minutes before the end of the cooking time, melt the ghee in a medium saucepan and sauté the garlic for a few minutes. Add the spring greens, Savoy cabbage, bay leaves, vinegar and asparagus, and season with salt and pepper. Cover and steam for 4–5 minutes.

4 Remove the salmon from the oven, then flake or cut it into chunks. Divide the veggies between your plates and serve with the baked salmon arranged over the top.

TIP
·

You can easily adapt this dish for the different seasons. In winter, simply substitute the spring greens with 3 medium turnips, cut into cubes, and 500g (5 cups) kale leaves, chopped.

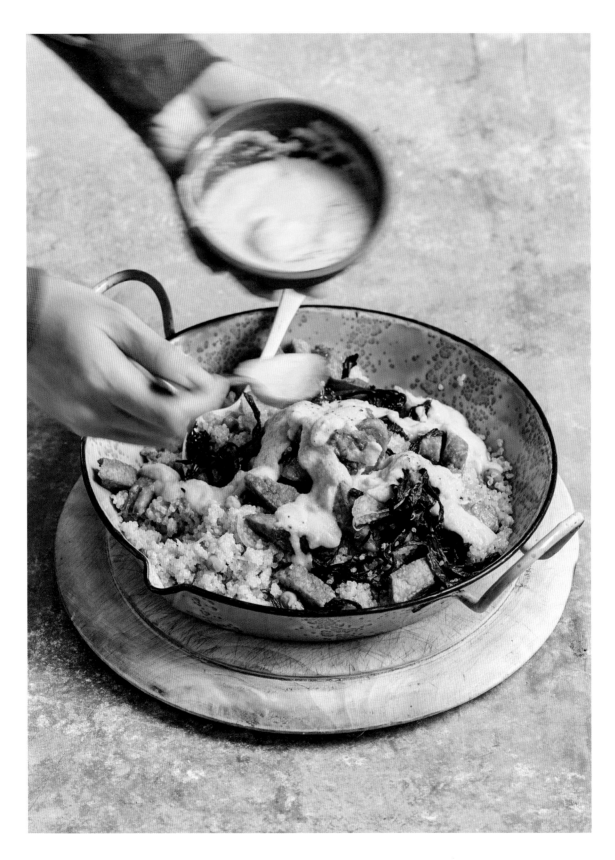

This exotic-sounding dish is pure comfort food – a spoonable pilaf made from quinoa, peas, leek and seaweed with a little garlic, teamed with crispy fried tempeh and a sweet carrot and ginger sauce. Unlike most of the recipes in this book, this one requires a few pans, but it's worth it for all of the textures.

Serves 6

Rich in iodine, which is often lacking in our diet, seaweed or sea vegetables are easy to enjoy once you've got the right recipes up your sleeve. Seaweed is popular in Asian cuisine, but once you get the hang of it you can start to pop it into other dishes for that umami flavour. Keep a stash of dried seaweed in the cupboard and add a little to a dish 10 minutes before the end of the cooking time to allow for it to rehydrate.

Tempeh is a high-protein, fermented soybean cake that you slice and cook a little bit like halloumi – in fact, depending on how you prepare it, it can often be mistaken for halloumi! You can marinate tempeh or coat it with spices, and grill or bake it, but my favourite way to enhance its natural nutty flavour is to slice it thinly and pan-fry in ghee or coconut oil until golden brown and crispy on the edges and chewy on the inside.

Tempeh, carrot, wakame, pea and quinoa pilaf

2 tbsp ghee, coconut oil or butter
½ medium leek or ½ onion, finely sliced
1 clove garlic, minced
150g quinoa, soaked for 6 hours or overnight
150ml (⅔ cup) water
sea salt and freshly ground black pepper
75g (½ cup) fresh or frozen peas
2 tbsp dried wakame
200g tempeh, cut into 5mm (¼ in) slices, then chopped into chunks

FOR THE DRESSING
2 large carrots, cut into thirds
5cm (2in) piece of fresh ginger, roughly chopped
1½ tbsp lemon juice or apple cider vinegar
4 tbsp extra-virgin olive oil
½ tsp unrefined toasted sesame oil
¼ tsp sea salt, plus more to taste
¼ tsp freshly ground black pepper, to taste
75ml (⅓ cup) water

TIP
·
You could toss in some shredded chicken or top with toasted cashews instead of using tempeh.

1 Melt 1 tablespoon of the ghee in a medium saucepan over a low-medium heat. Sauté the leek for 7 minutes until softened, adding the garlic after a few minutes.

2 Rinse and drain the quinoa. Add it to the pan with the water and a pinch of salt. Stir and simmer on a medium heat, lid on, for about 12 minutes. Add the peas and wakame to the pan, then quickly replace the lid and allow them to steam together for another 10 minutes.

3 For the dressing, put the carrot and ginger into a small saucepan. Cover with water and simmer for 12 minutes.

4 In a frying pan, melt the remaining ghee and fry the tempeh pieces in batches on both sides until browned. Add more fat as needed.

5 Meanwhile, add the cooked carrot and ginger to a blender with the rest of the dressing ingredients and blend to a smooth sauce. Taste and adjust the seasoning if necessary. Plate up the quinoa with the tempeh on top, then drizzle over the sauce.

Fragrant, delicate and served with a light gravy, mustard curries are everywhere in Sri Lanka. My favourite is with kingfish, which is gaining in popularity in the West, but any firm white fish will do. This version suggests swapping in a bay leaf for the traditional rampe (pandan) leaves to keep it practical while still tasting delicious. Serve this with broccoli and pea 'rice' to get your greens in, or you can mix it with some cooked basmati rice if you like.

Fish can be tricky to cook with, but I find poaching it in liquid one of the simplest methods – it doesn't go dry or stick to the base of the pan and it is usually easier to catch it at the right moment of 'doneness'. If you're cooking for a friend you could do the first few stages in advance, start poaching the fish when you're ready and finish with a swirl of coconut cream and fenugreek seeds.

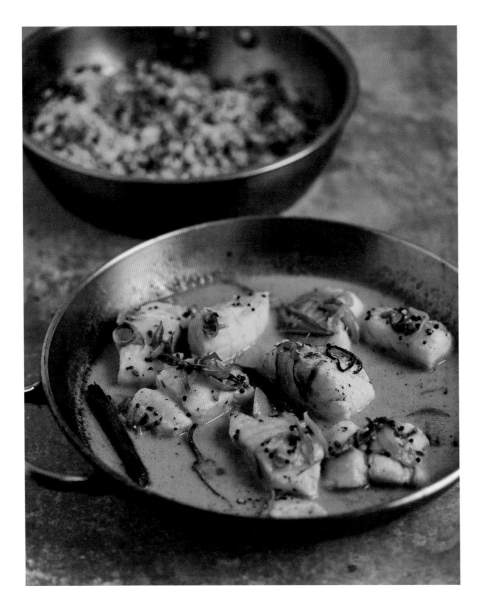

Sri Lankan mustard fish curry with broccoli pea 'rice'

1 tbsp ghee or coconut oil
1 tsp mustard seeds
1 medium onion, sliced
1 garlic clove,
    chopped finely
8 fresh or dried
    curry leaves
1 bay leaf
5cm (2in) piece of
    cinnamon stick
1 tsp fenugreek seeds
1 green chilli, slit
    lengthways
1 tsp ground turmeric
450g firm white fish, such
    as snapper, pollock,
    sea bream or cod, cut
    into chunks
150ml (⅔ cup) water
juice of ½ lime
100ml coconut cream
sea salt, to taste

FOR THE BROCCOLI
PEA 'RICE'
1 large head of broccoli
1 tsp ghee or coconut oil
50g (⅓ cup) peas
2 tbsp water
sea salt and freshly
    ground black pepper

1   Make the broccoli and pea 'rice' by removing the tough end of the broccoli stalk and roughly cut into chunks. Use a food processor (with the S-curved blade or grater attachment) or the coarse side of a grater to grate the broccoli into rice-sized pieces.

2   Melt the ghee in a large frying pan, add the grated broccoli and the peas with the water and stir to mix. Steam over a medium heat, lid on, for 4–5 minutes until tender but still with a little bite. Check after 3–4 minutes to make sure that there is still enough water in the bottom of the pan to stop it catching. Season with salt and pepper.

3   Meanwhile, melt the ghee in a separate heavy-bottomed pan. When it is hot, add the mustard seeds. As soon as the mustard seeds start to pop, add the onion, garlic, curry leaves, bay leaf, cinnamon, fenugreek and chilli. Sweat the ingredients until they are transparent and develop a pale golden colour.

4   Add the turmeric and cook for a further 30 seconds. Add the fish, water and lime juice, then cover and simmer for about 5 minutes until the fish is cooked through.

5   When the fish is cooked, add the coconut cream to the curry and cook for another minute. Season with salt and serve with the 'rice'.

Chicken adobo is a classic dish from my mum's country, the Philippines – it's the one that visitors remember most for its succulent chicken and rich and salty gravy, thanks to the soy sauce, and for the tart taste of vinegar. Growing up I used to ask my mum to cook extra of the adobo sauce to pour over veggies, so this is my re-creation of that meal.

Serves 4

As a vegetarian dish it can lack some of the lustre of the meat version so I've included plenty of ghee, aubergine for succulence and bite, and sweet potato to add sweetness. If you're not vegetarian then feel free to use homemade chicken bone broth (see page 261) as the gravy base for a more for authentic flavour. I use tamari (the Japanese version of soy sauce) as it's easy to find a good-quality brand and is typically gluten-free (check the label). If you're using bouillon to make the gravy base, then add tamari slowly as it is very salty. This is also a nice dish to throw bitter greens such as chard, into and if you can get them, use Chinese-style snake beans or English green beans, rather than the fine green beans. My favourite sweet potato for this is the Jamaican sort if you can find it at your local shops – pinky red skin and white flesh – and I love the small Asian-style aubergines for extra flavour.

Tamari, soy sauce and vinegar are all fermented so should only be eaten occasionally, in small amounts. This recipe also uses lots of garlic so be sure to pack this dish with enough vegetables to balance out such a strong-tasting salty gravy. You can also swap the apple cider vinegar for lime juice if you want. I've served this with basmati rice – for a nuttier combo go for brown basmati rice, soaked overnight and slightly overcooked to make it easier to digest.

Filipino vegetable adobo

3 tbsp ghee

1 medium onion, sliced

5 cloves garlic, sliced

500ml (2 cups) bouillon stock, bone broth (see page 261) or hot water

3 bay leaves

1 tsp black peppercorns

1 tsp ground white pepper

5 tbsp apple cider vinegar

1 large sweet potato, cut into 2.5cm (1in) cubes (about 640g prepared weight)

2 aubergines, chopped into 1cm (½ in) slices

2 tbsp tamari, to taste, add a dash more if using water instead of stock or bone broth

200g (1⅓ cups) green beans, halved on the diagonal

FOR THE RICE

200g (1 cup) white basmati rice, rinsed

370ml (1½ cups) water

½ tsp sea salt

1   Melt the ghee in a large heavy-bottomed saucepan over a medium heat and sauté the onion until soft. Add the garlic and sauté for another minute.

2   Add the remaining ingredients. Stir, bring to the boil, then simmer for 20 minutes, lid on. After 10 minutes, check there is enough water, then replace the lid. Do not stir too much to avoid mashing the sweet potato.

3   Meanwhile, in a medium saucepan with a tight-fitting lid, combine the rice with the water and salt and bring to the boil. Stir, then cover and reduce the heat to low. Simmer for 18 minutes, lid on. Remove from the heat and stand, covered, for 5 minutes, then fluff with a fork.

4   Add the green beans to the adobo and simmer, lid off, for another 5 minutes or until tender. Serve the rice in bowls with the adobo spooned over the top.

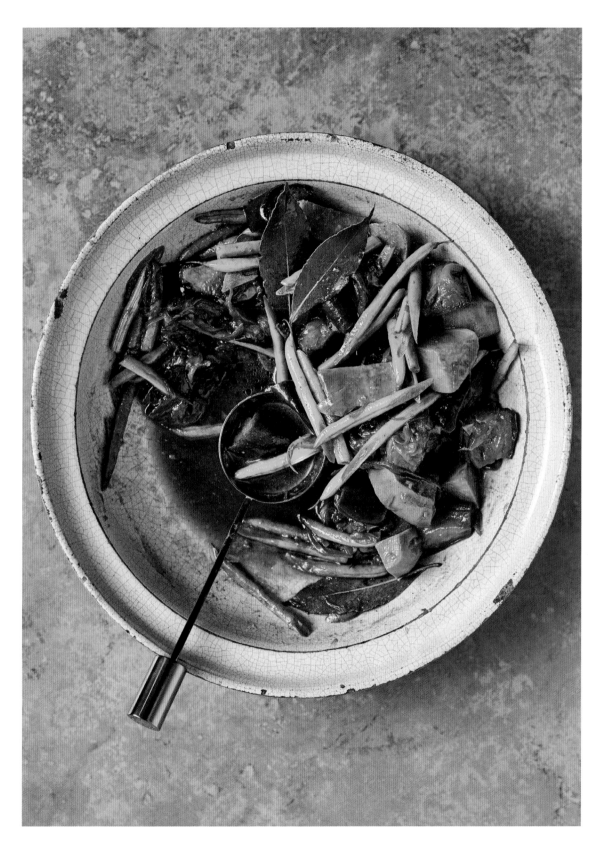

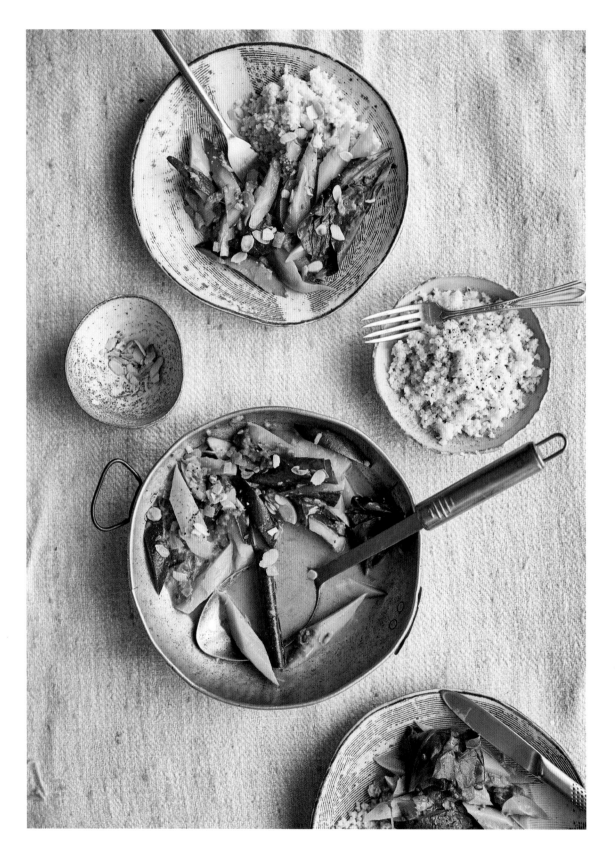

I remember the first time I tried curried parsnip soup as if it was yesterday – those big fluffy parsnips that usually only appeared in roast dinners in winter made the most beautiful sweet, creamy base for spices. Since then I've always liked parsnips in curried foods, from a creamy coconut Malaysian-style stew where I imagine they're as good as a plantain to this sweet-and-sour tamarind curry. I've mixed two veggies here – now that courgettes are available all year round, they can bring a little light-hearted juicy bitter crunch to the compact, sweet heaviness of the parsnips. This curry is both light enough for warm weather and stodgy enough for cold weather. Serve with cauliflower 'rice' for the former and white rice for the latter. To make the rice really special, toast some dessicated coconut and stir it through.

Serves 4

Tamarind courgette and parsnip curry on cauliflower 'rice'

2 tbsp flaked almonds

3 tbsp ghee, butter
  or coconut oil

1 large onion, chopped

1 large mild green
  chilli, sliced

2 cloves garlic,
  finely chopped

1cm (½ in) piece of fresh
  ginger, grated

1 tsp cumin seeds

1 tsp mustard seeds

1 cinnamon stick

about 3 medium–large
  parsnips parsnips
  (400g), peeled and cut
  into 3cm (1¼ in) chunks

1 tsp ground turmeric

½ tsp chilli powder

2 large tomatoes, skinned
  and deseeded (see page
  260), and chopped

1½ tsp tamarind paste
  (see page 260)

250ml (1 cup) water

2 medium courgettes,
  cut into 4cm
  (1½ in) chunks

1 x 400ml tin of full-fat
  coconut milk

sea salt and freshly
  ground black pepper

50g (1 cup) small chard or
  spinach leaves, washed

handful of fresh
  coriander, finely
  chopped, to serve
  (optional)

FOR THE
CAULIFLOWER 'RICE'

2 large cauliflowers

2 tsp ghee or coconut oil

4 tbsp water

sea salt and freshly
  ground black pepper

1 Heat a frying pan and dry-toast the flaked almonds until lightly browned at the edges. Set aside.

2 Melt the ghee and fry the onion, green chilli, garlic, ginger, cumin seeds, mustard seeds and cinnamon. Stir frequently until the mixture is golden. Add the parsnip chunks, turmeric and chilli powder. Cook for 1 minute then add the tomatoes, tamarind and water. Bring to a simmer and cook, lid on, for 15–20 minutes.

3 Add the courgettes, coconut milk and season well with salt and pepper. Cook for another 15–20 minutes, stirring until the mixture is simmering. Fold the green leaves through 5–10 minutes before the end, cooking gently until tender. Season to taste.

4 Meanwhile, for the cauliflower 'rice', remove the cauliflower leaves and the tough end of the stalk. Use a food processor (with the S-curved blade or grater attachment) or the coarse side of a grater to grate the cauliflower into rice-sized pieces. Melt the ghee in a frying pan, add the cauliflower and water and stir. Cook over a medium heat, lid on, for 4–5 minutes until tender but with bite. Check after 3–4 minutes to make sure that there is still water in the pan. Season to taste.

5 Plate up the cauliflower rice and serve with a generous portion of the curry on top. Scatter with the toasted almonds and the coriander, if using.

This is a proper plate of East by West! Fragrant with sesame, ginger and cardamom, it's Sunday roast with a twist. Serve it with a spiced tomato gravy, which lifts this usually heavy dish and makes it deliciously fresh. Other than the gravy, this all takes place in one big roasting tray, saving on the washing up and allowing the flavours to infuse a little for a chilled out lunch.

Serves 4

Sesame-roast chicken with Savoy cabbage and tomato gravy

2 tbsp ghee

sea salt and
    freshly ground
    black pepper

4 chicken thighs,
    bone-in and skin-on

2 small shallots,
    halved and peeled,
    or ½ leek or
    1 medium onion,
    roughly chopped

4 carrots (250g), cut into
    2cm (¾ in) lengths

4 small turnips (600g),
    cut into 2.5cm
    (1in) wedges

1½ tsp grated lemon zest

1 tbsp sesame seeds

½ Savoy cabbage,
    sliced into ribbons

FOR THE
TOMATO GRAVY

2 tbsp ghee

2–3 cloves
    garlic, minced

200g (1 cup) fresh
    tomatoes, skinned
    and deseeded (see
    page 260)

2 bay leaves

seeds of 4 cardamom
    pods, ground

1 tsp ground cumin

1.5cm (¾ in) piece of fresh
    ginger, chopped

85ml (just over
    ⅓ cup) water

1   Preheat the oven to 200ºC (fan 180ºC/gas mark 6). Place 1 tablespoon of the ghee in a large roasting tray. Add a pinch of salt and pepper and put it in the oven to heat for a few minutes.

2   In a large bowl, toss the chicken thighs, shallots, carrots and turnips with the remaining ghee, lemon zest and ¼ teaspoon each of salt and pepper.

3   Arrange the shallots, carrots and turnips in the roasting tray so that they are evenly spread out and place the thighs on top, skin-side up. Place the tray in the oven and roast for 15 minutes, then turn the vegetables over and continue roasting for another 15–20 minutes, until the chicken juices run clear and the vegetables are tender.

4   Meanwhile, toast the sesame seeds in a dry saucepan until golden and fragrant. For the last 10 minutes of cooking, scatter the cabbage ribbons and toasted sesame seeds over the chicken and vegetables and return it to the oven.

5   In the same saucepan, make the tomato gravy. Melt the ghee and stir through the garlic and tomatoes. Sauté for 2 minutes or so, then add the bay leaves, cardamom, cumin, ginger and water and bring to the boil. Cook for about 20 minutes, then remove the bay leaves and blend until smooth. Taste, adjust the seasoning, and keep warm until ready to serve.

6   Plate up the thighs, then toss the vegetables in the juices in the tray and serve drizzled with tomato gravy.

TIP
·

If you like your chicken
skin to be crispy, place the roasting
tray under the grill for a few
minutes before serving.

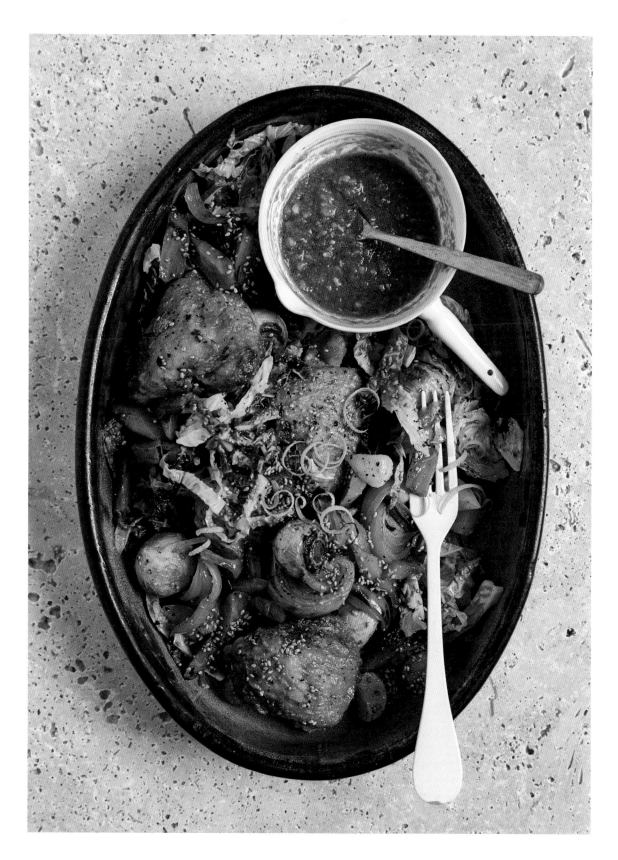

This is a slow-cooked dish that you can use to your advantage if you have a slowcooker – simply pop your soaked black- eyed beans in with everything else (there's barely any chopping) and come back to a hot evening meal. Otherwise, if I'm cooking it on the stove, I'll save it for lunch or supper on the weekend knowing that it will take 2–3 hours.

Serves 3–4

Melt in the mouth, well-cooked greens accompany this dish, making it a complete meal, providing you don't make it too spicy or salty. It's traditional to serve this with collard greens but they are only available in hotter countries such as southern USA, India, East Africa, Brazil and Portugal, so opt for spring greens, mustard greens or turnip greens instead, or try spinach, chard and Savoy cabbage, which are more widely available. Serve with basmati rice if you like, adding plenty of lime wedges and maybe a chutney or pickle (see pages 234–239) if serving to guests.

Creole black-eyed beans and 'collards'

1 tbsp ghee
1 medium onion, chopped
¼ tsp asafoetida
1 green pepper, chopped
3 sticks of celery, chopped
1 clove garlic, crushed
620ml (2½ cups) water
250g (1¼ cups) black-eyed beans, soaked overnight
2 tsp dried oregano
2 tsp coriander seeds, crushed
1 tsp smoked paprika

1¼ tsp sea salt, or to taste
1 tsp freshly ground black pepper
⅛ tsp cayenne pepper or more to taste
200g (2 cups) spring greens, chard, cabbage or spinach, any hard stalks removed and leaves chopped or cut into ribbons

1   Melt the ghee in a large heavy-bottomed saucepan. Add the onion and sauté until it begins to brown, then add the asafoetida, green pepper, celery and garlic and cook for 2 minutes, adding 1–2 tablespoons of the water if needed to prevent sticking.

2   Add the beans, remaining water, herbs, spices and ¼ teaspoon of the salt and bring to the boil, then simmer, lid on, for at least 2 hours until tender.

3   Around 10 minutes before you're ready to serve, and the rest of the salt to the saucepan. In a separate pan, steam your greens – they all have different cooking times. Spinach will cook faster, then chard, then cabbage, then spring greens. Serve the black-eyed beans with the greens on the side.

TIP
.

If you're using a slowcooker, place all the ingredients (apart from the greens) in the pot. Add ¼ tsp salt and cook on high for 8 hours, or until the peas are soft.

You could use dried cannellini beans instead of black-eyed beans – they take about 1½ hours to cook on the stove from soaked.

FEELING
PITTA

Reduce the amount of black pepper and paprika. Guests can sprinkle a little more on at the table.

FEELING
KAPHA

This is delicious with some added chilli or cayenne pepper.

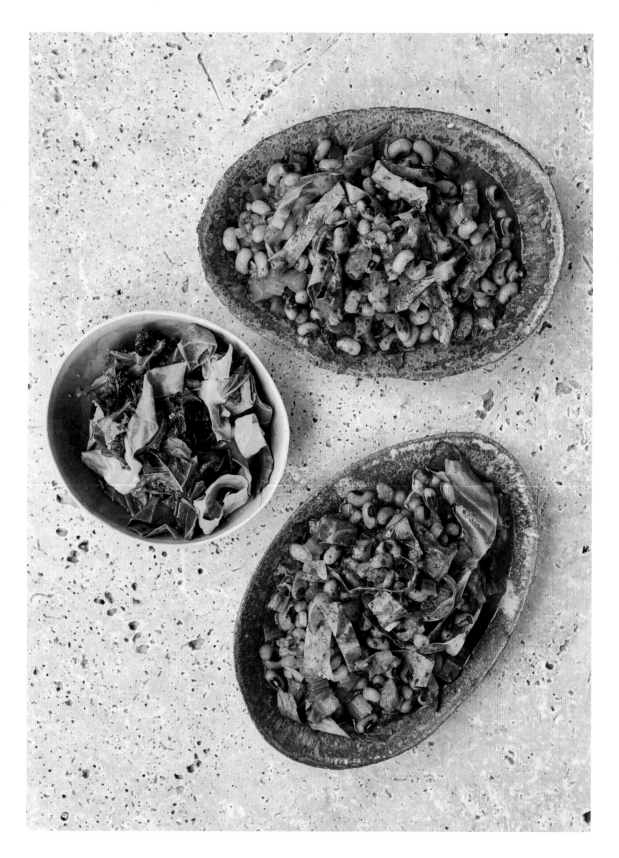

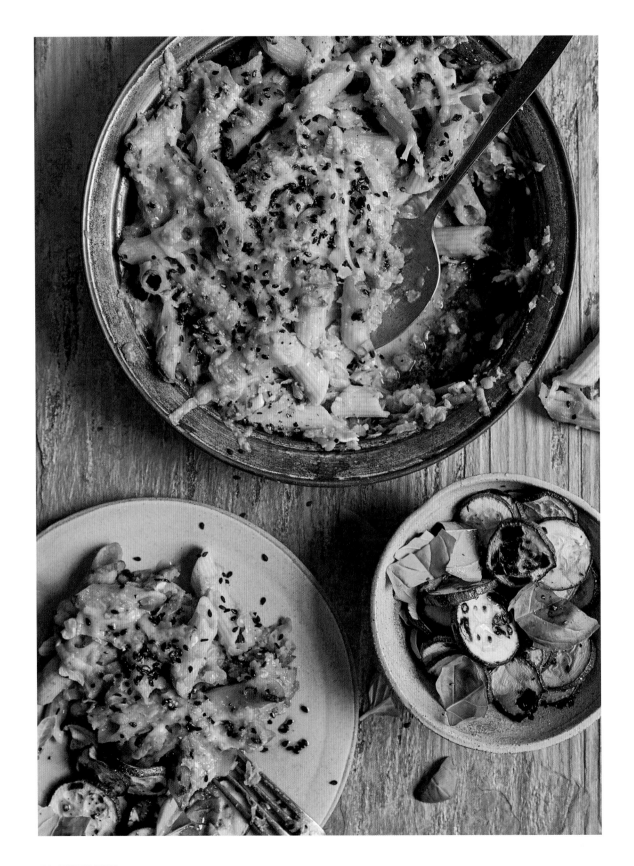

This is a really great meal to make from scratch – thanks to the red split lentils, it all comes together quickly without any advance prep. It's comforting, filling and just rich enough. Don't be put off by the long list of spices – it's worth it! The cottage cheese gives this a protein boost, along with the lentils, and makes a thick mellow sauce with the addition of carrots and smoked paprika. Eat this on a cool day in summer with the basil courgettes here or the Warm Green Salad on page 150, or team with sautéed cabbage in winter.

Serves 3

Zac 'n' cheese with basil courgettes

200g (2 cups) brown rice penne or other type of pasta
2 tbsp butter
2 cloves garlic, crushed
100g (½ cup) red split lentils, rinsed
500ml (2 cups) water
3 medium carrots (about 300g), grated
1 tsp smoked paprika
2 tsp Dijon mustard
1 tsp sea salt
1 tsp apple cider vinegar
200g (scant 1 cup) full-fat cottage cheese or homemade whole-milk ricotta (see page 254)
4 pinches of freshly ground black pepper

2 pinches of ground white pepper
2 pinches of ground nutmeg (optional)
65g (½ cup) sunflower seeds
40g (scant ¼ cup) Pecorino (or Parmesan), grated
black sesame seeds, to decorate (optional)

TO SERVE
2 large courgettes, sliced into rounds
extra-virgin olive oil, for drizzling
handful of fresh basil, torn

WORKS WITH

CABBAGE THORAN
page 228

SAUTÉED CUCUMBER,
GREEN BEANS,
BEETROOT AND
CARROT SALAD BOWL
page 143

FEELING
KAPHA

Swap the penne for cooked cauliflower – simply chop 1 head of cauliflower into florets, blanch and use it in place of the pasta.

1   In a medium pan, cook the pasta until just al dente (follow the packet instructions but reduce the cooking time by a minute or so). Drain and set aside.

2   In the same pan, melt the butter and sauté the garlic for a few minutes. Add the lentils, water, carrots and paprika and simmer, lid on, for 20 minutes until very soft. If the mixture is very runny, allow to simmer for a further few minutes with the lid off.

3   Add the Dijon mustard, salt, apple cider vinegar, cottage cheese, black and white pepper and nutmeg, if using. Blend until smooth, then taste and adjust the seasoning. The sauce should be really smooth and creamy – if it seems too dry, add a splash of water.

4   Fold in the cooked pasta and then transfer the whole thing to an ovenproof dish (about 20 x 16cm/8 x 6in in size), smoothing it out with the back of a spoon.

5   Sprinkle over the sunflower seeds and Pecorino evenly. Top with black sesame seeds, if using, and grill for 5 minutes until lightly browned.

6   Meanwhile, dry-cook the courgette slices in a ceramic-lined or seasoned cast-iron frying pan until tender and browned, then transfer to a dish, drizzle with olive oil, season lightly and cover with torn basil.

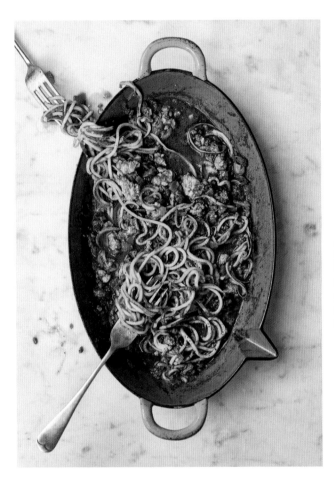

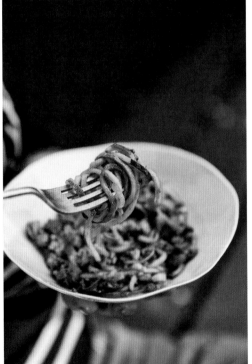

An excellent food for calming Vata, chicken livers are super-nutritious and tasty. As like increases like, eating livers supports the functioning of our own livers. A little goes a long way and they can be an acquired taste, so here the livers are mellowed with minced chicken and tomatoes, a mix of spices and herbs and fresh courgette noodles.

Serves 3

For a thicker sauce, and to ease in any newbies to liver, blend the livers with the passata first. When you get into this dish you can start to reduce the amount of tomatoes and up the spices.

Tuscan chicken livers and courgetti

2 tsp ghee
2 cloves garlic, crushed
1 onion, diced
pinch of ground
    cinnamon (optional)
1½ tsp fennel seeds
seeds of 4 cardamom
    pods, crushed
200g chicken breast
    or leg, minced
200g chicken
    livers, minced
150ml (½ cup) passata
    or 180g fresh tomatoes,
    skinned and deseeded
    (see page 260), or
    reduced bone broth
    (see page 261)

2–3 large courgettes
extra-virgin olive oil,
    for drizzling
¼ tsp sea salt
freshly ground black
    pepper, to taste
1 tsp dried or fresh
    sage leaves

1   Melt the ghee in a medium frying pan over a medium-high heat. Sauté the garlic, onion and spices, stirring frequently, for about 6 minutes until the onion is slightly soft.

2   Add the chicken and the livers and sauté for a few minutes before adding the passata and the tomatoes or bone broth. Cook for a few more minutes until everything is cooked through.

3   Meanwhile, use a spiraliser to make courgetti. Or use a julienne peeler or a knife to slice the courgettes into spaghetti-type strands. Add the courgetti to the centre of the pan and gently toss through the sauce, then top with a lid, allowing the courgettes to cook for a minute or two.

4   Divide between the serving plates. Drizzle with olive oil and season with salt and plenty of black pepper. For a fancy dinner date, fry fresh sage leaves in ghee or sunflower oil until crisp and scatter over the dishes.

FEELING
PITTA

Up the ratio of
chicken breast or leg
to chicken liver.

FEELING
KAPHA

Enjoy the sauce
served with plenty of
vegetables to balance the
nourishing qualities.

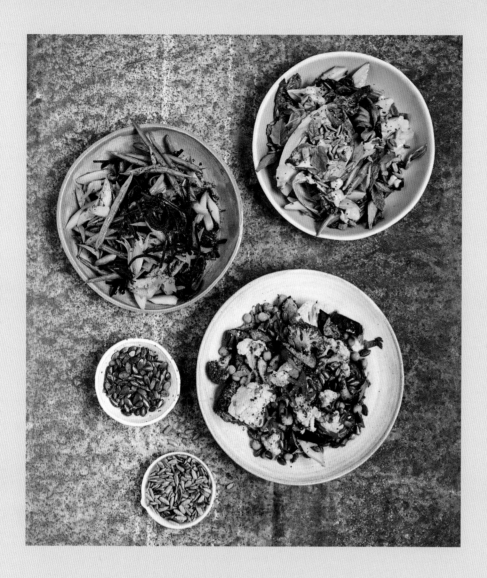

Pakti salad bowls

Raw salads are considered cold, rough and hard to digest in Ayurveda. They are okay in small quantities for Pitta types, but not great for anyone who is stressed-out or run-down, or Vata and Kapha types with wavering and slow digestion, respectively. Here are three Dosha-friendly salads, each lightly cooked so you still get the crunch of a salad without it flopping into a stew. All Dosha types can enjoy the other salads on occasion, unless they know they are feeling imbalanced that day. Asparagus is a Tridoshic wonder (see page 271) – whenever it is in season, make sure you stick it in your salad!

I've got warm green salads in this book (see page 150) and braised gem lettuce (see page 218) but sautéed cucumber? Yes, and it's delicious too! I love cucumber, but with its bitter seeds, hard-to-digest skin and cooling nature it's not a Vata favourite – until, that is, it's peeled and lightly fried to bring out more of that delicious sweetness. Cucumber is a great example of the way preparation changes the nature of foods, and of how cooking can give everything a little pre-digest magic fairy dust before it hits your tummy. The rest of the ingredients are very Vata-loving, too. For a more filling meal, top with shredded chicken or toss with cooked basmati rice.

Serves 2

VATA

Sautéed cucumber, green beans, beetroot and carrot salad bowl

1 tbsp ghee or butter
1 clove garlic, crushed
120g (just over ¾ cup) green beans
2 medium carrots, grated
½ cucumber, peeled and cut into 1cm (½ in) dice
1 medium beetroot, peeled and grated
sea salt and freshly ground pepper

FOR THE DILL AND MUSTARD DRESSING
1 tbsp apple cider vinegar
¼ tsp sea salt
2 tbsp fresh dill, finely chopped
½ tbsp Dijon mustard
60ml (¼ cup) extra-virgin olive oil

1 In a large frying pan, melt the ghee and gently sauté the garlic for 1 minute. Add the green beans and stir for 3–4 minutes, being careful not to burn the garlic.

2 Add the carrots and cucumber and continue sautéing for another 5 minutes. Set aside. In the same pan, sauté the beetroot for 3–5 minutes.

3 To make the dressing, add the vinegar and salt to a small bowl and whisk until the salt dissolves. Add the dill and mustard and whisk to combine. Slowly drizzle in the olive oil, whisking continuously, until the dressing is smooth and emulsified.

4 In two serving bowls, layer the beetroot and the cucumber and green bean mixture. Serve warm or at room temperature, drizzled with the dressing.

FEELING PITTA

Swap the beetroot and carrot for shaved, sautéed Brussels sprouts and peas and omit the garlic.

FEELING KAPHA

Swap the cucumber and green beans for mushrooms, leafy greens or peas.

TIP
·
For dinner parties, try roasting the carrot in small chunks or batons.

Avocado is a sweet, grounding and delicious food for Pitta types, and here it balances out the light, cooling and bitter radicchio leaves. The raw radicchio, chicory, endive (or even just a good lettuce) and mint with the avocado and lime dressing suits Pitta's strong digestive fire, but if you feel the need, braise or blanch the raw leaves first. Because it's hot and light, celery isn't usually good for Pitta but when it is caramelised in maple syrup it becomes deliciously bittersweet and adds another dimension to this dish while, interestingly, tasting like fennel!

If you like this salad bowl you could also top with shredded chicken or toss with cooked basmati rice for a more filling meal. PICTURED ON PAGE 142.

Serves 2

PITTA

Caramelised celery, avocado and radicchio salad bowl

4 tbsp sunflower seeds
½ tbsp ghee
1 radicchio, chicory, endive or gem lettuce, quartered and cut into wedges
½ tbsp maple syrup or jaggery
2 sticks of celery, cut into 5mm (¼ in) slices
½ avocado, de-stoned and cubed
handful of mint leaves

FOR THE AVOCADO
CREAM DRESSING
½ avocado, de-stoned
juice of ½ lime
2 tbsp extra-virgin olive oil
2 tbsp water
2 pinches of sea salt

1 In a large frying pan, gently dry-toast the sunflower seeds until golden, then set them aside.

2 In the same pan, add the ghee and fry the radicchio wedges for 5 minutes. Remove them from the pan and set aside.

3 Add the maple syrup and celery, then cook on a medium-high heat for 10–15 minutes, stirring occasionally, until coloured.

4 Add the dressing ingredients to a bowl and either blend or mash with a fork. Adjust the seasoning to taste.

5 Place the avocado and mint in a large bowl and toss with the dressing. Distribute between two plates or bowls, top with the caramelised celery and sunflower seeds and serve.

FEELING
VATA

Swap the veggies with sweet potato, courgettes and green beans.

FEELING
KAPHA

Serve this with dark chicken meat and cooked millet or barley.

This delicately smokey veg-packed salad is one of my favourites. The astringent brassicas, cauliflower and broccoli, are lightly roasted to add a little sweetness, along with the juicy aubergine and peas.

The dressing is sweet and pungent with plenty of fresh thyme, bitter parsley and a chilli kick if required. If you're feeling off balance, load it up with some leafy greens for extra bitter flavour. This is my partnerNick's favourite – he's definitely got Kapha tendencies and likes his meat and dairy. In his words: 'It's unusual for me to want to eat a plate of veg like that with nothing else!' For a more filling meal, toss with cooked barley and/or serve with scrambled egg. PICTURED ON PAGE 142.

Serves 2

KAPHA

Roasted broccoli, cauliflower and aubergine salad bowl

35g (¼ cup) pumpkin
    seeds
¼ head of cauliflower,
    cut into 2.5cm (1in)
    florets (about 150g)
¼ head of broccoli,
    cut into 2.5cm (1in)
    florets (about 150g)
1 aubergine, cut into 5mm
    (¼ in) thick half-moons
2 cloves garlic, left whole
2 tbsp ghee
sea salt and freshly
    ground black pepper
115g (¾ cup) peas,
    fresh or frozen
1 sprig of thyme
handful of parsley leaves
½ fresh red chilli,
    deseeded and
    chopped (optional)

FOR THE HONEY
MUSTARD DRESSING
juice and finely grated
    zest of 1 lemon
2 tsp wholegrain mustard
2 tsp raw honey
2 tbsp sunflower oil
fresh thyme, to taste
pinch of sea salt and
    freshly ground
    black pepper

FEELING
PITTA

Omit the chilli and swap
the honey for jaggery
or maple syrup.

1   Preheat the oven to 220ºC (fan 200ºC/gas mark 7). In a large frying pan, gently dry-toast the pumpkin seeds until golden, then set them aside.

2   On a large baking tray, toss the cauliflower, broccoli, aubergine and garlic cloves with the ghee and season with salt and pepper. Spread the vegetables out in an even layer and roast for about 20–25 minutes, stirring occasionally, until golden and tender. Remove the garlic cloves after 5–10 minutes and set aside.

3   For the last 3 minutes of cooking, add the peas and thyme to the baking tray, toss with the vegetables and return to the oven.

4   Meanwhile, make the dressing by putting all the ingredients into a jar or bottle. Shake until emulsified. Pop the roasted garlic cloves out of their jackets and mash into a paste, then stir into the dressing.

5   Toss the vegetables and parsley leaves in the dressing, then plate up and sprinkle with the toasted pumpkin seeds and chopped chilli, if using.

Though the method may be simple, there's plenty going on in this dish – everything you need is perfectly balanced with the creamy lemon-zest ricotta and the sweet aniseed of fennel taking centre stage.

The beauty of this is that you can eat with the seasons. Roasted veggies are often served as an autumn or winter warmer, so you'll find a selection of seasonal root veg in the recipe; however, adapt it with whatever you find, such as swede and Brussels sprouts. As the weather warms up, add in aubergine and summer squash. Remember to add one vegetable that softens as it cooks – such as sweet potato or courgette – to add stickiness and to stop things burning. Otherwise, you might want to add a little stock to make sure everything cooks evenly and the flavours mingle in the best way possible. Don't worry if you're not a huge fan of the liquorice flavour of fennel – it mellows as you roast it. When it's out of season, adjust the amount of fennel in the spice mix or just stick to coriander. If you love this flavour, check out the Beetroot Anise Millet Risotto (see page 150).

Serve with Ginger and Rhubarb Chutney (see page 235) to cut through the sweet root veggies and the creamy ricotta, or if you've chosen bitter brassicas, such as cauliflower and sprouts, then go with a sweet accompaniment, such as Black Pepper, Prune and Sesame Seed Chutney (see page 236).

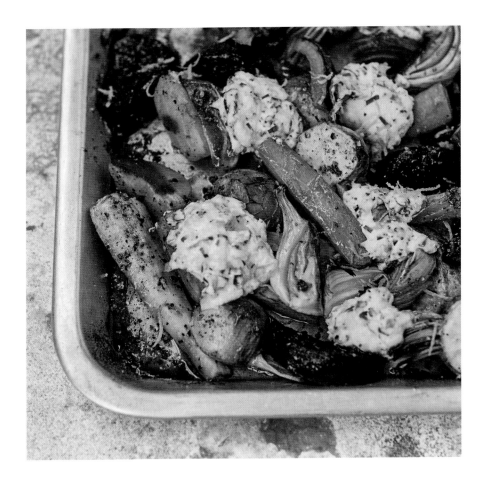

Serves 4,
or 6 as a side dish

One-pan baked veggies with roast fennel and herby ricotta

2 medium parsnips (about 300g), peeled and quartered lengthways

3 medium beetroots (about 350g), peeled and cut into 6 wedges

3 medium carrots (about 450g), cut into 3cm (1¼ in) lengths

6 small turnips (about 300g), cut into 8 wedges

½ celeriac (about 270g), peeled and cut into 3cm (1¼ in) chunks

1–2 baby fennel bulbs (about 400g), trimmed, cut lengthways into 1cm (½ in) slices, reserving fronds for garnish

6 garlic cloves, peeled

60ml (¼ cup) olive oil

¾ tsp sea salt

freshly ground black pepper, to taste

FOR THE FENNEL SPICE MIXTURE (OPTIONAL)

50g (½ cup) fennel seeds

2 tbsp coriander seeds

2 tbsp white peppercorns

1½ tbsp sea salt

FOR THE HERBY RICOTTA

225g (1 cup) homemade whole-milk ricotta (see page 254)

4 tbsp chives, chopped

4 tbsp basil, chopped

2 tsp grated lemon zest, plus extra for topping

big pinch of sea salt

TIP
.
Sprinkle this spice mixture on Kitchari (see page 184) and soups.

1 Start with the fennel spice mixture, if using. Dry-toast the fennel seeds, coriander seeds and peppercorns in a large heavy-based pan over medium-high heat. Watch carefully, tossing frequently so the seeds toast evenly, around 2 minutes. When fragrant, tip out the seeds onto a plate to cool. They must be cool before grinding, or they will clog up the blender blades. Blend to a fine powder with the salt, shaking the blender or scraping down occasionally. Store in a tightly sealed glass jar in a cool, dry place, or freeze.

2 Preheat the oven to 200ºC (fan 180ºC/gas mark 6). Combine the vegetables, garlic, oil, salt and lots of pepper in a large bowl. Add 1 tablespoon of the fennel spice mixture, if using, and get stuck in with your hands, tossing to combine and coat the vegetables.

3 Spread out the vegetables evenly in a large roasting pan. Roast them in the oven for 45 minutes, then use a large spoon to toss well. Return to the oven and roast for a further 15 minutes, or until just tender.

4 Meanwhile, combine the ricotta, chives, basil, lemon zest and salt in a small bowl with a fork. Dollop tablespoons of the ricotta on top of the vegetables and cook for a further 5 minutes in the oven. Serve immediately. Add fennel fronds to garnish.

Inspired by the English classic of Lancashire hotpot, this dish celebrates one-pot low and slow cooking. The recipe renders a medley of ingredients, including tougher cuts of meat, into a melt-in-the-mouth, easy-to-digest dish.

I've added pink peppercorns, which are one of my new favourite flavours in the spice pantry. From a medicinal perspective the pink berries are a great diuretic, which helps with bloating, and have antiseptic and disinfectant properties so act as a simple remedy for coughs and colds. Slightly sweet and reminiscent of juniper berries, they are often paired with mild-flavoured white fish and asparagus, but here they shine with sweet squash, turnips and lamb.

Because lamb is often fatty, I like to serve hotpot with a sautéed red cabbage salad, its pink colour offering a nod to the pink peppercorns that have disappeared into the layers of the hotpot. It's also perfect with mint for freshness and a chutney or two (my friend Alex from Lancashire swears by a pickle hotpot pairing!).

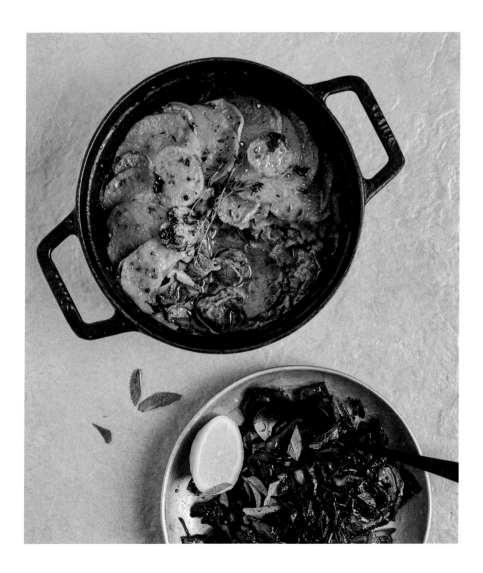

Serves 6

Pink pepper lamb hotpot with sautéed red cabbage and mint

500g diced lamb, mutton
 neck fillet or shoulder
sea salt and freshly
 ground black pepper
1½ tbsp butter, melted,
 plus extra to grease
½ large butternut squash
 (about 600g),
 peeled and cut into
 5mm (¼ in) slices
150g turnips, cut into
 5mm (¼ in) slices
1½–2 tbsp crushed pink
 peppercorns
4 sprigs of thyme,
 leaves picked
2 bay leaves

1 large leek, sliced into
 5mm (¼ in) rounds
500ml (2 cups)
 bouillon stock

FOR THE RED
CABBAGE
1 tbsp ghee
1 tsp black mustard seeds
300g (3 cups) thinly
 shredded red cabbage
15–20g (¼–⅓ cup)
 mint leaves, chopped
½–1 tbsp lemon juice
sea salt, to taste

1 Preheat the oven to 170ºC (fan 150ºC/gas mark 3).
 Season the meat lightly with salt and pepper.

2 Butter a 24cm (9½in) high-sided casserole dish and
 arrange one third of the sliced butternut squash and
 turnips in the bottom. Season with a little of the pink
 peppercorns and sprinkle with thyme. Top with the
 meat and bay leaves and season in the same way,
 followed by the leek, also seasoned in the same way.

3 Arrange the remaining slices of squash and turnips on
 top of the leek like overlapping fish scales, and season
 with salt and pepper. Pour enough stock over the top
 to come just up to the base of the topping (lift up a
 piece to check), then brush with the melted butter.

4 Cover and bake for 2 hours, then uncover and bake
 for another 30–40 minutes, until the top is golden
 and crisp.

5 Around 10 minutes before the end of the cooking time,
 make the sautéed red cabbage. Heat the ghee in a
 large frying pan and add the mustard seeds. Sauté
 until they pop and are fragrant. Add the cabbage and
 sauté for 10–15 minutes until just tender, adding one
 or two tablespoons of water if needed. Toss through
 the other ingredients and serve immediately with
 the hotpot.

WORKS WITH

CABBAGE THORAN
page 228

SRI LANKAN
CELEBRATION PICKLE
page 237

Millet is one of my favourite grains. It contains more vitamins, minerals and protein than rice, and has a mellower flavour than quinoa, but you can use it in much the same way as you would the other grains. Its cheaper price tag also wins a place in my heart! The roasted beetroot adds another level of indulgence to this deliciously warming risotto. This is a very Kapha-friendly recipe – great for winter when you want to feel warm and hibernate, but don't want to feel too sluggish.

This risotto also works well with a warm green salad. Digesting raw salad can be tricky, but when heated the food starts to break down, allowing us to digest it more easily. I also love how heated salad greens take on a whole new flavour profile, too: bitter edges get rounded out and nuttiness is amplified.

If you're lazy about chopping beetroot you can always use a food processor to grate it, or if your oven is on, you can bake or roast it in the oven to get a head start. Another tip is to pour half the stock into the pan and let it simmer away with an occasional stir. It's the last stage of cooking that's important to get the perfect texture for you, whether you prefer a wet risotto or a dry one.

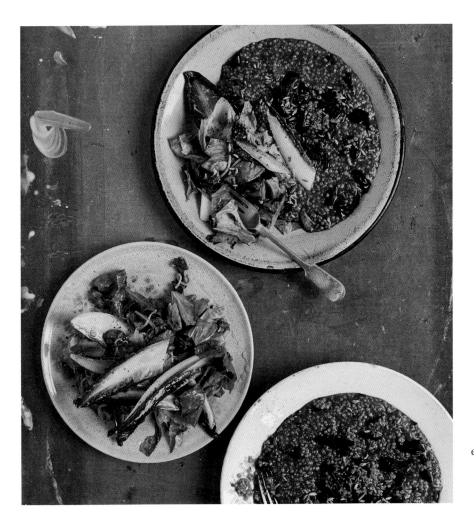

WORKS WITH

GREEN CHUTNEY
page 229

WHOLE-MILK
RICOTTA
page 254

FEELING
VATA

Enjoy more of a wet texture. Add plenty of extra-virgin olive oil, and serve with a little salad. Stick to rice or soaked well-cooked oat groats.

Beetroot anise millet risotto with warm green salad

450g beetroot, peeled
and cubed
1 litre (4 cups) bouillon
stock or bone broth
(see page 251)
250ml (1 cup) water
3 tsp fennel seeds, plus
1 tsp extra to decorate
3 tbsp ghee
1 small white onion, diced
2 cloves garlic, finely
chopped
200g (1 cup) millet,
soaked overnight,
rinsed and drained
sea salt and freshly
ground pepper
25g (¼ cup) grated
Parmesan (optional)

FOR THE WARM
GREEN SALAD
1 tbsp ghee
1 shallot or ½ leek, sliced
2 tbsp Dijon mustard
½ tbsp apple cider vinegar
sea salt and freshly
ground black pepper,
to taste
½ head of red chicory,
leaves separated
3 handfuls of
mixed greens
(such as spinach,
romaine and rocket)
1 tbsp chopped parsley

1 Place the beetroot in a saucepan with the stock and water. Bring to the boil and simmer for 10 minutes until tender.

2 Meanwhile, in a large saucepan, dry-toast 1 teaspoon of the fennel seeds until fragrant (be careful not to burn them) and set aside.

3 In the same saucepan, melt the ghee and sauté the remaining 3 teaspoons of fennel seeds for a few minutes until fragrant. Add the onion and garlic and continue to sauté over a moderate heat for about 5 minutes, until softened. Rinse and drain the millet, then add to the pan and cook for 2 minutes – making sure that you keep stirring.

4 Add 500ml (2 cups) of the beetroot stock and simmer. Stir occasionally. When most of the stock has been absorbed, add as much stock as needed, a ladleful at a time. Cook, stirring often, for about 12 minutes or until the millet is well cooked.

5 Meanwhile, make the salad. The key here is to barely wilt it. Add the ghee to a frying pan over a medium heat. Add the shallot and cook for 3 minutes. Mix in the mustard, vinegar, salt and pepper, and cook for a further minute. Add the chicory and mixed green leaves and toss with tongs. Cook for 2 minutes, tossing the whole time.

6 Season the risotto, if needed, making sure to taste it first as bouillon stocks are already well seasoned. Stir through the beetroot cubes from the stock and the Parmesan, if using, and serve with the warm green salad.

FEELING
PITTA

Make this with
asparagus or broccoli
and barley or rice.

FEELING
KAPHA

Serve with more salad and
add a little homemade
chilli oil if you like.
Enjoy more of a dry
risotto texture.

Once upon a time, making my own cheese and finely dicing vegetables would not have been my thing. I loved homemade food but I saw cooking as a chore and washing up even more so. Now I've relaxed into the tasks so much more, I actually feel uplifted rather than depleted from trying to rush it all through.

This recipe sums up the beauty of seeing a dish through from start to finish with a little bit of skill and precision, while remaining a hearty meal rather than a restaurant-style display! So go all Little Miss Muffet and strain those curds and whey to make paneer and make an art out of chopping and prepping your veggies. Do it to classical music if you like, and make the preparation of your food the most sacred act that you have.

When you can get them, go for the bigger green beans (English bobby beans!) – but the most common beans in the supermarkets now are the fine green beans, which I like to halve on the diagonal. This is best eaten for lunch, rather than dinner, as the cheese makes it a bit tricky to digest. The sauce is also delicious with a little cumin for variation.

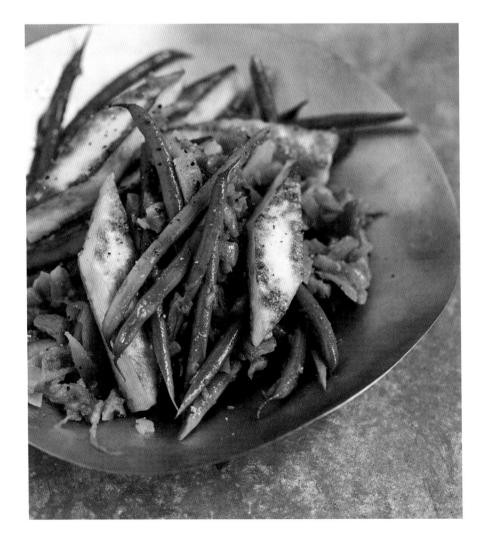

Golden paneer with tomato-y green beans and carrots

1 quantity of homemade
  paneer (see page 254),
  patted dry and sliced
  on the diagonal
1 medium onion,
  diced small
3cm (1¼ in) piece of
  fresh ginger, finely
  diced or grated
4 cloves garlic, finely
  chopped
½ tsp ground coriander,
  or 1 tsp coriander
  seeds, ground
¼ tsp ground turmeric

6 large tomatoes,
  skinned and deseeded
  (see page 260)
2 large carrots, finely
  diced or grated
sea salt and freshly
  ground black pepper,
  to taste
200g (1⅓ cups)
  green beans
1 tbsp ghee
portion of cooked
  basmati rice, quinoa
  or your favourite pasta,
  to serve

1   You can make the paneer a few days or couple of
    hours ahead and store it until you're ready to serve.
    It will keep for 4–7 days in the fridge but it is best
    enjoyed in the first 2 days. The drier and more
    compact the paneer is, the better it is for frying.

2   Heat a large ceramic-lined or seasoned cast iron
    frying pan and fry the onion until it starts to brown.
    Add the ginger and garlic and stir, then add the spices.
    Throw in the tomatoes and carrots, season to taste
    and simmer, lid on, for 10 minutes. Add the green
    beans and simmer for 3 minutes, lid off, until tender.

3   Meanwhile, melt the ghee in another pan on a medium
    heat. Add the paneer and fry until golden on one side,
    being careful not to burn it. Turn the paneer over and
    fry on the other side until it has a golden crust. Serve
    with the tomato-y green beans.

**FEELING
VATA**

Sub in tempeh instead of
paneer occasionally.

**FEELING
PITTA**

Reduce the onion, garlic
and ginger a touch or
enjoy less of the sauce.

**FEELING
KAPHA**

Up the ginger and reduce
the quantity of the cheese
(or swap for sautéed
cooked chickpeas). Add
¼ teaspoon chilli powder.

TIP
·

If you want to dice the
carrots, top and tail them, then
cut in half lengthways. Half again.
Cut into batons or carrot sticks that
are around 5–7.5cm (2–3in) long
and 1cm (½ in) thick. Then cut
them across into equal-sized dice.
For perfectly square dice, trim the
rounded parts off each side of the
carrot to square the edges before
cutting the sticks.

A real biryani is the crème de la crème of culinary skill. It's the lasagne of the Indian kitchen – everyone's got their own style and everyone's grandma makes the best one. Experience is necessary for learning how much to par-cook the rice, and then how long it needs in the oven to give you those lovely long strands. The trick is to achieve the perfect balance between chewy, bitty undercooked biryani and overcooked stodge.

This recipe avoids the stress while still giving you a biryani-style experience. Biryanis are traditionally very spicy and loaded with onions – this one is fragrant, mild and comforting. You won't find many recipes that mix high-starch ingredients and animal proteins in this book, but here the lamb adds a lovely unctuousness.

For a veggie-only biryani (a great dish to clear out the fridge in one go!), double the veggies and raisins, add a few carrots and increase the cumin very slightly. Serve the veggie version at lunchtime, with yoghurt and nuts.

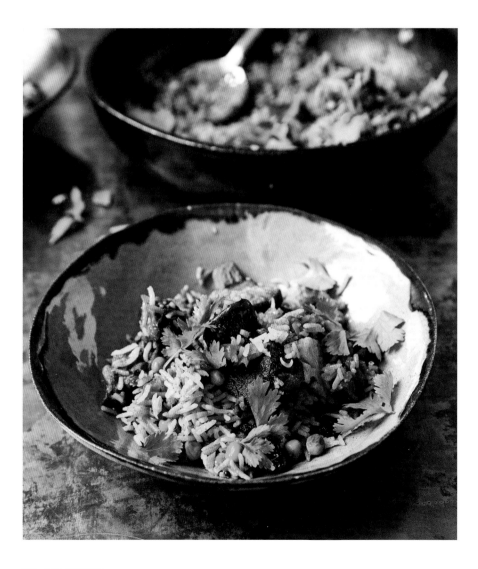

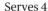
Lamb and vegetable biryani

3 tbsp ghee

750g lamb (neck or
shoulder) cut into
5cm (2in) cubes

1 tsp coriander seeds

1 tsp black peppercorns

1 tsp cumin seeds

2 tsp garam masala

1 tsp ground turmeric

5cm (2in) piece of fresh
ginger, finely chopped

½ large leek,
finely chopped

¾ tsp sea salt

seeds of 5 cardamom
pods, ground

1 bay leaf

1 large cinnamon stick

200ml water

½ large head of
cauliflower (300g),
cut into florets

1 aubergine, cubed

150g (1 cup) fresh
or frozen peas

30g (¼ cup) raisins

320g (1⅔ cups) white
basmati rice, rinsed

butter, for greasing

handful of coriander
or mint leaves, plus
extra for serving

TIP
·

For some flair at a dinner party
I like to fry off an onion slowly
until soft and then on a higher
heat until browned, adding some
raisins and cashews to sauté at the
end. Use to garnish the top along
with some extra fresh herbs.

1   Heat 1 tablespoon of the ghee in a large ceramic-lined
or seasoned cast-iron frying pan. Add half the lamb
and brown it all over. Remove and repeat with the
second batch. Set aside.

2   In the same pan, melt the remaining ghee over a
medium heat. Sauté the coriander seeds, peppercorns
and cumin seeds for a few minutes until they start to
pop. Add the garam masala and turmeric and sauté
for a few minutes. Add the ginger and leek and fry
for a minute before adding the lamb, salt, cardamom,
bay leaf, cinnamon stick and water.

3   Bring to the boil, cover and cook for 1–1 hour 10
minutes. Check that the lamb is tender. Add the
cauliflower and aubergine, and cook for another
10 minutes. Add the peas and the raisins.

4   Meanwhile, cook the rice according to the
packet instructions.

5   Preheat the oven to 200ºC (fan 180ºC/gas mark 6).
Grease a large lidded baking dish (around 25 x 40cm
/10 x 15in in size) with butter. Spoon in one third of
the rice, cover with half of the lamb curry and sprinkle
with half of the fresh coriander. Repeat these layers
again. Finally, add the remaining rice to the dish and
dot with a little more butter. At this stage, the dish can
be refrigerated for a few hours, then cooked when
you're ready.

6   Place in the oven and heat through for 15 minutes
if it is freshly prepared, or up to 40 minutes if you
are cooking from cold. Serve hot, garnished with
extra coriander and mint.

This is inspired by a childhood favourite of mine. My childminder Sonia's husband, Lew, was an amazing cook and the food was always hearty and belly-warming; this is my version of one of my favourite dishes – mince on mash with broccoli. The mince was cooked with baked beans and onions and served runny, around a mound of mash, and I used to stand the broccoli florets on the mound like they were trees on a white hill surrounded by a muddy river. We even gave it a drizzle of tomato sauce before we tucked in. Not sure what that symbolised! In this version I add some spices to gently flavour the mince while making it easier to digest. I've swapped out the baked beans for carrot and tomato, which makes up for the sweetness and adds a little acidity.

I like to make this in my slowcooker on a wet and wintry day. Of course, winter is not really the season for broccoli so when that's not around, swap for seasonal greens. Serve it on a pile of mashed swede, which adds a delicious flavour dimension and makes a less starchy accompaniment to meat than potato mash. This recipe calls for 1½ average-sized swedes, which can feed four. Save the other half of the swede for the Quinoa Minestrone on page 190.

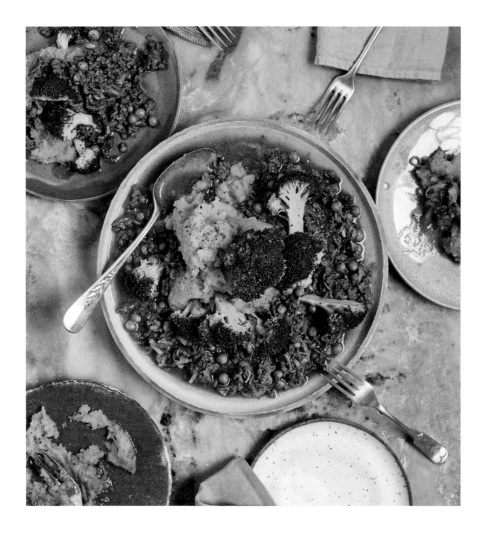

Serves 4

Spiced mince and gravy on swede mash with broccoli trees

1 tbsp ghee

1 tsp mustard seeds

2½ tsp ground cumin

1 tsp ground coriander

1 tsp ground turmeric

1½ tsp ground ginger

½ tsp ground cinnamon

5cm (2in) piece of fresh ginger, grated

1 medium leek or 1 medium–large onion, finely sliced

350g lamb mince

3 carrots, grated

4 large tomatoes (about 300g), skinned and deseeded (see page 260)

400ml bone broth (see page 261) or bouillon stock

½ tsp sea salt and ½ tsp freshly ground black pepper, to taste

450–500g broccoli

100ml water

100g (⅔ cup) peas

handful coriander leaves (optional)

FOR THE MASH

2 swedes, topped and tailed, peeled and cut into 2cm cubes

200ml water

2 bay leaves

½ tsp sea salt

1½ tbsp butter

¼ tsp ground nutmeg

generous pinch of ground white or black pepper

1 In a ceramic-lined or seasoned cast-iron frying pan, melt the ghee, add the mustard seeds and fry them until they start to pop. Add the rest of the spices and fry for a few minutes before adding the fresh ginger, leek and mince, sautéeing over a high heat for 5–7 minutes and breaking up the mince as you go.

2 Stir in the grated carrots and the tomatoes, then pour in the bone broth, and bring to the boil. Reduce to a rapid simmer and cook for 25 minutes, lid off, until the gravy has reduced to your desired thickness.

3 Meanwhile, make the mash. Pop the swede into a large saucepan with the water, bay leaves and a pinch of salt. Gently bring the water to the boil over a medium heat. Then place the lid on tightly and cook for about 30–35 minutes, or until tender, keeping an eye on the water level.

4 Drain well, removing the bay leaves and reserving the cooking water. Return the swede to the pan over a very low heat, add the butter, nutmeg and white pepper and mash coarsely, adding more of the cooking water if needed. Replace the lid and remove from the heat.

5 When there is 7 minutes left of the mince cooking time, place the broccoli in a medium saucepan with 100ml water and bring to a simmer, lid on. Remove the lid and cook for another 3 minutes, or until tender.

6 Around 2 minutes before serving, add the peas to the pan of mince. Divide the mash between the plates, pour the mince around it, then top with the broccoli. Garnish with the coriander, if using, and serve.

TIP
·

If you like, try blending the mash in a food processor to give you a smoother purée – but I prefer the rough texture of the mash with the mince.

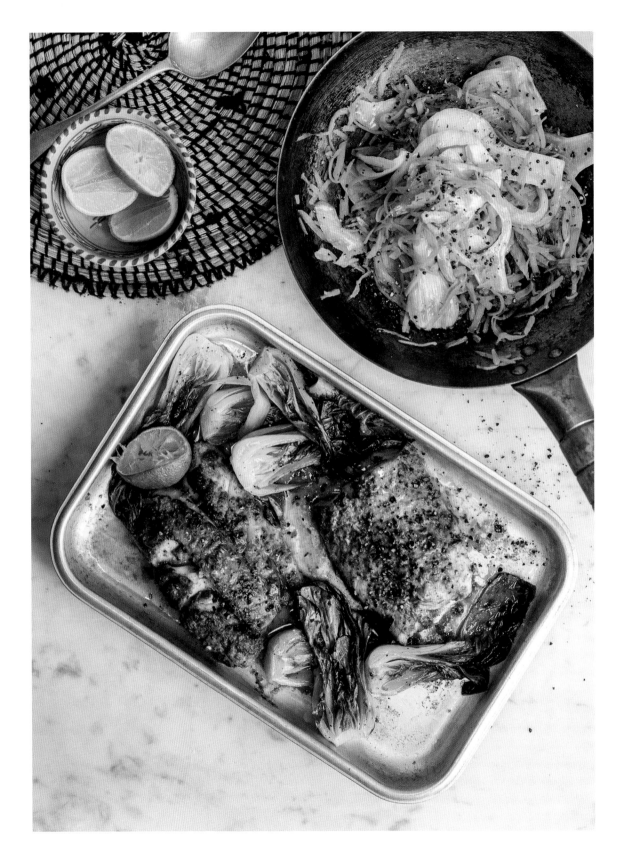

I don't have a tandoor (a type of clay oven), but I do like tikka – usually small pieces of meat or fish in a spicy marinade, baked in said oven. This adaptation is a deliciously easy fish dish that I can pop in the oven while I prepare a stir-fry of veggies, making it perfect for entertaining. In India the tikka marinade is made with yoghurt and spices, but since yoghurt with fish is an Ayurvedic 'no-no', I've swapped it with ghee, which helps to activate the spices as well as baste the fish. Marinate the fish in advance for the best flavour, then bring to room temperature before cooking. The whole dish comes together really easily and looks the business.

Serves 2

Tikka fish and pak choi with carrot, fennel and mustard stir-fry

1 tsp ground ginger

1 tsp ground turmeric

1½ tsp garam masala

½ tsp freshly ground black pepper, plus extra to taste

½ tsp sea salt, plus extra to taste

½ tsp toasted cumin seeds or ground cumin

2–3 tbsp ghee

1 lime or lemon

½–1 tbsp water (optional)

2 fillets (about 300g) firm white fish such as pollock, cod, haddock, coley, tilapia

1 pak choi, quartered lengthways

1 fennel, trimmed and cut into long slices

1 tbsp black mustard seeds

¼ tsp chilli powder (optional)

2 large carrots, grated

sea salt and freshly ground black pepper, to taste

1   Mix the ginger, turmeric, garam masala, black pepper, salt and cumin together. Combine with 1 tablespoon of ghee and the juice of ½ lime to make a paste, adding ½–1 tablespoon of water if necessary.

2   Coat the fish in the paste and marinate in the fridge for at least 2 hours or overnight. When you are ready to cook, bring the fish to room temperature.

3   Preheat the oven to 180ºC (fan 160ºC/gas mark 4). In a large pan, melt 1 tablespoon of the ghee over a medium heat and sear the pak choi until golden, then season with a little salt and pepper and set aside.

4   Place the fish on a baking tray and bake for about 15 minutes or until the fish is cooked, adding the pak choi for the last 5 minutes.

5   Meanwhile, melt the rest of the ghee in the same pan, if needed, and sauté the fennel. When it is lightly browned, add the mustard seeds and cook until they start to pop (be careful not to let them burn and become bitter). Add the carrot, season and stir-fry for a few minutes, until just tender. Plate everything up and squeeze over the juice of ½ lime.

FEELING
VATA

Slightly overcook the vegetables and add plenty of fresh ginger to the stir-fry.

FEELING
KAPHA

Add the chilli and increase your portion of veggies.

This makes a gorgeous summer party recipe. It's a bit like a Thai papaya salad, which is one of my favourites when I'm travelling, but instead of the raw unripe green papayas, which are hard to find and tricky to digest even if you do find them, I use a combination of white radish, mung bean noodles and cabbage – this gives you a lovely white backdrop to the bright colours of the chilli, green beans and of course the bright yellow and pink boiled eggs!

You can also try this with tempeh, tofu, shredded chicken or a piece of pan-fried fish. In the summer you could add sautéed mung bean sprouts for protein. In the winter, make a delicious dashi stock (see page 222) or bone broth (see page 261) and use to simmer the salad ingredients for a lovely Thai-style soup, topped with the eggs as per the recipe, or you could even just poach them in the soup. Save the beetroot pickling liquid to add some sour flavour to a dal.

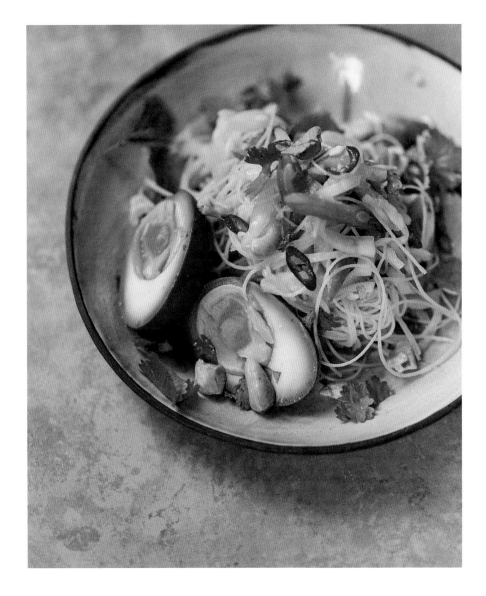

FEELING
VATA

Use more oil and
make sure the veggies
are well cooked.

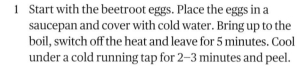

Serves 2–3

Thai white radish and glass noodle salad with beetroot egg

1 x 80g packet mung-bean glass noodles
1 tbsp ghee
3 garlic cloves, minced
¼ white cabbage (about 200g), shredded
100g (¾ cup) green beans
2 pinches of sea salt
1 large white radish (mooli), grated or julienned
small bunch of fresh coriander, chopped
2 spring onions, very thinly sliced
40g (¼ cup) cashews or almonds, coarsely chopped and toasted, to serve
1 red Thai chilli, thinly sliced, to serve

FOR THE BEETROOT EGGS
3 medium eggs
120ml (½ cup) water
60ml (¼ cup) apple cider vinegar
big pinch of salt
½ small beetroot, peeled and grated

FOR THE DRESSING
4 tbsp lime juice
1½ tbsp raw honey or light jaggery (best for colour)
2½ tbsp sunflower oil or macadamia oil
½ tbsp fish sauce
pinch of sea salt

1 Start with the beetroot eggs. Place the eggs in a saucepan and cover with cold water. Bring up to the boil, switch off the heat and leave for 5 minutes. Cool under a cold running tap for 2–3 minutes and peel.

2 Mix together 120ml (½ cup) water, vinegar, salt and beetroot in a small bowl and leave the eggs in there for around 30 minutes until pink in colour, turning occasionally for even coverage. Remove the eggs, give them a quick rinse and pat dry.

3 Cook the glass noodles according to the packet instructions, then leave to drain and dry out a little.

4 Place the ingredients for the dressing in a jam jar and shake well until emulsified and thickened.

5 Melt the ghee in a large saucepan and gently sauté the garlic, cabbage and green beans with the salt until tender, then at the last minute add the white radish and sauté for a further minute.

6 Take the pan off the heat, then allow to cool a little before tossing through the noodles, coriander, spring onions and half of the dressing.

7 Pour over the rest of the dressing, cut the pink eggs in half lengthways, season and arrange alongside. Sprinkle with the chopped nuts, decorate with the sliced chilli and serve.

FEELING
PITTA

Skip the chilli and opt for jaggery to sweeten the dressing.

FEELING
KAPHA

Increase your portion of all the veggies and have less of the egg.

This dish has been part of my recipe repertoire for years. If someone is coming over and I get a complete blank about what to cook, or I just don't know what I fancy eating, I make this. Sometimes I go with the bare bones – butternut squash, lentils, coconut, garlic and ginger. Other times I throw in the greens and the spices and garnish with the coriander and lime. If I'm feeling really adventurous, I'll start off sautéeing my favourite spice mix (see page 247) in coconut oil before continuing with the recipe – or if I've already started the cooking and my taste buds are saying they want something more, then I'll sauté the spice mix with oil in a separate pan to make a tarka (see page 265) and drizzle it over the finished dish.

My friends tell me this is a winner with the kids – it's amazing how coconut can help veggies and lentils go down and soften their first introduction to Eastern spices – and it's also become a staple recipe to personalise with whatever ingredients they have to hand. You could set it up in your slowcooker, omitting the greens, and cook it lovingly for 12 hours on the lowest heat – either in the morning before you go to work or overnight (as this is also great for breakfast!). Simply cook the greens separately or throw them in for the last hour.

Serves 4–6

Coconut, squash, lentil and leek curry with rainbow chard

1 medium butternut squash
¼ tsp asafoetida
1 large leek, sliced
7.5cm (3in) piece of fresh ginger, finely chopped
½ bar creamed coconut plus 750ml (3 cups) water, or 1 x 400ml tin of full-fat coconut milk plus 850ml (scant 3½ cups) water

250g (scant 1½ cups) red split lentils
½ tsp freshly ground black pepper
2 tsp ground turmeric
200g rainbow chard or spring greens
1 tsp sea salt
75g (1 packed cup) fresh coriander, chopped
1 lime, sliced

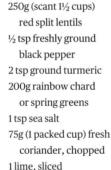

FEELING
VATA

Reduce your portion of greens. Skip the creamed coconut and use bone broth (see page 261) with plenty of ginger and ghee.

FEELING
KAPHA

Use bone broth instead of creamed coconut. Increase the greens and add some chilli.

1 Peel the squash and cut it into 2.5cm (1in) chunks.

2 Put the asafoetida, leek, ginger and squash into a pan with the creamed coconut. Put the lid on and bring to a medium simmer.

3 After 15 minutes, add the lentils, pepper and turmeric and stir. Allow to simmer on medium for a further 15–20 minutes, lid on, until the lentils are soft and the squash is tender. Add more water if necessary to reach your desired consistency (you may need to add up to 500ml/2 cups).

4 Add the greens, stalks removed, in the last 5–15 minutes of cooking (chard needs about 7 minutes, spring greens need about 15 minutes). Garnish with coriander and lime slices and serve.

TIP
·

You could cook the squash for 15 minutes in the oven, then cool – this makes it easier to chop.

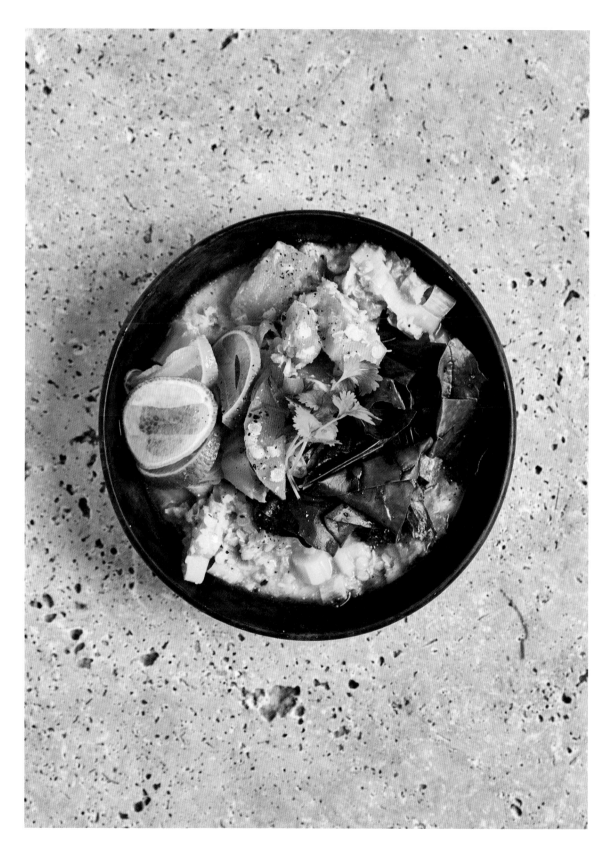

This recipe has done the rounds with my friends, who have taken to falling back on this when they have a busy or very fun week with barely a green thing on their plates. Inspired by an Ayurvedic cookbook I've had for years by Amadea Morningstar, it is a real back-to-basics soup recipe, without any garlic, onion, sautéing or fuss. It is perfect for using up broccoli stalks – if I have a whole head of broccoli I favour the stalk first, then add enough florets to make up to 250g and save the rest for something like the Veg Masala for the Brain (see page 198).

The cashews or sunflower seeds are soaked to make them easier to blend, and you can choose to blend the soup to creamy or textured, depending on how you like it. Alternatively, you can add ghee instead. The flavour comes from the leeks, and the bright green colour looks fantastic with a sprinkling of black sesame seeds and some dehusked watermelon seeds for extra crunch.

Serves 2

Cream of broccoli soup with black sesame and watermelon seeds

250g broccoli (mostly
    stalks), chopped
¼ leek, sliced
250ml (1 cup) water
8 whole cashews or
    1 heaped tbsp
    sunflower seeds,
    soaked for 1 hour and
    drained, or 1 tbsp ghee
½ tsp sea salt
freshly ground
    black pepper, to taste

TO SERVE
extra-virgin olive oil,
    for drizzling
handful of dehusked
    watermelon seeds
    (I love Mello brand)
handful of black
    sesame seeds

1   Simmer the broccoli, leek and water until the vegetables are tender and bright green. Blend with the soaked cashews, and add the salt.

2   Season with freshly ground black pepper. Serve with plenty of extra-virgin olive oil and a generous sprinkle of watermelon seeds and black sesame seeds.

FEELING
VATA

Enjoy this at lunch rather
than dinnertime. For
dinner, make it a cream of
pea or asparagus soup.

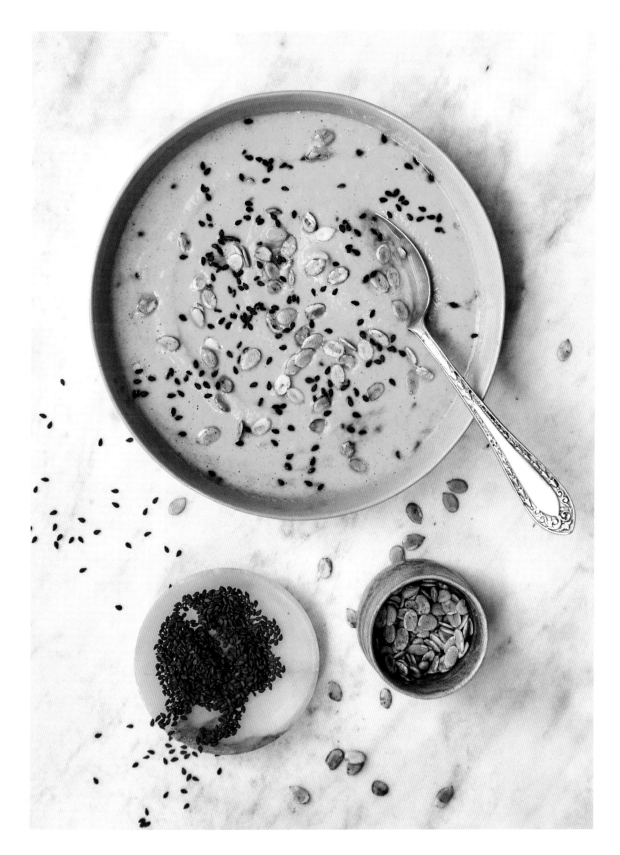

Dal is an absolute Indian classic – it's cooked every day in most households. Everyone needs a good dal recipe up his or her sleeve; often my go-to dish, this one is nourishing, easy to make and gentle on a stressed digestive system. Make sure the lentils are cooked very well – old chana dal doesn't cook well, so make sure your packet is fresh. If you didn't soak the lentils overnight, use split red lentils or split mung dal that can be cooked straightaway.

I love my dal with something green and fresh – if I'm eating this for supper, I usually sauté the courgettes to gently cook them, but for lunch I sometimes enjoy them raw. Feel free to add your choice of greens, remembering to cook them for evening meals.

Tarka refers to the technique of adding spices to hot oil, which helps to bring out their flavour (as well as their properties). Everyone has their favourite way of serving tarka – it can either become the base of the dal, or for a really fresh flavour you can pour the tarka over the freshly cooked dal, top with a lid and then leave to infuse for 5 minutes before serving.

Serves 3

Tarka Dal with grated courgette

200g (1 cup) chana dal, soaked in water overnight
750ml (3 cups) water
2 tbsp ghee
1 tsp cumin seeds
1 tsp black mustard seeds
10 curry leaves
1 large spring onion or 1 medium onion, sliced
1 green chilli, finely sliced
1 medium tomato, skinned and deseeded (see page 260), finely chopped
½ tsp ground turmeric
½ tsp sea salt
2 garlic cloves (use wild garlic leaves in summer), crushed
¼ tsp asafoetida
1 large courgette, grated
freshly ground black pepper
handful of fresh coriander leaves, chopped

1 Simmer the chana dal in the water for about 45 minutes until very soft. Adjust the consistency to your taste, adding more water if you like it more soupy and lighter to digest.

2 To make the tarka, melt the ghee in a pan and fry the cumin and mustard seeds on a medium heat until they start to pop. Add the curry leaves, spring onion and chilli and stir for a few minutes.

3 When the chana dal is cooked, stir in the tomato, turmeric, salt, garlic and asafoetida. Add the tarka to the dal and remove from the heat, placing a lid on top.

4 Meanwhile, in the same pan that was used for the tarka, sauté the grated courgette for a couple of minutes with a pinch of salt.

5 Garnish the dal with freshly ground black pepper and a scattering of coriander leaves, then serve with a handful of sautéed courgette.

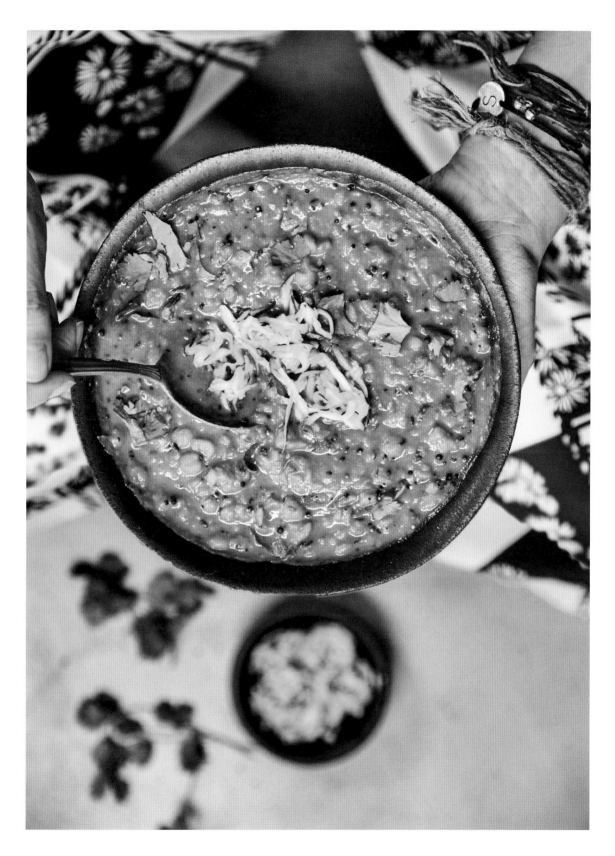

I made this soupy stew with my Mexican (and Swiss!) friend Jeanine, adding an Ayurvedic twist with asafoetida rather than epazote, the fresh herb used in Mexico to help make beans more digestible.

Black turtle beans are deliciously tasty – so much so that you don't even need stock for this. In Mexico the onions and garlic are often roasted whole, which adds a smokey, rich flavour. We're sautéing them with ghee instead – not traditional but given the thumbs up by Jeanine when she tried it.

This dish is super-basic but you can 'soup' it up as you wish. I love guacamole but the extra garlic and onion can add to the Rajasic nature (see page 14) of the dish, so this version uses avocado, coriander, lime and extra-virgin olive oil – mash it together if you like and make 'veda-mole'!

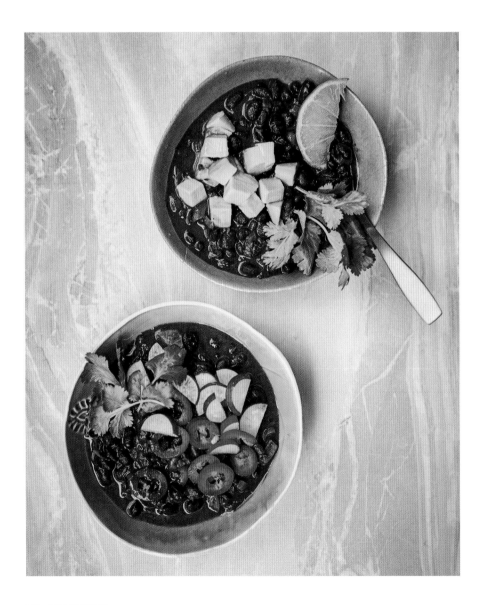

Black bean soup with avocado and lime

210g (1 cup) black turtle beans, soaked overnight, rinsed and drained
370ml (1½ cups) water
1 tbsp ghee
¼ tsp cumin seeds
1 small onion, finely chopped
1 garlic clove, finely chopped
½ tsp asafoetida
¾ tsp sea salt

FOR THE TOPPING
1 avocado, de-stoned and chopped (for Vata and Pitta)
½ red chilli, chopped (for Kapha)
4 radishes, roughly chopped (optional)
juice of ½ lime
1 small handful of coriander, roughly chopped
extra-virgin olive oil, to serve

1 Place the soaked beans in a pan and cover with the water – you want it to sit about 2cm (¾ in) above the beans, so add a little more or less as needed. Bring to the boil, then turn down to a simmer and partially cover pan. Gently simmer for about 1–1½ hours until the beans are really soft and tender. Top up with a little water as needed.

2 When the beans are almost cooked, melt the ghee in a large saucepan and fry the cumin seeds and the onion until the onion is soft. Add the garlic and the asafoetida and sauté until fragrant.

3 Stir the garlic mixture into the beans and allow the flavours to mingle for 5 minutes. Add water to reach your desired consistency.

4 Serve topped with avocado or chilli slices, radish (if using), lime juice, coriander and extra-virgin olive oil.

FEELING
VATA

FEELING
PITTA

FEELING
KAPHA

Enjoy the avocado, as this makes it nice and heavy.

The coriander and lime keeps it cool for you.

Thin this out with more water, and add more garlic and cumin for flavour. Avoid avocado and instead enjoy some chilli and radish.

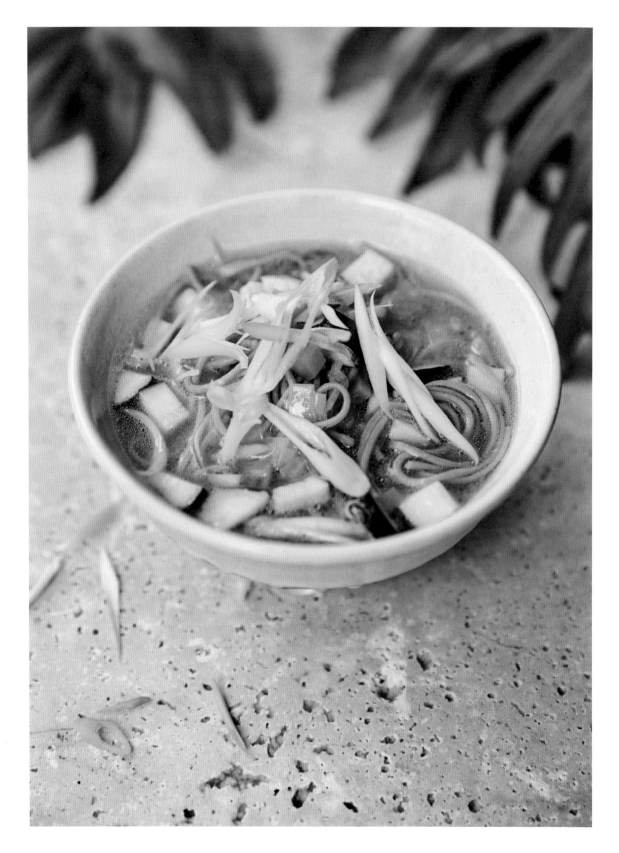

This is a clean-flavoured dish that's reminiscent of a lot of simple Japanese cuisine – this kind of dish balances out the more unctuous dishes that I love. It's like an Asian version of my Spring Clean Vegetable Brown Rice Soup (see page 196), made using buckwheat soba noodles and miso and ginger for flavour.

In the summer, add some skinned and deseeded tomatoes to this and maybe some fresh oregano for an Italian–Japanese fusion. You could even add some cooked cannellini beans for a Japanese minestrone! In the winter, swap in some diced root vegetables. Add your choice of miso to taste, stirring it at the end so as not to cook away the probiotics if you bought the unpasteurised stuff. Throw in an egg or some poached chicken, or use bone broth as the base for a more hearty meal. Try making a dashi stock for this too (see page 222).

This makes a good soup for cleanse and reset (see page 290) and works well in your insulated flask for work if you slightly undercook the noodles before bottling it up.

Serves 3–4

Vegetable soba noodle soup with miso bone broth

3 tbsp ghee
½ medium leek, finely chopped
1 clove garlic, finely chopped
5cm (2in) piece of fresh ginger, grated
1 medium carrot, diced
1 stick of celery, diced
100g of soba (buckwheat) noodles, snapped in half
1 litre (4 cups) bone broth (see page 261), water or dashi stock (see page 222)
1 medium courgette, diced
1 bunch spring onions, sliced, plus extra for serving

1 tbsp brown rice miso, plus extra depending on miso strength
1 tsp freshly ground black pepper

TO SERVE (OPTIONAL)
1 tsp unrefined toasted sesame oil
juice of ½ lemon or lime
1 tbsp Braggs Liquid Aminos or tamari, depending on miso strength
handful of watercress

1 Melt the ghee in a pan over a low-medium heat, then sweat the leek, garlic and ginger. Add the carrot and celery and sweat for another minute or so.

2 Add the noodles and bone broth and simmer for 10–12 minutes. Add the courgette and spring onions, then remove from the heat and stir in the miso and black pepper. Taste and season, then serve with the extras, if desired.

This is what I eat when I've just got home from travelling – whether that's been up and down the UK on trains, over the UK on flights, or just in a studio shooting all day. Basically wherever there has been some green lacking and I'm in need of something easy to digest that's quick so I can get to bed and catch up on some zzzs.

Serves 3–4

I've based this on spinach and green peas, because they are the easiest to get hold of. Both can be pulled out of your freezer if necessary – not the best, but certainly better than many of the alternatives. This is easy to make and so flavoursome that you don't need any dairy or broth to make it sing. If you have some bone broth, by all means add it to boost the nutrients, but there's definitely no need for bouillon.

I love how quick this soup is to make. From simmering the spinach and peas to puréeing – it's 15 minutes tops, from start to finish. Enjoy with Ragi Rotis (see page 62), if you want something more filling, or throw in some cooked basmati rice if you want to take this up a level for guests. Keep it interesting for yourself with the choice of toppings below – a simple swirl of olive oil and some toasted pumpkin seeds with a grating of Parmesan, a spicy tarka to get some spices in there or add some smoked paprika and cinnamon or Aleppo chilli and a bit of yoghurt for a Moroccan take.

Quick green simmer soup

1 tbsp ghee, plus extra for serving (optional)
1 clove garlic, finely chopped
400g (generous 2½ cups) frozen peas
500ml (2 cups) water or homemade bone broth (see page 261)
200g (4 cups) spinach leaves
½ tsp sea salt

TO SERVE (OPTIONAL)
2 tsp lime juice, plus ghee and Parmesan
1½ tbsp ghee, plus 1 tsp each cumin and coriander seeds and pinch of asafoetida
spoonful of homemade yoghurt (see page 259), plus 1 tsp smoked paprika, ½ tsp ground cinnamon or Aleppo chilli

1   Heat the ghee in a medium saucepan over medium-high heat and sauté garlic for 1 minute. Add the peas and water and bring to the boil. Reduce the heat and simmer for about 2–3 minutes, stirring occasionally, until the peas are tender and bright green. Stir in the spinach, cover and cook for 2–3 minutes, stirring occasionally, until the spinach has wilted.

2   Blend in batches until smooth, adding a little water to reach your desired consistency. Season with salt.

3   I like to top this soup in different ways. One option is to squeeze in a little lime juice, swirl with ghee and grate over some Parmesan. Otherwise, to make a tarka, heat the ghee in a saucepan on a medium-high heat and fry the cumin seeds, coriander seeds and asafoetida for 1 minute until fragrant. Pour the tarka over the soup. Another option is to add a dollop of yoghurt (best at lunchtime), sprinkle with smoked paprika and top with cinnamon or Aleppo chilli to serve.

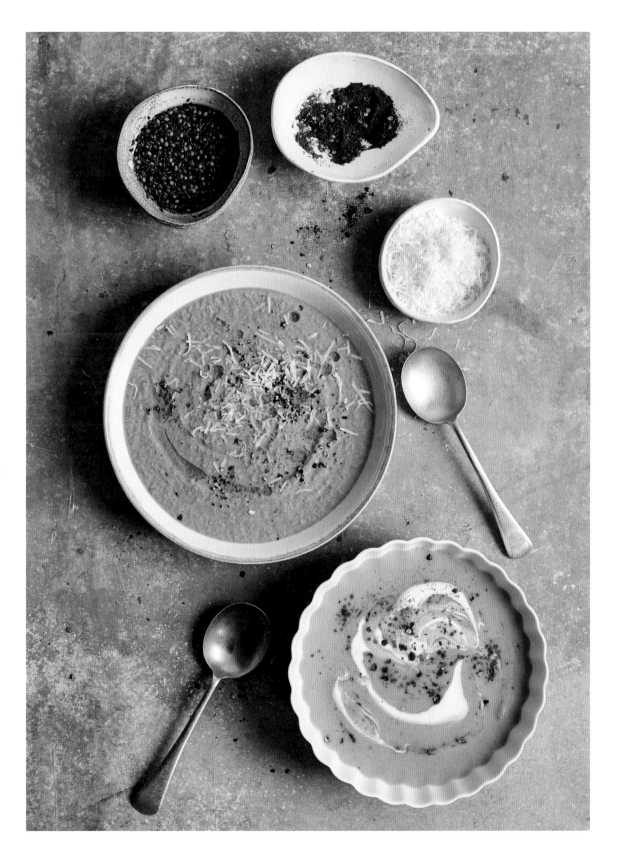

This simple carrot soup is ideal when you want something rich, soothing, light and sweet. Carrot and ginger would be the obvious choice here – and, as you can tell, I love ginger! Or carrot and coriander, which is very good for Pitta. But I love this soup – with a delicious sour note from the lime, it's lip-smackingly good. It makes the perfect starter for four or light meal for two.

For a treat I like to serve this with orange zest on top or Aleppo pepper and some toasted crushed pistachios. Want something more filling? Throw in 135g (1 cup) cooked basmati rice or toast some Ragi Rotis (see page 62). PICTURED ON PAGE 173.

Serves 2

Moroccan carrot soup

2 tbsp butter
1 medium onion, chopped
500g carrots, cut into
    1cm (½ in) chunks
720ml (2½ cups)
    homemade chicken
    broth or bouillon stock
2 tsp cumin seeds
1–2 tbsp fresh lime or
    lemon juice
¼ teaspoon ground
    allspice
sea salt and freshly
    ground black pepper

TO SERVE
125g (½ cup) homemade
    yoghurt (see page 259),
    stirred to loosen
small handful of mint
    leaves, chopped
orange zest (optional)
1 tbsp pistachios
    (optional)
1 tsp Aleppo pepper
    (optional)

1   Melt the butter in large saucepan over medium-high heat. Add the onion and sauté for 2 minutes, then mix in the carrots. Add the broth and bring to the boil. Reduce the heat, cover and simmer until the carrots are very tender, about 20 minutes.

2   Toast the cumin seeds in a dry frying pan over medium-high heat until fragrant, about 4–5 minutes, then allow to cool. Finely grind in a spice mill or a pestle and mortar.

3   Remove the soup from the heat. Carefully use a handheld blender in the pan or purée in batches in a blender until smooth. Return to the pan and whisk in the lime juice and allspice. Season with salt and pepper to taste.

4   Ladle the soup into bowls, and drizzle the yoghurt over the top, then sprinkle generously with the ground toasted cumin plus the mint, orange zest, pistachios and Aleppo pepper (if using).

FEELING
VATA

Add some jaggery
and ghee.

FEELING
PITTA

Add some jaggery
and fresh coriander.
You could use 250ml
(1 cup) coconut milk and
370ml (1½ cups) water
instead of the broth.

FEELING
KAPHA

Add some chilli,
ginger and black pepper
and leave out the yoghurt.

All over the world, chicken soup is known for its healing properties. The anti-inflammatory properties of a good bone broth are excellent for the gut and packed with immune-supporting minerals. Both restorative and therapeutic, this one-pot meal with aromatic vegetables and herbs is slow-cooked so that it can deliver the nutrients in a super easy-to-absorb form. And then, of course, there's that comforting taste of nostalgia …

Serves 6

This is a great recipe for an easy Sunday lunch – all you need is a really big pan or pot to fit the whole chicken, veggies and extras. The recipe is inspired by the 'Jewish penicillin' way of making this classic feel-better soup, complete with dill, dumplings and noodles. Rather than matzo crackers, I'm using gram flour to make my 'matzo balls' – lovely egg and gram flour dumplings that bob about in the soup.

If you have any digestive problems, it is best to eat the chicken and the dumplings at separate meals. Unless I'm entertaining and want to serve the complete works, I usually make the chicken soup and enjoy the chicken and vegetables, then pop the carcass into my slowcooker for 24 hours, adding a fresh batch of vegetables and aromatics halfway through to make a second batch of chicken soup cooked with dumplings – it makes for a week of delicious food.

If you love these dumplings, enjoy them with Wahay Soup (see page 202).

PICTURED ON PAGE 177.

Chicken soup for the soul with gram dumplings

FOR THE SOUP

1 x 1.8kg chicken

2 medium onions, peeled and roughly chopped

3 carrots, roughly chopped

3 sticks of celery, roughly chopped

3 cloves garlic, peeled, but left whole

4 bay leaves

few sprigs of thyme

2 handfuls of Jewish fine egg noodles or spaghetti, broken into bits (I also like quinoa, corn and rice spaghetti), optional

small bunch each of flat-leaf parsley and dill, roughly chopped

sea salt and freshly ground black pepper, to taste

FOR THE GRAM DUMPLINGS

90g (¾ cup) gram flour

1 tsp baking powder

½ tsp sea salt

freshly ground black or white pepper

2 medium eggs

1½ tbsp extra-virgin olive oil, ghee or chicken fat

2 tbsp chopped dill

1 Rinse the chicken and place in a very large saucepan. Cover with water until it reaches at least 8cm (3in) above the surface of the chicken. Bring to the boil, then turn the heat down and simmer for 30 minutes. Skim off any froth that comes to the surface.

2 Add the rest of the soup ingredients (apart from the parsley, dill and noodles, if using) and bring everything back to the boil, then turn down the heat and leave to simmer for 1 hour. If you want to make your gram dumplings with chicken fat, then reserve 1½ tablespoons of the fat by skimming the surface regularly into a bowl – the fat will start to solidify at the top as it cools.

RECIPE CONTINUES…

3 Meanwhile, to make your gram dumplings, whisk together the gram flour and baking powder in a bowl. Beat the eggs in a large bowl with the olive oil or ghee (or your reserved cooked chicken fat), dill and the salt and pepper. Slowly stir in your gram flour until well blended to make a thick, sticky batter. Leave in the fridge for 30 minutes, covered with cling film, then wet your hands with cold water and roll the dough into about twelve small balls (roughly 1 teaspoonful each) – or make them slightly bigger, if you like. Don't roll them too large, though, because they double in size when cooked!

4 Carefully remove the chicken to a large dish and leave to cool slightly. Using two forks, shred the chicken from the bones and set aside, reserving the skin and bones to make another stock (see page 261).

5 Bring the soup back to the boil and gently drop in the dumplings. When they rise to the surface, turn the heat down to a simmer and cover the pan. Cook for 20–25 minutes, until the dumplings are cooked through and the centres are light. Cut one open to check – if the centre is hard and dark, cook for another 3–5 minutes, until cooked through.

6 About halfway through the dumpling cooking time, add in the noodles, if using, to the pan and cook gently for the final 10 minutes.

7 Add all your shredded chicken meat to the soup, along with the parsley, and warm through for 3 minutes. Season with salt and pepper, sprinkle with the dill and serve.

TIP
·

If you find it hard to shape your dumplings, then chilling the batter for about 3 hours will help. Don't worry if you can't get the hang of shaping them, though, as you can simply use teaspoonfuls of the mixture – they might not be the perfect shape but will be lovely and rustic.

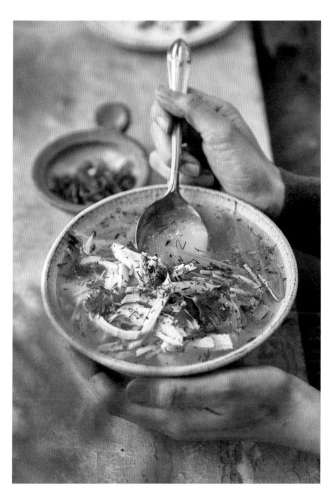

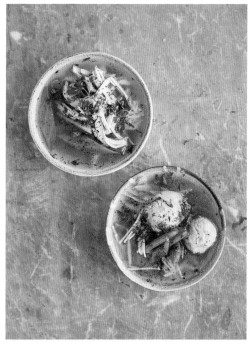

Winter Dosha soups

A soup can do what medicines can't! Warm and soothing soup in the chill of winter can help you relax in an inexplicable way. Especially when you've come down with a cold, cough or fever. It's by far the most comforting food, not to mention healthy and delicious too, and on a bitterly cold winter day nothing warms you up as much as a hearty bowl of soup.

Ayurveda recommends healthy soups for the lighter evening meal, as well as for children and convalescents. Fresh seasonal vegetables, grains, pasta, beans, lentils, herbs and spices can all make flavoursome additions to the soup pot.

When everything is cooked together first in a pot, it means the ingredients are already very familiar with each other by the time they reach your tummy, which is what makes soups and stews so effective for your digestion – especially if you cook them slowly over a long time.

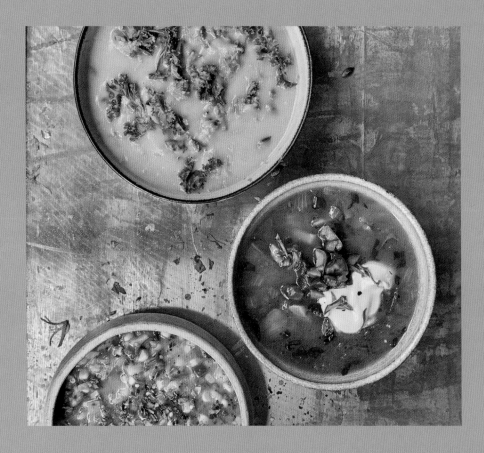

Chestnuts are warm, sweet and nourishing – which suits Vata to a 'T'! When in season in autumn and winter, they are perfect to help build up Vata body types. Chestnuts nourish the kidneys and build Agni (see page 278). They are one of the few astringent (and therefore more drying) foods that Vata types can enjoy, in moderation.

Serves 4

I love this delicious soup, which looks just like a mushroom soup and fools everyone I've ever given it to! I really like the ingredients chopped up and floating in the sweet broth so you get a different taste in every mouthful and can really appreciate the sage, but feel free to blend it until smooth. For a bigger hit of green, add some chard, cabbage or kale, on occasion, or load it up with green beans – if you try this, serve with crème fraîche, almond milk or cashew cream to make it creamy.

VATA

Winter chestnut, cream and sage soup

1–2 tbsp ghee (use 2 tbsp if using bouillon stock)
1 medium onion, chopped
6 fresh sage leaves, roughly chopped, plus extra to garnish, or 1½ tsp dried sage
1 litre (4 cups) chicken or bouillon stock, or water

400g cooked, peeled chestnuts
handful of chard, cabbage or kale, chopped (optional)
sea salt and freshly ground black pepper
100ml crème fraîche, almond milk or cashew cream (optional)

1 Melt the ghee in a saucepan over a medium-low heat and sweat the onion for about 10 minutes, until soft and translucent. Add the sage and and sauté for 1 minute, then add the stock.

2 For a chunky soup, finely chop the chestnuts or add them whole – reserving a small handful to decorate.

3 Season with salt and pepper to taste, then increase the heat and simmer for 15 minutes, stirring from time to time, and adding the greens for the last 5–10 minutes of cooking, if using. Simmer until tender.

4 For a smooth soup, remove from the heat and cool slightly, then blend until very smooth. Return the soup to the pan, add the crème fraîche, almond milk, if using, and adjust the seasoning if necessary. Warm through gently. Sprinkle with the reserved chestnuts – and chopped fresh sage, if you have it – then serve.

This soup is light and refreshing enough for warmer weather too. Add a splash of coconut milk, if you like, and it's positively tropical. Try it it first without the coconut milk, though, because it's so good anyway – instead, save the milk for when you need extra cooling foods or fancy something more creamy and filling.

Serves 4

Bright orange butternut squash becomes even brighter with a touch of zingy orange zest. Oranges aren't very good for Pitta, but here the zest adds flavour without the need for juice or pungent spices, which are also aggravating. Cooked kale is the best green for this dish as, unlike spinach, it's cooling for Pitta. All that fibre and bitter taste helps to stimulate peristalsis, which is great to keep things moving, making it an excellent cleansing spring tonic too.

I don't like preparing butternut squash much – it's time-consuming and cumbersome. To help I always make this soup when I'm baking, which means that I can pop the squash in the oven to help soften it, then go from step 2.

Vata types can enjoy this by skipping the kale (or enjoy a little, very well cooked) and adding the coconut milk. Kapha types vice versa – you don't need your kale cooked quite so well, and leave out the coconut milk. PICTURED ON PAGE 178.

PITTA

Butternut squash, kale and orange zest soup

1 small butternut squash (about 800g)
1 tbsp coconut oil
1 medium onion, diced
1 litre (4 cups) bouillon stock or bone broth (see page 261)
200g (1½ cups) kale, chopped
1 tbsp full-fat coconut milk (optional)
zest of ½ orange

½ tsp sea salt, plus more to taste if using bone broth rather than bouillon stock
⅛ tsp pepper

TO SERVE (OPTIONAL)
1 tbsp parsley leaves, chopped
1 tbsp toasted pumpkin seeds

1   Peel the squash, then slice in half vertically and remove the seeds and stringy bits. Slice it into 2.5cm (1in) cubes. Melt the oil in a large saucepan over a medium heat. Sauté the onion for 3–4 minutes, until translucent. Add the squash and cook, stirring for 5–8 minutes, until it starts to stick to the bottom.

2   Add the stock and bring to the boil. Use a wooden spoon to scrape any bits stuck to the bottom of the pan. Turn the heat down to a simmer, partially cover, and cook for 35–40 minutes, until the squash is soft.

3   For a chunky soup, add the kale for the last 7 minutes, or blend the soup and serve sautéed kale on top. Stir in the coconut milk, if using, zest and seasonings. Serve topped with the parsley and pumpkin seeds, if using.

Anyone feeling Kapha may often get short-changed on the more creamy (as well as stodgy) recipes. Potatoes are usually heavy to digest, but in this recipe Kapha types can enjoy them because they are blitzed up with corn to make a creamy chowder-style soup, which is fragrant with herbs and spiced with cumin, smoked paprika and chilli.

Vata types can also enjoy this occasionally by using less potato, blending well and adding some Vata Churna Spice Mix (see page 247) and a little lime juice. For Pitta, remove the chilli and add a dash of coconut milk and some of your spice mix too, if you like. PICTURED ON PAGE 178.

KAPHA

Corn, potato and chilli soup

1 tbsp sunflower oil

½ leek, finely chopped

2 cloves garlic, crushed

1 large green or red pepper, finely chopped

2 medium potatoes, scrubbed and diced (leave the peel on if organic)

750ml (3 cups) bone broth (see page 261) or bouillon stock

150g (1 cup) fresh corn kernels, or frozen corn kernels, allowed to thaw

1 jalapeño, or poblano chilli, deseeded and finely chopped

2 tsp ground cumin

1 tsp dried oregano

sea salt and freshly ground pepper

½ tsp smoked paprika

handful of parsley or coriander leaves, finely chopped

chilli flakes, to garnish

1 Heat the oil in a saucepan. Add the leek and sauté over a medium heat until translucent. Add the garlic and green pepper and sauté until the mixture begins to turn golden.

2 Add the potatoes and broth. Bring to a boil, then lower the heat and simmer gently, covered, until the potatoes are tender, about 15–20 minutes. Mash about half the potatoes roughly in the pot, or just enough to thicken the soup slightly.

3 For a chowder-style soup, remove half the soup mixture and blend until smooth with half the corn and then return everything to the pan along with the rest of the ingredients. Or give it all a blast in the pan with a handheld blender.

4 Otherwise, keep it chunky and add the corn in one go with the chilli, cumin and oregano. Add additional water as needed to give the soup a thick but not overly dense consistency. Stir together, return to a simmer, then simmer gently for 10–15 minutes, or until the corn is done.

5 Season with salt and pepper and simmer over a very low heat, stirring frequently, for another 5 minutes. Taste to adjust seasonings and garnish with the parsley and chilli flakes to serve.

I love sweet and sour flavours and, thanks to the tang of tamarind, this South Indian dal and veggie stew is one of my favourites. Sambhar, also known as sambar is a staple in some parts of India and Sri Lanka, and is considered very Sattvic (see page 14) thanks to its soft, easy-to-digest lentils and its high veg content.

The 'real' sambhar depends on family tradition. However, for the most part, there are two types: either made with sambhar powder (which I've used here) or roasted coconut. There are also two serving styles: as a gravy for dipping your dosas or uttapams, or as a thick stew. Nearly any vegetable you like can go into a sambhar.

For the lentils, you can use chana dal, toor dal (as used in the Tamilnadu Vegetable and Lentil Stew, see page 200), whole mung beans or mung dal. I tend to use the latter, which are digestible for all Doshas and quicker to cook.

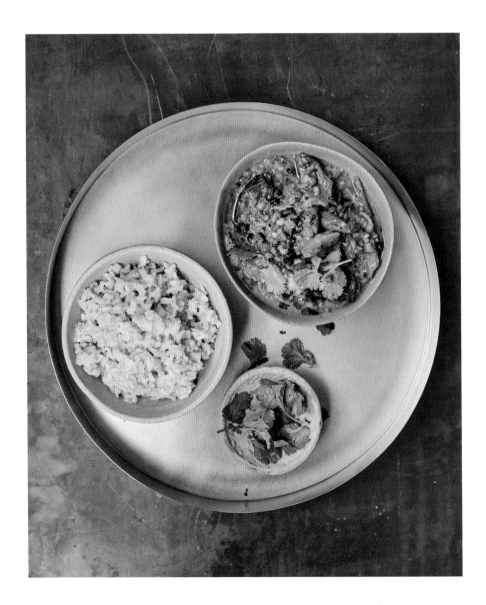

South Indian Moong Sambhar

1 tbsp ghee or coconut oil

200g (1 cup) okra, tops removed and halved if large (or swap for green beans)

1 medium carrot, cut lengthways into 2.5cm (1in) pieces

½ tsp ground turmeric

1 medium onion, sliced

1 green chilli, chopped

100g (½ cup) mung dal, or toor dal or chana dal (or mung beans, soaked overnight, rinsed and drained) – see Tip below

1 litre (4 cups) water

2 small Asian aubergines or 1 small European aubergine, cut into 2.5cm (1in) pieces

1 tbsp tamarind paste (see page 260) or juice from 50g tamarind block

1 tbsp Sambhar Powder (see page 266)

sea salt, to taste

FOR THE TARKA

1 tsp ghee or coconut oil

½ tbsp mustard seeds

¼ tsp asafoetida

8–10 fresh curry leaves

1 dried red chilli, broken into pieces (optional)

1 Melt the ghee in a large saucepan and fry the okra (no need with green beans) for 5 minutes, then set aside. Add the carrot, turmeric, onion, green chilli, mung dal and water to the saucepan. Stir, bring to the boil and simmer for at least 20 minutes until the lentils are soft.

2 Add the aubergines, okra, tamarind paste and sambhar powder and allow to simmer for 10 minutes or until all the vegetables are tender. Add hot water to reach your desired consistency and season to taste.

3 Make the tarka. In a small frying pan, melt the ghee and add the mustard seeds, asafoetida, curry leaves and dried red chilli, if using. Quickly pour the tarka into the sambhar, then stir well and serve.

TIP
·

The cooking times for the other dals and whole mung beans will vary and take longer. It is easier to cook the lentils separately in one pan until just tender, and cook the vegetables in a separate larger saucepan, adding in the cooked dals or mung beans halfway through the cooking so they finish cooking together. Then add your tarka.

FEELING
PITTA

Leave out the chillies and add plenty of fresh coriander leaves.

BREAKFAST DOSAS
page 80

DHOKLA
page 229

Kitchari (also spelled kitcharee, khichadi, kitchadee, kitchari and in many other variants) is one of the staple healing foods in Ayurveda. It is believed to balance the Doshas, support the tissues, detoxify the body and purify the digestive system. In India, it is used to nourish the elderly and sick, and it is often a baby's first food since it is easy to digest. It also used for mono-diet fasting at retreats and cleanses, where participants eat kitchari for every meal for a couple of days to give the digestive system a much-needed rest while still providing the essential nutrients.

This Ayurvedic 'chicken soup' is perfect for when you are feeling under the weather, exhausted after a long trip or in need of a cleanse or a comforting hug. It's a simple one-pot dish that makes it quick and easy to add a thousand-year-old healing food and all of its benefits to our modern diet. You can easily customise it with your Dosha's pacifying herbs, spices and vegetables. Lightly spiced, it makes a delicious breakfast porridge and a staple for the cleanse reset (see page 290).

Mung beans are one of Ayurveda's superfoods: Tridoshic (see page 271) and Sattvic (see page 14), easily digestible and great for removing toxic residues from the intestines. Similarly, basmati rice is also considered balancing and Tridoshic, making them a perfect match. When combined, mung dal and basmati rice provide a 'complete' meal with all the fibre, protein and nourishment the body needs in a very soothing and digestible form. You can make it with brown basmati rice and whole mung beans (just make sure you soak them overnight!), but if you are feeling unwell or have a weak digestion, I recommend following this recipe to keep it soothing and nourishing. This makes one very generous portion; to enjoy this the Ayurvedic way – without waste and without reheating – start with the measurements below and tweak to suit. For example, you can reduce the basmati and mung beans to 50g (¼ cup) each and add a touch less of the flavourings.

Serves 1–2

Kitchari

70g (⅓ cup) white basmati rice, soaked for 1 hour

70g (⅓ cup) mung dal (or mung beans, soaked overnight)

2 tbsp ghee

1 bay leaf

pinch of asafoetida

370ml (1½ cups) water

1 tsp cumin seeds

5cm (2in) piece of fresh ginger, finely chopped, or ¼ tsp ground ginger

1 tsp ground turmeric

¼ tsp black pepper

pinch of sea salt, to taste

fresh coriander, to serve (optional)

TIP
·

For weak digestion, skip the tarka and cook the ginger, cumin and turmeric in the first stage, then add more water to make it soupy and overcook for another 10 minutes.

1 Rinse the rice and mung dal three times.

2 In a heavy-bottomed pan, melt half the ghee and sauté the bay leaf and asafoetida. Add the mung dal, rice and water and simmer for 20–25 minutes, lid on, until tender. Add more water as necessary.

3 In a separate pan, make a tarka. Melt the remaining ghee, then add the cumin seeds and cook gently until they start to pop. Add the ginger and sauté until golden brown. Add the turmeric and sauté for a few more minutes.

4 Add the tarka to the rice and dal mixture. Cook for 5–7 minutes, stirring often. Season with salt and pepper and serve with fresh coriander, if desired.

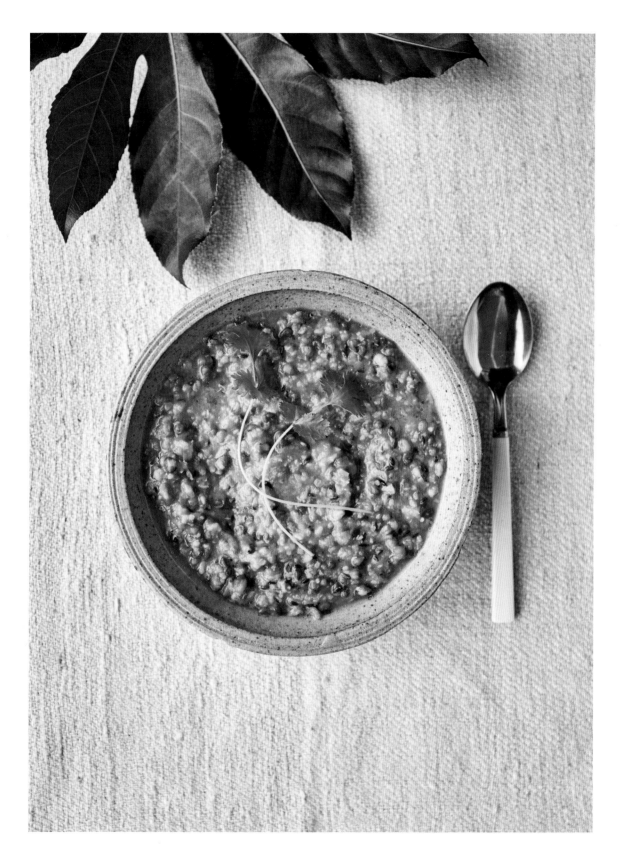

Back in 2010, I celebrated my 30th birthday by learning Vedic meditation on Bondi Beach with Gary Gorrow, who is now a good friend. Gary has been instrumental in dropping little seeds of knowledge all around me to grow. I wanted to include one of his recipes in this book (as with my other cookbooks). He shared this – one of his favourite dals, which originally came from a Rastafarian, hence the name. It captures the taste buds of all newbies to Ayurveda because it is absolutely delicious and tells a great story, which is that Ayurvedic food is not necessarily Indian, but rather food that adheres to the principles of Ayurveda. The only slightly questionable ingredients here are the mustard and the tinned coconut milk – you could swap the wholegrain mustard for ¾ tablespoon of mustard seeds if you like, and use fresh coconut milk if you can find it.

Serves 4

Gary Gorrow's
Rasta dal

1 tbsp ghee
1 onion, finely chopped
2 cloves garlic, minced, or a pinch of asafoetida
3cm (1¼ in) piece of fresh ginger, chopped
1 tbsp ground cumin
1 tbsp wholegrain mustard
½ tbsp ground turmeric
1 tsp ground cinnamon
pinch of chilli powder
1 carrot, chopped
250g (scant 1½ cups) red split lentils, rinsed
500ml (2 cups) water
1 x 400ml tin of full-fat coconut milk

4 fresh tomatoes, skinned and deseeded (see page 260), very finely chopped
juice of 1 lime or lemon
sea salt and freshly ground black pepper
fresh coriander leaves and toasted cashews, to serve (optional)

1   Melt the ghee and gently fry the onion until soft. Add the garlic, if using, and cook until soft. Add the ginger, cumin, mustard, turmeric, cinnamon and chilli and cook for 30 seconds. Add the asafoetida (if not using garlic), then the carrot, and stir through.

2   Add the lentils, water and coconut milk. Bring to the boil, then simmer for 20–30 minutes, lid on, but stirring from time to time, until the lentils are cooked.

3   Add the tomatoes and cook for few more minutes until they are soft. Add the lime juice, salt and pepper to taste. Serve with coriander and toasted cashews on top, if you like.

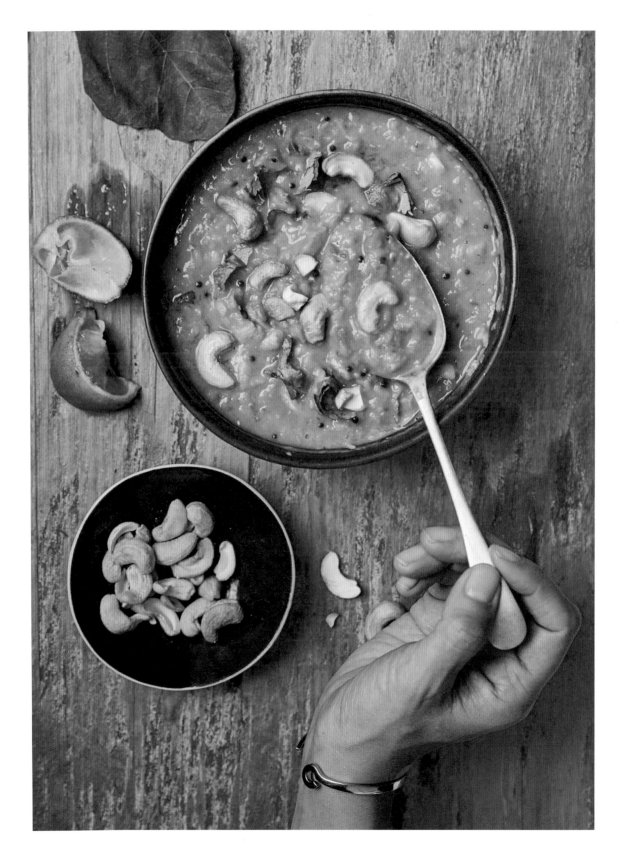

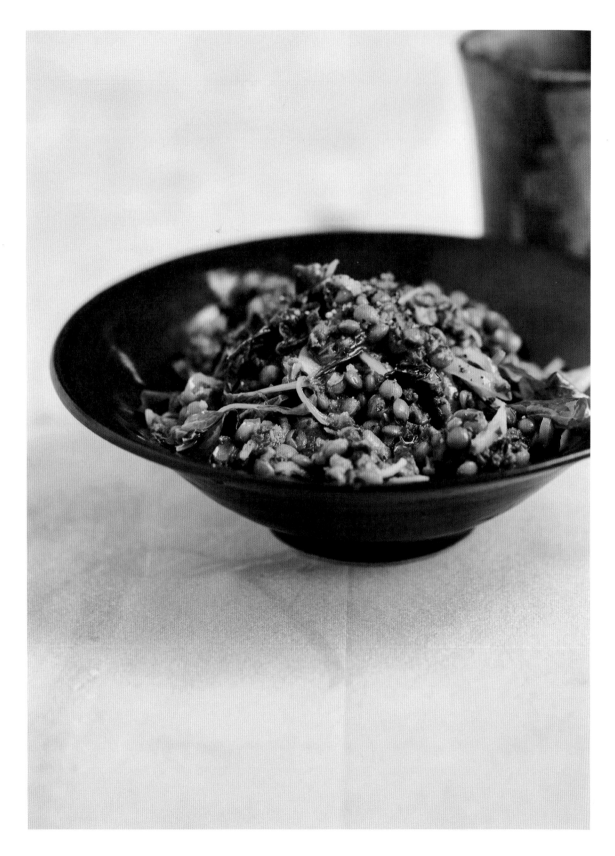

'Hippy comfort food' is how my sleep-when-you-die friend described this dish when he came round for dinner – but after sampling it, he wanted the recipe! I'd whipped this up for him when he said 'I didn't grow up cooking and so I've never bothered.' To show him how easy it is to make something from the pantry, I'd soaked a cup of brown lentils in the morning, then, that evening, added it with the other ingredients to the pot and simmered for 20 minutes. With fresh greens thrown in and cooked until tender, this is comfort cooking at its easiest. 'So where do I get the greens from then?' he asked. Your freezer, of course!

Serves 2–3

Brown lentil, spinach and coconut hotpot

200g (1 cup) brown lentils, soaked for 8 hours or overnight, rinsed and drained
1 x 400ml tin of full-fat coconut milk
1 small onion, sliced
1 large garlic clove, finely chopped
250ml (1 cup) water
¾ tsp ground cumin
½ tsp ground coriander
4cm (1½ in) piece of fresh ginger, sliced
sea salt and freshly ground black pepper, to taste
6 nuggets of frozen spinach or 200g (4 cups) fresh spinach or other leafy greens
dash of tamarind paste (see page 260), or lime or lemon juice

1   Throw the lentils, coconut milk, onion, garlic, water cumin, coriander and ginger into a medium saucepan and allow to simmer, lid on, for 20 minutes. Season to taste with salt and pepper.

2   Add the spinach, bring to a simmer and cook for another 5–10 minutes, until tender. Add the tamarind paste and serve.

TIP
·

To turn this into an intense-flavoured curry to serve alongside rice, quinoa or bread, double all of the ingredients apart from the lentils and leave out the water.

This is a deliciously light and brothy minestrone with a hint of tomato. The sweetness of swede, caraway, carrot and oregano really make this dish. Because this soup is broth-based, the flavour is best with stock, but if you're looking for something extra subtle to combat excesses then use water and add more herbs to keep it really fresh. I love it when the quinoa is nice and soft and floating in the broth – quinoa is packed with protein, as are the red split lentils, which dissolve quickly to enrich the dish and give it that tomato-y feel. When tomatoes aren't in season, I sometimes revert to tomato purée.

This recipe is perfect for the lunchbox insulated flask because all the ingredients keep well, despite the heat retention – not such a great plan with soups or stews that include leafy greens, which tend to go mushy and brown with overcooking. The quinoa will continue to swell and soak up that lovely brothy liquid, so it won't necessarily look the same as when it went in!

Serves 2–3

Quinoa minestrone

½ tbsp ghee

½ medium leek, finely sliced

1 stick of celery, finely chopped

¼ tsp caraway seeds

¼ tsp dried oregano

1 large carrot, finely diced

1 large courgette, roughly diced

75g swede, celeriac or parsnip, finely diced

50g (⅓ cup) quinoa, soaked overnight, rinsed and drained

25g red split lentils

6 fresh tomatoes, skinned and deseeded (see page 260), or 2 tbsp tomato purée

600ml (scant 2½ cups) chicken stock or bouillon stock

large pinch of sea salt

freshly ground black pepper

½ tbsp tamari (or extra sea salt)

½ tsp smoked paprika

1   In a medium pan, melt the ghee. Sweat the leek and celery with the caraway seeds and oregano until soft.

2   Add the carrot, courgette and other root veg and sweat for a little longer, then add the rest of the ingredients. Simmer for about 20 minutes, until the carrot loses its crunch and the quinoa is cooked, adding a little more water to reach your desired consistency. Season to taste.

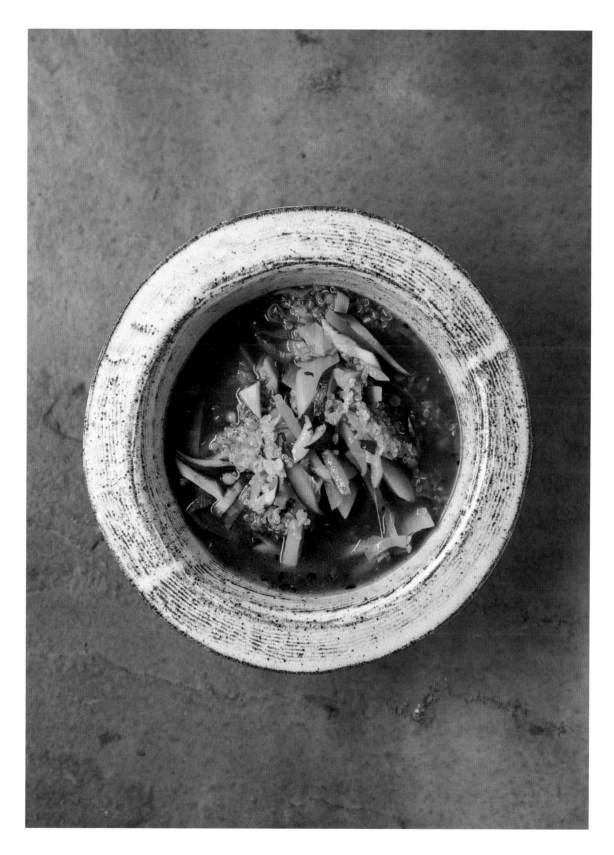

I knew I'd love this soup from the moment I first saw it. Not too thick but not too thin, it's a flavourful big bowl of warmth. Invented by the Berbers (nomadic north Africans), harira has been adopted as a traditional breakfast meal during Ramadan. Traditionally it is made with chickpeas and mung beans but I've used all mung beans (noticed a theme yet?) because they are better for all Doshas and easier to cook from scratch. It's not common to mix proteins in Ayurveda, but a small amount of lamb gives the mung beans a rich flavour – you could always use lamb broth for the base instead.

This soup is great for the slowcooker and cheaper cuts of meat – I use middle neck or scrag end of lamb, although the scrag end is not for anyone who doesn't like fiddling with bones! For a treat, enrich the soup with egg yolks and serve it with a squeeze of lemon juice or lemon wedge, but it's also delicious without.

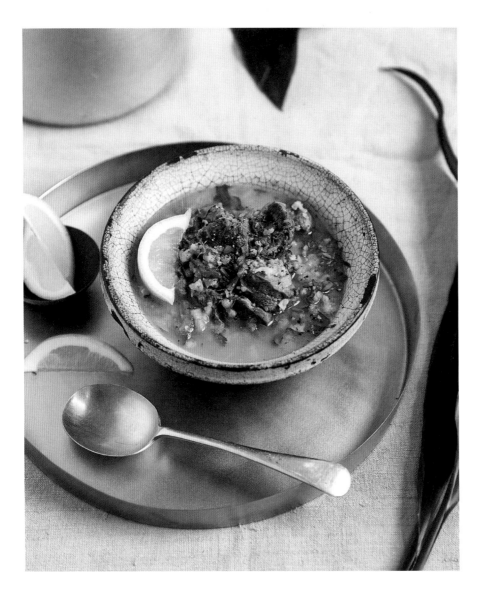

○◑●

Serves 6

Harira – lightly spiced lamb and mung bean soup

200g (1 cup) whole
    mung beans, soaked
    overnight, or split
    mung dal
1 tbsp ghee
200g lamb neck
    (middle not best end),
    roughly chopped into
    small cubes
1 medium onion, chopped
1 stick of celery, chopped
3 tbsp gram flour
450g tomatoes, skinned
    and deseeded (see
    page 260), chopped
2 tbsp parsley leaves,
    chopped
1 tbsp coriander leaves,
    chopped

5cm (2in) piece of fresh
    ginger, finely chopped,
    or 1 tsp ground ginger
½ tsp ground turmeric
1 tsp ground cinnamon
sea salt and freshly
    ground black pepper,
    to taste
1.75 litres (7 cups) water

TO SERVE (OPTIONAL)
2 egg yolks
juice of 1 lemon,
    plus extra wedges
    for serving
handful of coriander
    leaves, chopped

1   Drain the mung beans, then rinse them under cold water and set aside.

2   Melt the ghee in a large saucepan and fry the lamb, onion and celery for 2–3 minutes, stirring until the lamb is just browned. Add the gram flour, tomatoes and all the herbs and spices. Season well with salt and pepper and cook for about 1 minute, then add the mung beans and the water.

3   Slowly bring to the boil and then leave on a rolling boil for 10 minutes. Reduce the heat and simmer very gently for up to 1 hour until the mung beans are very tender. Season with salt and a little bit more pepper. Taste and add more water to reach your desired consistency.

4   To add the egg yolks, beat them with the lemon juice and stir into the simmering soup. Immediately remove from the heat and stir until thickened.

5   Pour the soup into warmed serving bowls and serve garnished with coriander and wedges of lemon.

FEELING
VATA

Make sure to add the
the egg yolks for
extra nourishment.

FEELING
PITTA

You could use dried
chickpeas instead of mung
beans as a variation.

FEELING
KAPHA

Try dried chickpeas
instead of mung beans,
add lots of greens, skip the
yolks and thin out the
stew to keep it light.

This classic dish is usually made of chicken, egg and sweetcorn in a rich broth; however, Ayurveda recommends only one type of protein per dish to ease digestion. You don't hear much about mushrooms in Ayurveda (unlike traditional Chinese medicine where the reishi, shiitake and cordycep are big hitters), but their healing properties are recognised as being powerful. A little like garlic, mushrooms are considered good in small quantities, otherwise they become Tamasic (see page 14), but much less so than meat and fish.

In this simple soup, dried shiitake mushrooms are simmered for half an hour to make a flavoursome broth while providing a meaty bite. If you don't have shiitakes, then use homemade chicken bone broth for a rich flavour or the dashi stock from the Proper Miso Soup (see page 222) and throw in some rice noodles or cook in some basmati rice instead to bulk out the soup. Ayurveda advises against reheating mushrooms, or eating them cold, so this soup is best when freshly made and piping hot. You could make this with shredded chicken, if you like – just leave out the egg.

Serves 2

Chinese-style shiitake and sweetcorn soup

2 medium corn
  on the cobs
750ml (3 cups) bone broth
  (see page 261), bouillon
  stock or water
10g dried shiitake
  mushrooms,
  or 40g fresh, sliced
5mm (¼ in) piece of
  fresh ginger, grated
  (optional)
1 tsp sea salt, plus more
  to taste
large pinch of ground
  white pepper

1 tbsp apple cider vinegar
  or lemon juice
½ tbsp unrefined sesame
  oil, to taste
¾ tbsp arrowroot or
  ½ tbsp cornflour
  (optional)
1 medium egg, beaten
1 spring onions,
  finely sliced
tamari or soy
  sauce (optional)
½ tsp jaggery (optional)

FEELING
KAPHA

Favour dried shiitake
rather than fresh for
this soup.

1 Grate the corn from the cobs and add to a large saucepan with the broth, shiitake mushrooms, ginger, if using, and salt. Bring to the boil, lid off, and then leave to simmer gently for at least 30 minutes.

2 Add the white pepper, apple cider vinegar and sesame oil. Bring back to the boil.

3 Mix the arrowroot, if using, with just enough cold water to form a paste. Add this in a thin stream to the soup, stirring constantly, and cook for 3–5 minutes until the soup has thickened slightly.

4 Very gently stir in the beaten egg in a thin stream until just cooked, then sprinkle with the spring onions and remove from the heat.

5 Season to taste. If you like, add a little tamari (this will make the soup darker) and jaggery, if it needs sweetness.

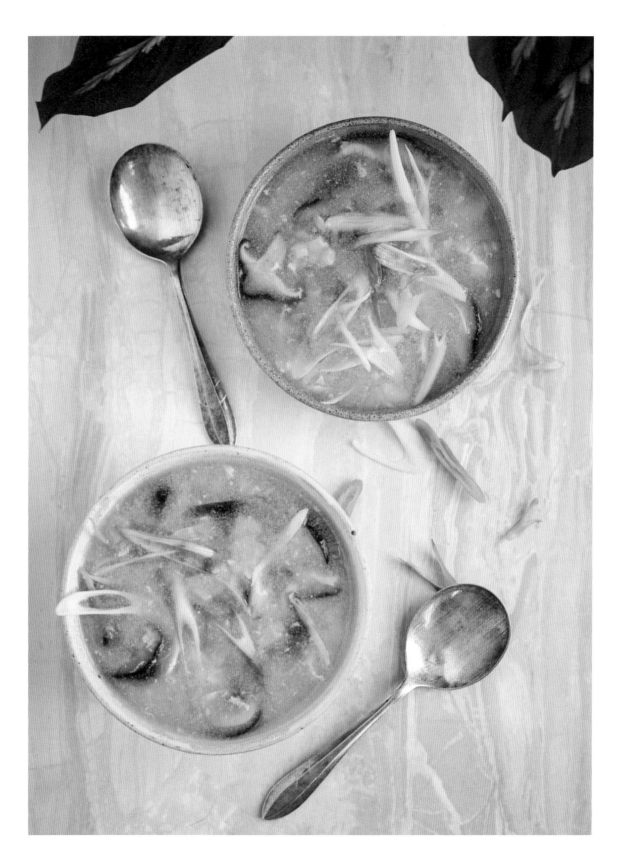

Seasonal change is big news in the world of Ayurveda. It makes sense that when your environment changes, so too does your body as you strive to come into alignment with the natural world. Springtime signifies new beginnings as the land wakes up from the cold and wet and moves through to warmer promises.

Serves 2–3

After the stodgy heavier foods favoured in winter you might be looking for lighter, fresher foods, choosing brothy rather than unctuous dishes. To support this change it's a good time to cut back on fats and oils, fried foods and dairy and make use of spring vegetables, which have plenty of the astringent, pungent and bitter tastes. I like to team spring veggies with long-cooked brown basmati rice that's been soaked overnight – tender enough to chew easily but still retaining bite and texture – either as a light stir-fry or an even lighter soup.

Start the day with Stewed Apple (see page 76), then enjoy this vegetable brown rice soup for lunch and dinner, topped with plenty of fresh herbs, and teamed every now and then with fish or eggs. If you need more oomph or are still feeling the cold, add a taste of the East with even more pungent ingredients such as onions, garlic, ginger, black pepper and small amounts of cayenne pepper.

Spring-clean vegetable brown rice soup

1 tbsp ghee

7.5g (¼ cup) fresh parsley, rough chopped

¼ tsp dried rosemary

½ tsp dried oregano

½ tsp dried thyme

1 stick of celery, diced

1 medium carrot, diced or grated

1 litre (4 cups) chicken stock, bouillon stock or water

45g (scant ¼ cup) brown basmati rice, soaked overnight, rinsed and drained

1 turnip or potato (170g), cut into pieces

1 bay leaf

200g (1⅓ cups) green beans

sea salt and pepper to taste

½ tsp chopped fresh basil (optional)

1 Melt the ghee in a large saucepan and sauté the parsley, rosemary, oregano, thyme, celery and carrot slowly for 10 minutes over a medium heat.

2 Add the stock, brown rice, turnip and bay leaf. Bring to the boil. Cover and lower the heat, then simmer for 1½–2 hours, adding the green beans 20 minutes from the end. Season to taste with salt and pepper and add more water if you prefer a lighter soup. Serve, garnished with a little basil, if desired.

FEELING VATA

Top with ghee and transition from winter to spring very gradually.

FEELING KAPHA

Cut back the grains and use whole barley (avoid pearl barley)

TIP

Mix it up with the following spring veg: asparagus, red or green peppers, beetroot and beetroot greens, broccoli, Brussels sprouts, cabbage, cauliflower, celery, chard, corn, dandelion greens, endive, kale, leeks, lettuce, mushrooms, peas and radishes.

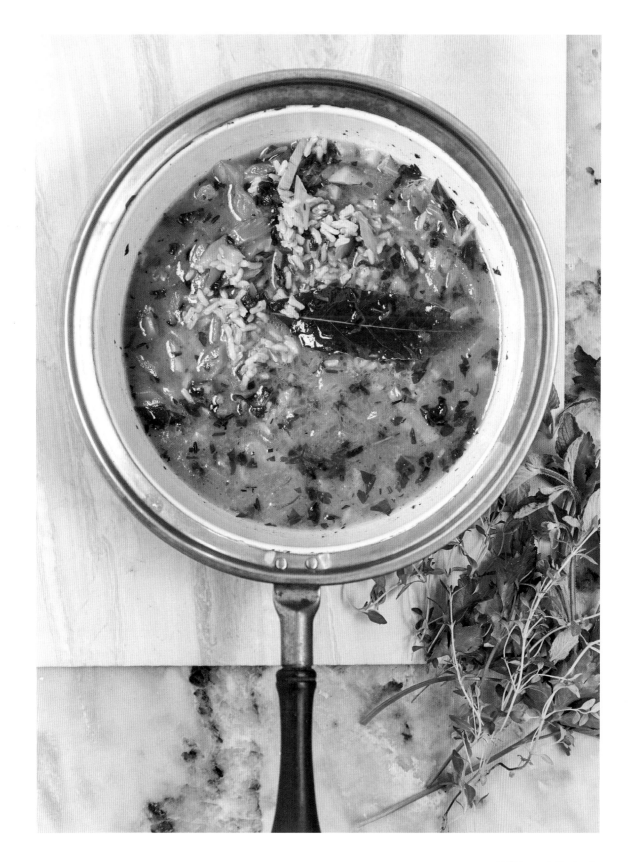

My friends at the Alliance of Natural Health (ANH) are scientists, nutritionists and dieticians who work tirelessly to promote and support natural and sustainable approaches to healthcare around the world. Little did I know, when I shyly told Rob Verkerk Ph.D., the organisation's founder, about my interest in Ayurveda, that he too is a long-standing fan. In fact, he's been directly involved in protecting this medicinal culture against the European Union's strict legislative system that's threatened not only Ayurveda, but all traditional systems of medicine.

This is Rob's East by West Ayurveda-style recipe for improving mental clarity, full of antioxidant and nutrient-rich veggies and nuts. From a Western perspective, we know a lot about the synergistic power of the nutrients found in superfoods. That includes brightly coloured veggies, herbs and nuts. From an Ayurvedic perspective, many of these big-talking superfoods are pungent and astringent – which can aggravate Vata and 'annoy' the brain, rather than support it. To counter this effect, the recipe also includes creamed coconut or whole organic double cream, to give sweetness or unctuousness, and to aid the absorption of fat-soluble vitamins and bioactive compounds in the herbs. For the omnivores out there wanting to further increase mental clarity with some proteins and peptides, serve this dish with fish, such as baked trout or gently pan-fried sea bass.

The recipe includes two Ayurvedic herbal powders – Shankhpushpi and Brahmi powder. These are among the most potent herbs for cognition, memory and brain health. They are readily available from Ayurvedic herb suppliers, but could be omitted if you can't find them, or don't mind doing without some cognitive benefits!

Those with weaker digestion might want to cook the vegetables a little longer for less crunch, and choose fewer ingredients, mixing it up every time you make the dish – for example, leaving out the walnuts or almonds, broccoli or green beans and maybe just using one of the two brain herb powders at a time.

Serves 4

Veg Masala for the brain

1 tbsp ghee
½ tsp Shankhpushpi powder (optional)
½ tsp Brahmi powder (optional)
½ tsp ground turmeric
¼ tsp asafoetida
5mm (¼ in) piece of fresh ginger, grated
1 red chilli, finely chopped
sea salt, to taste
200g (4 cups) baby spinach leaves

4 fresh tomatoes, skinned and deseeded (see page 260), coarsely chopped
350g (6 cups) broccoli florets
300g (3 cups) green beans, chopped into 2.5cm (1in) lengths
115ml (½ cup) double cream, crème fraîche or creamed coconut

1 Gently melt the ghee in a frying pan over a low heat and stir in the Shankhpushpi and Brahmi powders, if using, with the other ground spices. Add the ginger and chilli along with a pinch of sea salt. Heat and stir for 2 minutes over a medium heat.

2 Slowly add the spinach over a medium-high heat and stir until wilted. Add the tomatoes, broccoli and beans, then place the lid on the pan and simmer for 3–4 minutes until the beans and broccoli are still bright in colour but sufficiently tender.

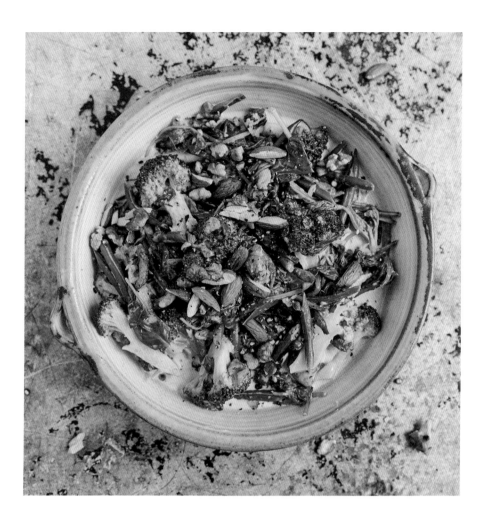

juice of ½ lemon

50g (⅓ cup) skin-on
almonds, toasted and
roughly chopped

50g (½ cup) walnuts,
toasted and roughly
chopped

2 tbsp coriander leaves,
chopped

cooked basmati rice,
to serve

3 Stir through the cream and heat for a couple of
minutes. Remove from the heat. Add additional salt
to taste, if needed.

4 Transfer to a serving dish, drizzle with lemon juice
and sprinkle with the almonds, walnuts and chopped
coriander. Serve with basmati rice.

FEELING
VATA

Favour green beans
instead of broccoli.

FEELING
PITTA

Choose creamed coconut
over double cream.

FEELING
KAPHA

Use a small amount of
coconut milk instead
of creamed. Go wild with
the ginger and chilli.

Ananda Spa in the Himalayas was one of the first luxury Ayurvedic spas. Years ago I was lucky enough to experience a yoga nidra (conscious sleep meditation) with one of their teachers in London and I've been in contact with their managers ever since. Recently, I met up with senior vice president Mahesh Natarajan on his last day of a whirlwind tour of Europe. As is the Filipino way (or maybe just my way!) I asked him what he missed from home. You could see his imagination stir and the excitement on his face at the thought that soon he'd be able to enjoy home cooking again. He immediately told me about this stew, also known as Mulagootal, which has been passed down the generations in his family. This is a traditional Tamilnadu lentil recipe prepared by the Brahmin community. It is a wholesome dish, typically served with a cooling yoghurt preparation to balance the spices, both to be eaten alongside hot steamed rice.

Mahesh's family traditionally uses snake gourd, which I love, but it is hard to find. Other alternatives are chayote squash or bottle gourd, but easier-to-source replacements include spring greens, chard and kale. Cucumber is cooling and sweet with bitter skin, which gives a nice flavour balance, but if the skin is too thick then peel it first. If you can't find toor dal (also known as split pigeon peas), then use overnight-soaked mung beans, or split mung dal – the taste of mung dal is a little different but it takes about 20–25 minutes to cook on the hob (without soaking).

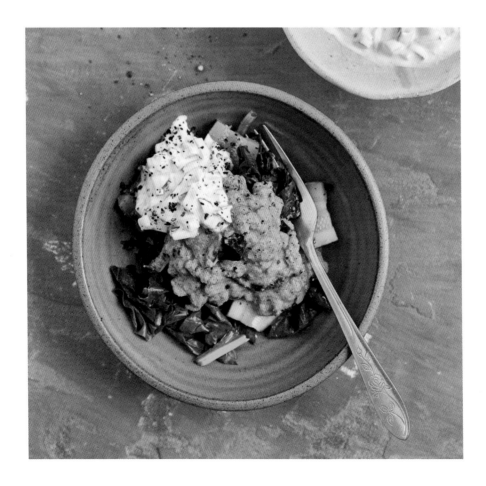

Tamilnadu vegetable and lentil stew with cucumber raita

100g (½ cup) toor dal, soaked overnight, rinsed and drained
370ml (1½ cups) hot water
½ tsp ground turmeric
2 bottle gourds, cut into 2.5cm (1in), or 200g (2 cups) spring greens, chard or kale
½ tsp sea salt
½ tsp Sambhar Powder (see page 266)
¼ tsp asafoetida
½ tsp jaggery

FOR THE TARKA
1 tsp ghee
¼ tsp black mustard seeds

½ tsp urad dal
12 fresh curry leaves

FOR THE SPICE PASTE
½ tsp cumin seeds
½ tsp black peppercorns
20g (¼ cup) desiccated coconut
1 tbsp water

FOR THE RAITA
¼ tsp ghee
¼ tsp black mustard seeds
½ green chilli, finely chopped
3–4 fresh curry leaves
pinch of sea salt
1 medium cucumber, finely chopped
125g (½ cup) homemade yoghurt (see page 259)

FEELING
KAPHA

Both the cucumber and the yoghurt in this recipe can provoke Kapha, so eat only occasionally, with extra asafoetida and mustard seeds.

TIP
·

If you don't have time to soak the dal overnight, you could soak it for 15 minutes in 370ml (1½ cups) hot water – Mahesh's mum likes to do this, to make sure the dish keeps some coarse texture.

1   To make the tarka, melt the ghee, then add the mustard seeds and allow them to pop. Add the urad dal and curry leaves. Toss, then remove from the heat and set aside.

2   To make the spice paste, add half of the prepared tarka to the spice paste ingredients with the water. Grind or pulse into a coarse wet mixture and set aside.

3   In a pan, soak the toor dal and ¼ teaspoon of the turmeric in the hot water for 15 minutes. Put the pan over a medium heat and cook until soft and slushy – this can take 35 minutes to an hour depending on how ong the toor dal was soaked.

4   Simmer the bottle gourd in a pan of water for 5 minutes with a pinch of salt until lightly cooked, then drain and set aside. If using greens, remove any tough stalks. Sauté the leaves with a splash of water until tender.

5   Add the toor dal, sambhar powder, ½ teaspoon of salt and the asafoetida and bring to the boil. Reduce the heat, add the spice paste and bring to the boil again, then mix in the jaggery. Remove from the heat, add the remaining tarka and stir.

6   For the cucumber raita, start by making another tarka. Heat the oil, then add the mustard seeds. Allow them to pop, then add the chilli and curry leaves. Stir together and set aside. Add a pinch of salt to the cucumber in a bowl and set aside for 10 minutes. Drain the excess water from the cucumber, then mix through the yoghurt and the tarka. Serve the stew with the cucumber raita.

This soup is pronounced 'Wa-Hay'! Because it started with wahay moment using whey. My mum and I were making ricotta with whole milk (see page 254). Usually the leftover whey – which is nutritious and body-building – goes into a jug, to be added to smoothies, dips, sauces and curries, bit by bit. This time we decided to try and make the real whey ricotta, which skilled cheesemakers make from the whey left behind when making other types of cheese. We simmered it and did all the right things but it only made one or two curds. We added more lemon juice to see if that did the trick but we were left with a tart lemony broth. While I researched and found out that you can't actually make ricotta from ricotta whey (only the whey from harder cheeses, which leave behind much more of the milk solids), my mum got busy turning our lemony whey into a delicious, light soup with some garlic, onion and ginger, along with some fresh thyme and some chopped bottle gourds.

To give it oomph we made some quick gram dumplings and sat down to probably one of my favourite lunches. You could also serve this with pasta or potatoes, if you prefer. This has reignited my love of marrows, which are delicious instead of the bottle gourds. If you're making whole-milk ricotta (see page 254) then you must make this.

Serves 4

Wahay soup

1.3–1.5 litres whey, left over from making one batch of whole-milk ricotta (see page 254)
1 medium onion, finely chopped
2 cloves garlic, finely chopped
3cm (1¼ in) piece of fresh ginger, finely chopped
3 sprigs of thyme
1 tsp sea salt
¼–½ tsp freshly ground black or white pepper
4 tbsp lemon juice
1 medium marrow, cubed, or 2 bottle gourds

1 whole pointed hispi cabbage or handful of softer leaves like beetroot greens

FOR THE DUMPLINGS (OPTIONAL)
90g (¾ cup) gram flour
1 tsp baking powder
sea salt and freshly ground black pepper, to taste
2 medium eggs
1½ tbsp extra-virgin olive oil or melted ghee
2 tbsp chopped dill

TIP

If you find it hard to shape the dumplings, try chilling the batter for about 3 hours beforehand. Otherwise you could simply drop the batter in teaspoonfuls at a time without shaping – they will look lovely and rustic.

1   Start by making the dumplings, if desired. In a bowl, whisk together the dry ingredients, adding salt and pepper to taste.

2   In a separate bowl, whisk together the eggs and oil until just combined. Make a hole in the centre of the flour mixture and add the egg mixture. Fold together with a rubber spatula until thoroughly incorporated; the batter will be very thick and sticky. You can make this ahead of time and keep in the fridge until you're ready to go.

3   For the soup, put the whey, onion, garlic, ginger and thyme in a large pan and bring to the boil, then simmer for 20 minutes. With wet hands, roll the dumpling dough into eight balls. Bring the soup to the boil then add the dumplings, marrow and cabbage. Cook for 5 minutes, until the dumplings bob on the surface. Cut one in half to check they are cooked all the way through.

4   Reduce to a simmer, add the salt and pepper and the lemon juice and continue to cook for about 5 minutes more, then add any really soft leaves (spinach, chard or beetroot greens). Remove from the heat and serve immediately.

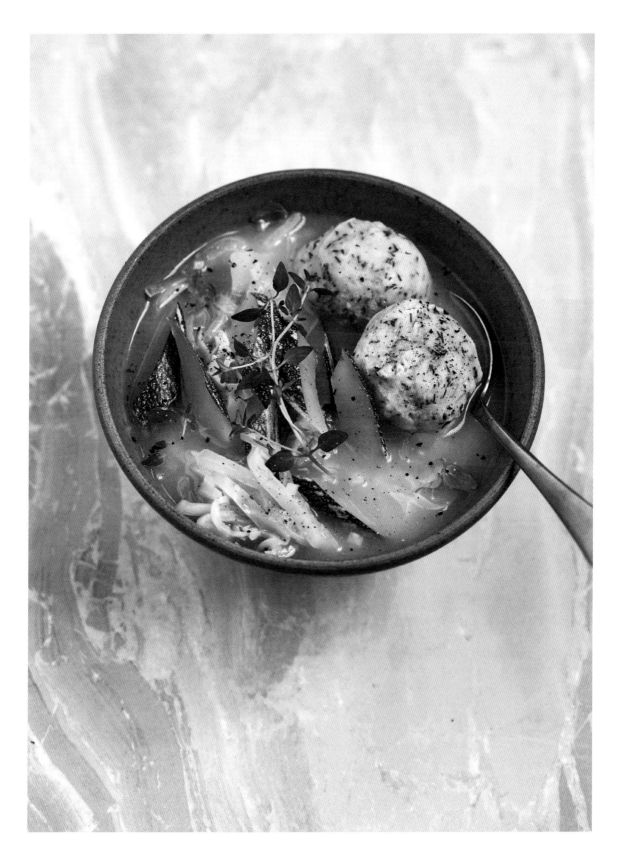

Pudas, or pudlas as they are known in northern India, are easy Indian-style vegetable pancakes. I smothered these simple gram flour bases in a range of different toppings and pizza pudas were born. Parents take note – this is a great way of hiding veggies or at least making them go down a bit easier!

Makes 2

You could choose to add nigella seeds and asafoetida to the pancake batter, along with your choice of Dosha Churna Spice Mix (see page 247). Despite the Indian flavours, these pizza pudas team well with Italian toppings, so feel free to experiment with any fresh ingredients you have. I love mine with baby spinach or sautéed chard, anchovies and roasted red peppers, but then again, nothing beats a margherita! The recipe for this garden-fresh no-cook pizza sauce couldn't be more simple – just blend and go. Same with the delicious basil oil – drizzle this on anything and everything. For a no-bake pizza you can simmer the tomato sauce first before spreading over the pudas, then cover with your choice of fresh ingredients such as rocket and ricotta and serve.

The pudas are also great as garlic bread, or ripped up for dunking in soups. Cooking them in a dollop of coconut oil or ghee makes them crispy on the outside and soft on the inside and you can also thin them out more to make quesadillas or pancakes, sliced into wedges and drizzled with extra-virgin olive oil.

Pizza pudas

FOR THE BASES
120g (1 cup) gram flour
½ tsp cumin seeds
  or ground cumin,
  or more to taste
½ tsp sea salt
pinch of asafoetida
  (optional)
1 tsp nigella seeds
  (optional)
1 tsp Dosha Churna Spice
  Mix (see page 247;
  optional)
175ml (¾ cup) water
115g (1 cup) shredded
  courgette, carrot
  or cucumber
1 tbsp coriander,
  finely chopped
6 tsp melted coconut
  oil or ghee
rocket and ricotta, to serve

FOR THE SAUCE
6 plum tomatoes, skinned
  and deseeded
  (see page 260)
3–4 garlic cloves,
  roughly chopped
1 tsp balsamic vinegar,
  plus more to taste
4 tsp sea salt
freshly ground
  black pepper
3 tsp extra-virgin olive oil

FOR THE BASIL OLIVE OIL
leaves of 1 small bunch
  of basil (about 30g)
75ml (⅓ cup) extra-virgin
  olive oil
pinch of sea salt

1 To make the bases, mix the gram flour, cumin and salt, asafoetida, nigella seeds and Dosha churna spice mix (if using). Slowly add the water and whisk to make a smooth batter. Add the grated courgette and chopped coriander and mix well.

2 Place a ceramic-lined or seasoned cast-iron frying pan on a medium-high heat. Test to see if it's hot enough by sprinkling a few drops of water on it – the water should sizzle right away. Pour half of the mixture onto the pan and spread quickly and evenly with the back of a spoon. Starting from the centre, spiral the batter evenly outwards to form a 22cm (8½ in) circle.

RECIPE CONTINUES...

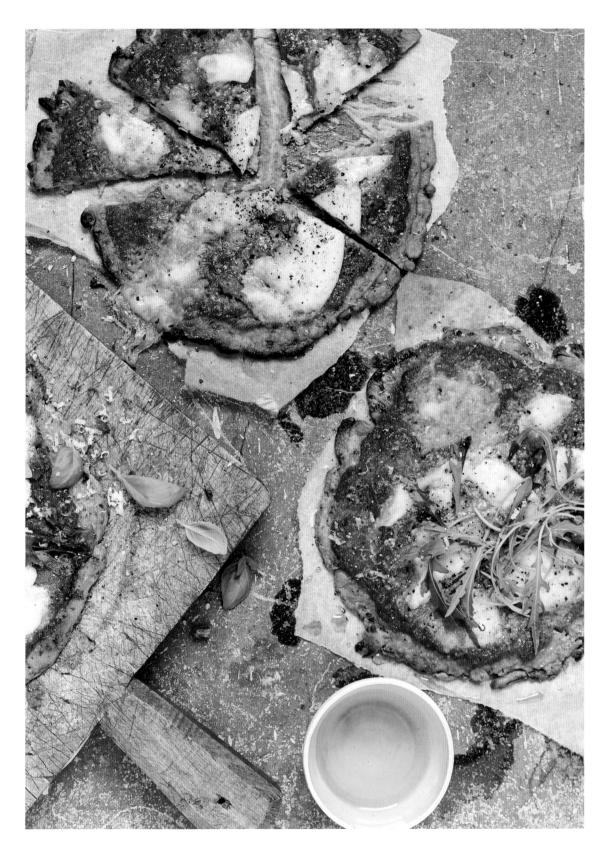

3   After about 6 minutes, the batter will have almost cooked, so gently spread 1 teaspoon of coconut oil over the top. Wait for about 30 seconds, then flip the puda using a flat spatula. Press down lightly with the spatula to help it to cook evenly. Turn the puda three or four times for another 4–5 minutes, until crisp and brown on both sides. Repeat for the remaining puda and oil and set aside until you're ready to serve.

4   To make the basil oil, bend the basil with the olive oil. This keeps for 3 days in the fridge, but make sure to bring it to room temperature before use.

TIP

·

You can refrigerate leftover sauce for up to a week. Alternatively, freeze it for up to 3 months. The easiest way to do this is to spoon it into muffin tins and freeze until solid. Pop the frozen cubes out of the moulds and transfer to a freezer container. Thaw overnight before using on pizza pudas.

5   To make the sauce, roughly chop the tomatoes and put them into a blender or food processor, adding the garlic, vinegar, salt and black pepper. Blend until smooth, and then add further seasoning to taste.

6   For a fresh pizza you can cook the sauce at this point for about 8 minutes and then spoon a dollop onto your pizza pudas, using the back of the spoon to smooth it out. Pile on rocket and ricotta and drizzle with the basil oil. Otherwise spread the raw sauce onto the pizzas, top with your favourite ingredients, then pop it into an oven, preheated to 180°C (fan 160°C/gas mark 4) or under a hot grill and cook to your liking.

FEELING
VATA

Stick to cooked pizza toppings.

FEELING
PITTA

Use less garlic in the tomato sauce and more basil oil. Raw toppings work well for you.

FEELING
KAPHA

Cut back on the amount of oil used to cook the pizza bases and swap the basil oil for fresh basil. Add some chilli flakes or fresh chilli.

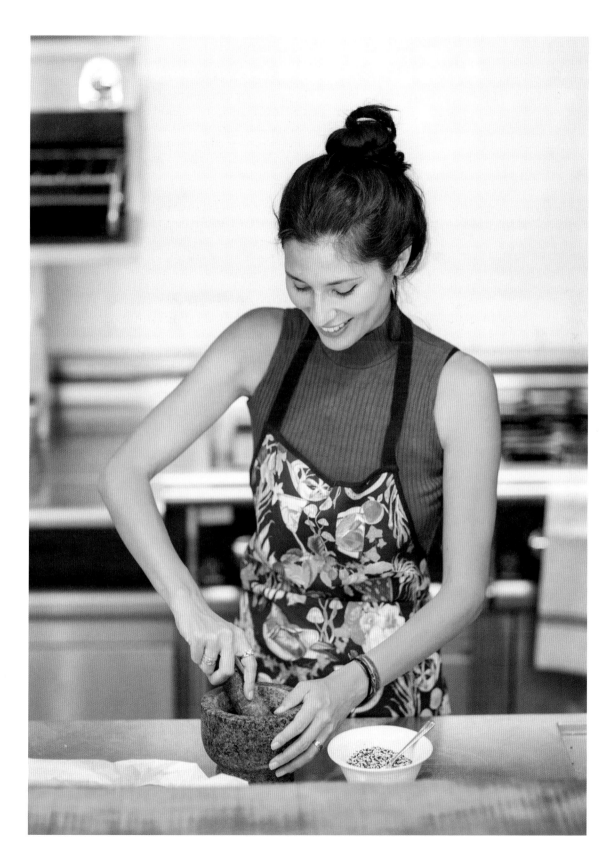

CELEBRATION AND SHARING PLATES 207

A thali is a complete meal composed of various little dishes (sometimes up to fifteen!) on a single plate. Usually saved for special occasions, thalis are said to have originated in southern India and have their roots in Ayurveda, where they are a representation of the six Tastes (as well as so many textures), making them not only a balanced and delicious meal but also great for supporting our Doshas and bodies.

For many people, making thali is a full-time job, which is why it's so special when you get to eat a homemade one. Here are seven basic categories which you can use to build a decent thali from the recipes in the book – this number certainly makes things a bit more doable! You can easily make a sizeable batch of chutney or pickle in advance, then you know it's also good for other meals. If your digestion is especially tricky, it's best not to go full steam ahead – so many different ingredients might just be a bit much for you to handle, so take it easy and build up that stomach fire first with a little cleanse reset (see page 290) and some balanced eating for a while. A nice idea is using a thali as a 'pot luck' with friends. Divide the dishes between you all, then get together to feast and make merry.

Serves 1–2

Thali time!

Roti

Ragi Roti
(see page 62)

Curry

Tamarind Courgette
and Parsnip Curry
(see page 133)

Salad

Braised Gem Lettuce Wedges with
Fennel and Sesame Gomashio
(see page 218)

Rice Dish

Lamb and
Vegetable Biryani
(see page 154)

Raita/Chutney/Pickle

Achucharu – Sri Lankan
Celebration Pickle
(see page 237)

Soup

Spring Clean Vegetable
Brown Rice Soup
(see page 196)

Dal

Gary Gorrow's Rasta Dal
(see page 186)

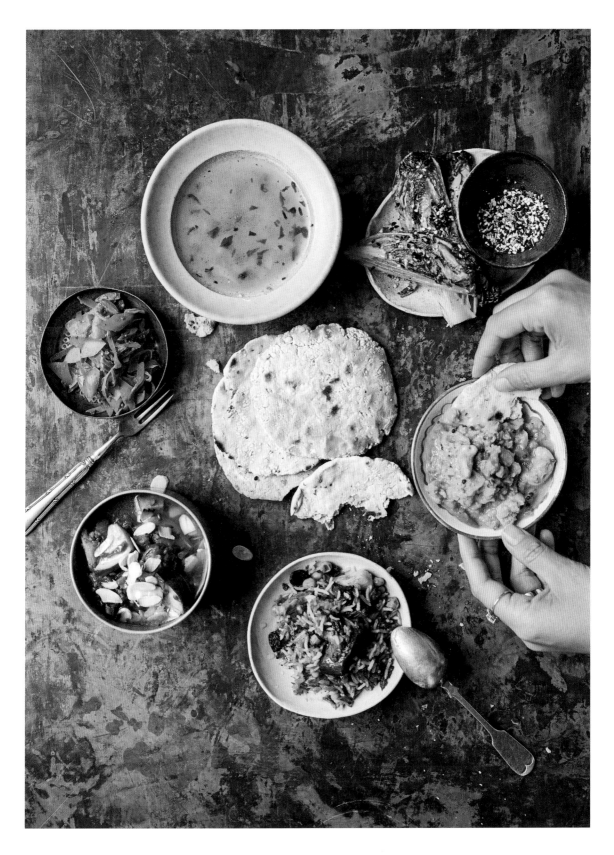

There is something wonderful about a pie and its promise of delicious filling inside. I've gone for a Greek-inspired recipe of spinach, feta and herbs here, but instead of encasing it in the usual wheat pastry I've teamed it with a golden chickpea pastry made in a similar way to shortcrust. It brings back memories of 'rubbing' flour into butter during one of my only cooking lessons at school. This also works with rice flour, but you need patience as it's tricky to work with and tends to break, but you can easily patch up the cracks.

You can use chard or any of your favourite seasonal greens instead of spinach, but make sure you adjust the cooking times accordingly.

Since it's more time-consuming and fiddly then your average bowl of dal, I like to make this when I have guests – everyone gets their own pastry pie. The recipe makes four large hand pies, perfect with veggies or salad.

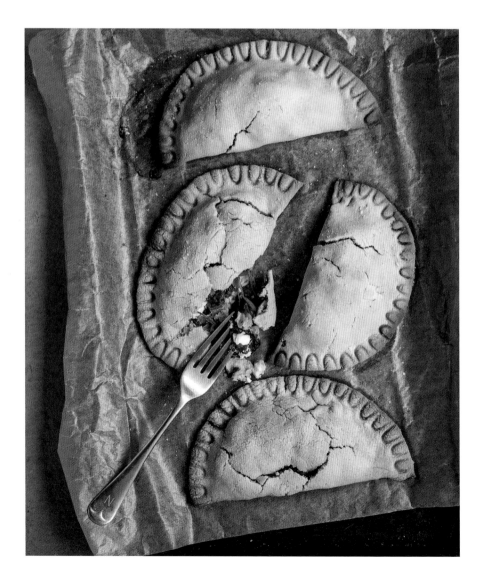

Spinach and feta hand pies

1 tbsp ghee

½ small onion
or leek, diced

1 clove garlic, finely
chopped

300g (6 cups)
spinach leaves

2 tbsp parsley, chopped

2 tbsp mint, chopped

¼–½ tsp ground nutmeg

¼ tsp freshly ground
black pepper

75g feta cheese,
cut into small cubes
or crumbled

extra-virgin olive oil,
for brushing

FOR THE PASTRY

220g (scant 2 cups) gram
flour, or 220g (1½ cups)
rice flour, plus more
for dusting

½ tsp sea salt and freshly
ground black pepper,
to taste

80g unsalted
chilled butter

75ml (⅓ cup) cold water,
plus more if needed

1 Start with the pastry. Mix the flour, salt and pepper in a bowl. Grate in the butter. Rub the butter into the flour until you reach fine crumbs. Pour in the water, adding more if necessary, until you reach a workable dough. Knead it for a few minutes, then keep at room temperature until you're ready to use.

2 Melt the ghee in a frying pan over medium heat. Sauté the onion for about 5–7 minutes, until soft. Add the garlic and cook for another minute. Add the spinach and allow it to cook down for about 5 minutes, until fairly dry. Remove from the heat, leave to cool, then squeeze out any excess water. Place in a bowl and stir through the remaining ingredients, apart from the olive oil. Set aside in the fridge until ready to use.

3 Preheat the oven to 200ºC (fan 180ºC/gas mark 6) and line a baking sheet with baking parchment.

4 Cut the pastry dough into four pieces. Dust a clean work surface with flour, and working with one at a time, press or roll the dough out into a flat disc that's about 15–18cm (6–7in) across.

5 Divide the filling evenly across half of each disc (about 3 tablespoons of filling per round), leaving a border around the edge. Fold the other half of the dough over the filling, and use a fork to seal the edges well. Repeat with the remainder of the pies.

6 Transfer the hand pies to the lined baking sheet. Brush the tops with olive oil and sprinkle with a pinch of sea salt. Bake for 15 minutes, then rotate the baking sheet and bake for another 10–15 minutes until the hand pies are lightly browned on top and around the edges. Cool for a few minutes and serve warm, or allow to cool completely.

FEELING
VATA

Try chopped green
beans and/or grated
carrots instead of spinach.
Add an egg to the mix to
make it more filling.

FEELING
PITTA

Throw in some fresh
coriander, if you like.

With a crunchy base and a sweet creamy topping, this is about as East by West as it gets! The earliest incarnation of a cheesecake is said to date back to ancient Greece. I like a German-style cheesecake, oven-baked and not too sweet.

Perfect for a special occasion, my version incorporates the beautiful Indian spices of cardamom and saffron to provide a refreshing alternative to the more traditional options of chocolate, vanilla or lemon. If you're sensitive to the flavour of cardamom, try adding less the first time you make this. The base is made from toasted gram flour, which makes it deliciously nutty, without the heaviness of nuts. This base is also used for making the Cardamom Millionaires (see page 104).

In terms of a new taste sensation, this is possibly my favourite cheesecake recipe ever, and it tastes as good as it looks! It is beautifully rich and full in flavour so is best served in small slices – with plenty of gratitude and mindfulness.

Serves 8–10

Saffron cardamom cottage cheesecake with a millionaire crust

4 medium eggs, separated
100g (½ cup) light jaggery, finely chopped
400g full-fat cottage cheese or homemade paneer (see page 254)
1 tsp vanilla extract
generous pinch of sea salt
seeds of 12 cardamom pods, ground
1 large pinch strands of saffron, infused in 1 tbsp very hot water
edible flowers, to serve (optional)

FOR THE MILLIONAIRE CRUST
150g (1¼ cup) gram flour
seeds of 6 cardamom pods, ground
100g (½ cup) jaggery, finely chopped, or coconut sugar
100g (½ cup) ghee or butter, plus extra for greasing
pinch of sea salt

1   Grease and line an 18cm (7in) springform tin with baking parchment. Make the millionaire crust by following the method on page 104. Spread the mixture into the tin, and press it down evenly using the back of a metal spoon. Let the mixture cool for about an hour in the fridge.

2   Preheat the oven to 170ºC (150ºC fan/gas mark 3). To make the filling, place the egg yolks and jaggery in a food processor and blend for about 2 minutes until pale and well combined. Add the cottage cheese, vanilla, salt, cardamom and saffron mixture and blend again until completely smooth.

3   Whisk the egg whites to stiff peaks and gently fold them into the mixture in four stages, using a metal spoon.

4   Bake in the preheated oven for 1 hour 15 minutes until golden and just set. Loosely cover the cheesecake with baking parchment for the last 30 minutes if it's turning very dark. Remove and leave to cool to room temperature. The base is a little crumbly but beautiful. Decorate with flowers, if desired, and serve.

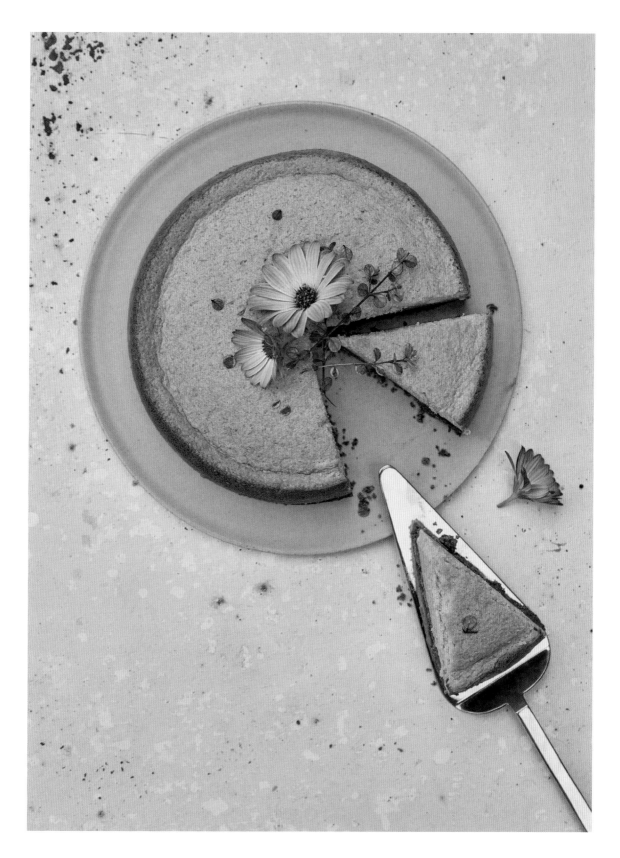

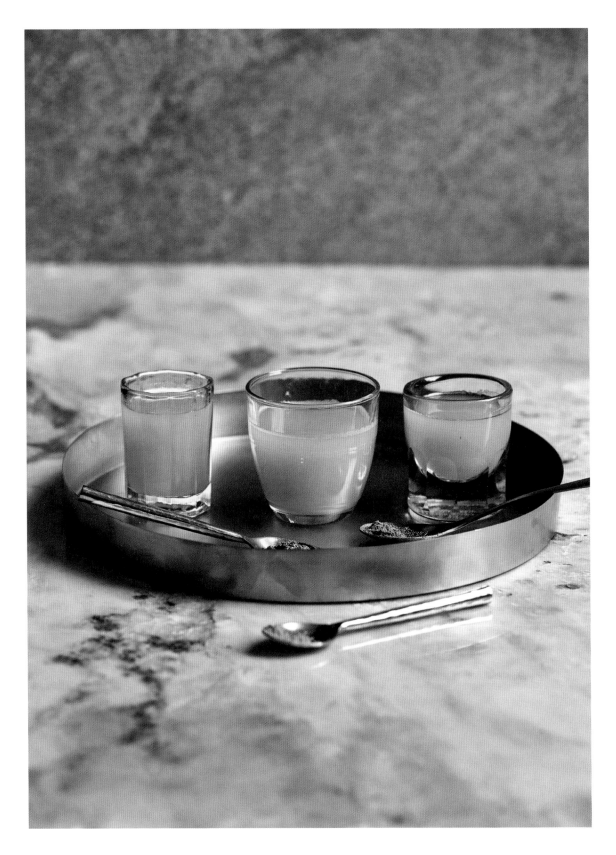

This little tumbler of warm, spiced apple juice served with a tiny teaspoon of Dosha churna (or 'choona') spice mix is definitely a conversation starter.

Serves 3–4

The idea came from my stay at Vana Ayurvedic Retreat, where they had two restaurants: the day-to-day one that we mostly favoured; and the fancy one where we could choose from a Dosha-specific Thali menu, which always started with this drink. The gingery sweet liquid coats your tongue, then the spices hit your tongue like a sherbet bomb before they infuse your body and tell you that it's time to eat!

Choona spiced apple juice

500ml (2 cups) freshly pressed apple juice

100ml water

½ tsp lemon zest

2.5cm (1in) piece of fresh ginger, finely sliced

½ cinnamon stick or ¼ tsp ground ginger

⅓ tsp Dosha Churna Spice Mix per serving (see page 247), or more to taste

1 Pour the apple juice and water into a saucepan with the lemon zest, ginger and cinnamon.

2 Bring the mixture to the boil and then leave to simmer gently for a few minutes. Strain into heatproof glasses and serve with a very small spoon of the Dosha Churna Spice Mix.

I first tasted this drink during Holi (the festival of colour and love celebrated in the spring) in India. Served in little earthenware mugs and as delicious as a milkshake but with other worldly flavours, thanks to all the spices, it was a flavour I would never forget! Apparently it's usually spiked with a very happy marijuana called bhang, making it particularly celebratory.

This traditional drink, known as kesar pista or thandai, is traditionally served chilled, but Ayurveda recommends serving warm or at room temperature and sipping very slowly. It's for celebrations rather than every day, and is particularly good if you're feeling imbalanced or in need of a helping hand.

Serves 3–4

Celebration pistachio and saffron milk

250ml (1 cup) whole milk or non-dairy milk, such as drinking coconut milk, almond milk or rice milk (see pages 256–257)

120ml (½ cup) water (optional)

8–10 strands of saffron

FOR THE SPICE MIX (7 TBSP)

2 tbsp raw pistachios, plus extra for garnish

1 tbsp raw cashews, plus extra for garnish

3 tbsp jaggery or raw honey

¼ tsp ground cinnamon

seeds of 5 cardamom pods, ground, or ¼–½ tsp ground cardamom

⅛ tsp cloves

⅛ tsp fennel seeds (optional)

¼ tsp ground ginger

¼ tsp freshly ground black pepper

¼ tsp poppy seeds

1 Start by making the spice mix. Dry-toast the pistachios and cashews in a pan until fragrant. Allow to cool and then grind them to a coarse powder. Add the jaggery and the rest of the ingredients and grind until well blended. Store in an airtight container.

2 If you're using dairy milk, pour it into a small saucepan with the water and simmer for 10 minutes. If you are using other milks you can skip this step.

3 Pour your choice of milk into a blender and add 2 tablespoons of the spice mix. Blend, then taste and add more spice mix if needed. Chill for a few minutes or leave to stand. In a small bowl, dissolve the saffron in 2 tablespoons of the milk mixture.

4 When you are ready to serve, take the glasses and very carefully spread the dissolved saffron on the walls of the glass with the help of a spoon. Immediately pour the milk into the glass – you should see the orange colour from the saffron on the walls of the glass, contrasting with the light yellow or pale yellow milk. Garnish with chopped pistachios or almonds.

FEELING
PITTA

Skip the ginger and black pepper and add some mint.

FEELING
KAPHA

Use rice milk (see page 257) as the base and cut down on the nuts.

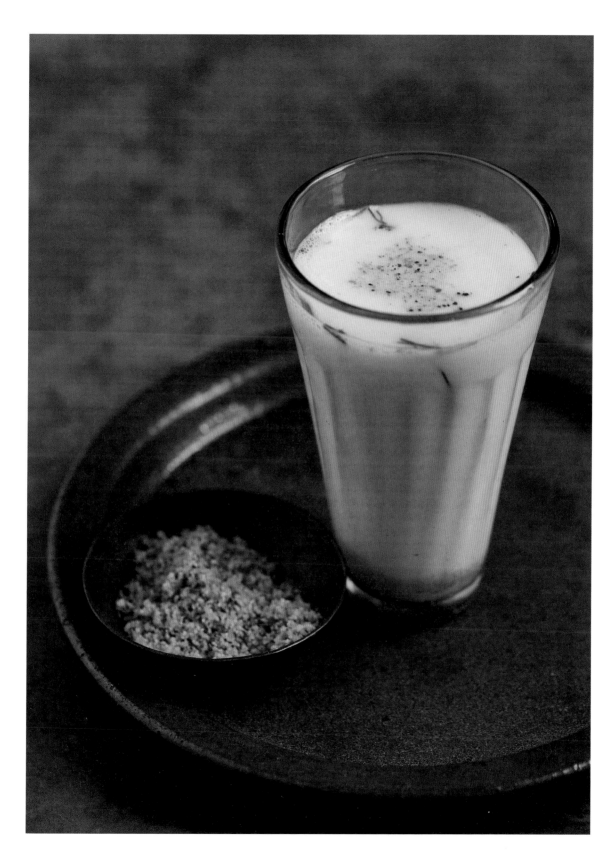

I first discovered cooked lettuce during my art foundation course, when a friend of mine, who is half-Chinese, said he'd cook supper for a few of us and dashed to the supermarket to buy a lettuce. I remember thinking – who goes out to buy only one lettuce?! He made the most delicious Asian stir-fry dish and, yes, that lettuce made it. Since then I've loved eating lettuce cooked as much as raw – and so does my digestion. Serving griddled wedges of lettuce always looks great on the table and requires minimum work in the kitchen. Some hot ghee and a sprinkle of Japanese-inspired salty sesame condiment takes it to the next level. This is a much easier-to-digest side than your average bowl of side salad.

Serves 1

Braised gem lettuce wedges with fennel and sesame gomashio

1 baby gem lettuce,
cut lengthways
into 4 pieces
melted ghee, for brushing
and dipping

FOR THE FENNEL AND
SESAME GOMASHIO
75g (½ cup) black
sesame seeds
75g (½ cup) white
sesame seeds
1 tsp fennel seeds,
or more to taste
1½ tbsp sea salt
1 tsp ground cumin
(optional)
1 tsp coriander seeds
(optional)

1   To make the fennel gomashio, toast the black and white sesame seeds in a dry frying pan over a medium heat, until the white sesame seeds begin to brown and pop – be very careful not to burn them. Transfer to a bowl and allow to cool completely.

2   In the same pan, toast the fennel seeds with the salt and allow to cool completely. Mix everything together, then roughly blend using a spice grinder or pound in batches in a pestle and mortar to give an uneven texture. If using a powerful blender, try not to blend too much or you'll end up with tahini!

3   Preheat a griddle pan over a high heat. Brush the lettuce wedges with melted ghee and griddle for 1 minute on each cut side. Arrange the lettuce on a plate and scatter with fennel and sesame gomashio. Serve with a small side of hot ghee.

TIP
.
Take care when toasting black sesame seeds as it's harder to see if they burn.

4   You can store leftover gomashio in a jar with a tight-fitting lid in a cool dry place for up to 1 month.

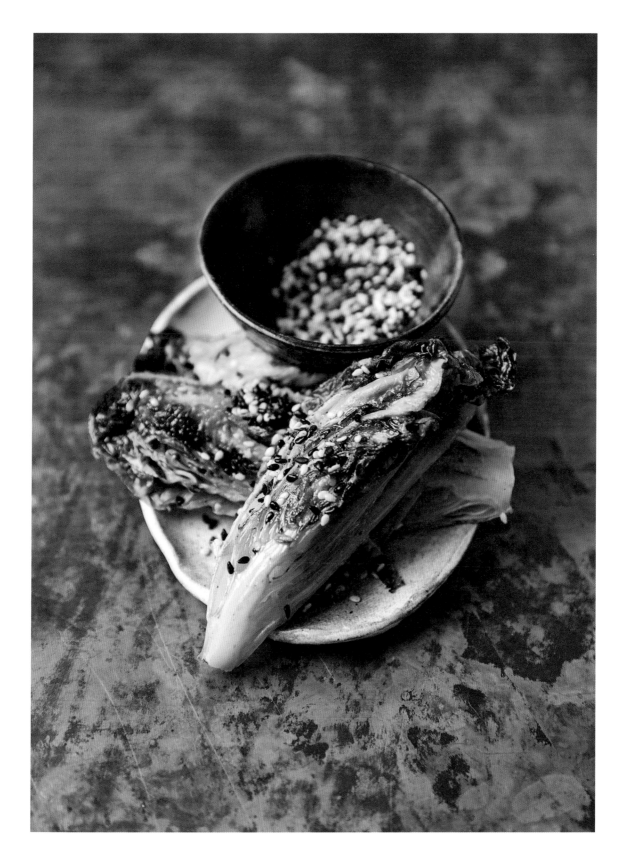

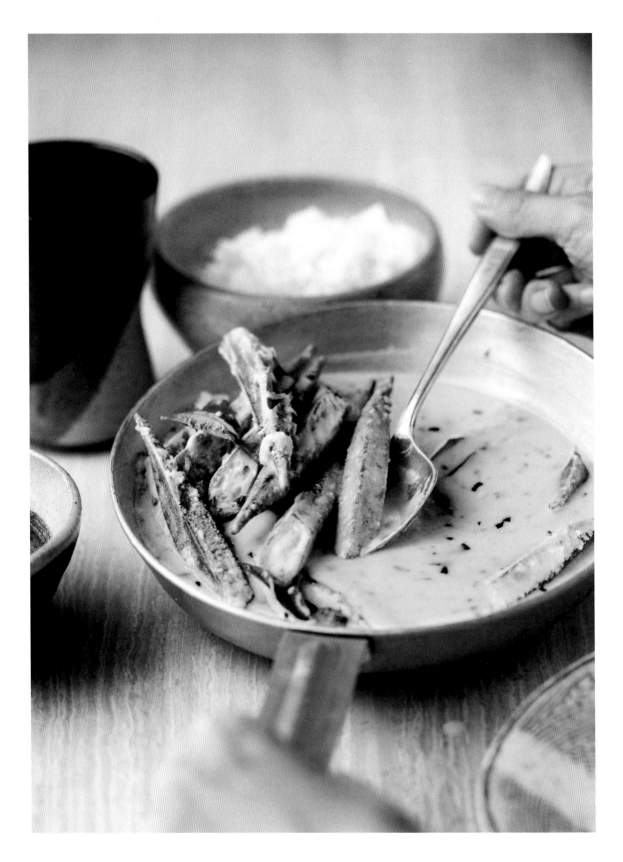

Okra is a super-nutritious vegetable that's popular in West Africa, Ethiopia, South Asia and Turkish and Greek cuisines – but not one that we are particularly used to seeing on British menus. Also known as ladies' fingers, the pods are cooked in stews, fried, pickled or eaten raw in salads. I like okra when it is slow-cooked with onions, garlic and tomatoes, à la Greek or Turkish cooking, but I also love this Sattvic (see page 14) version, which is creamy and spiced. It's a delicious side dish for four people or a good main for two when teamed with a Ragi Roti that's fresh off the griddle (see page 62).

After tempering the spices, the okra is sautéed in ghee to caramelise it – this works well for people who are not used to the texture of okra. Right at the end I add some cream or coconut cream. My friend Mr Todiwala of the Indian restaurant Mr Todiwala's Kitchen and Spice Cafe Namaste taught me that this dish could be classified a 'curry' because it contains coconut milk or cream and is saucy – everything else we call curry in the UK is actually just Indian food!

Serves 4

Spiced okra with cream

1 tbsp ghee

2 tsp black mustard seeds

½ tsp fenugreek seeds

½ tsp cumin seeds

2 pinches of asafoetida

6 curry leaves

5cm (2in) piece of fresh ginger, grated or finely chopped

½ green chilli, finely chopped

¼ tsp ground turmeric

250g okra

250ml (1 cup) water

4 tbsp full-fat cream or coconut milk cream (from the top of a tin)

2 sprigs of coriander leaves, finely chopped

just under ½ tsp sea salt

1   Melt the ghee in a large saucepan on a medium heat. Add the mustard seeds. As soon as they start to pop, add the fenugreek seeds, cumin seeds, asafoetida and curry leaves and cook for another minute.

2   Add the ginger, green chilli, turmeric and okra. Sauté for 5–10 minutes on a medium-high heat, stirring frequently to prevent it from catching.

3   Add the water and simmer for 10 minutes, lid off, until the okra is tender, adding a little more water if necessary to ensure there is a sauce. Turn down the heat and stir in the cream and the coriander, being careful not to let it boil otherwise the sauce will curdle. Season with salt and serve immediately.

FEELING
VATA

Add an extra tablespoon of cream, if you like, or use more ghee in the frying process.

FEELING
PITTA

Cool off by sticking to the coconut cream; leave out the chilli and cut back on the spices slightly if you like.

FEELING
KAPHA

Add more chilli, if you like, and only use 1 tablespoon of cream and ghee.

Misoshiru is one of the staples of Japanese cuisine. Whether you are eating the simplest fare or the finest of feasts, you will find a little pot of hot miso soup for sipping. Meaty and brothy, it's brimming with that all-important umami taste, which has been labelled as the fifth taste in the West (where pungent and astringent have not yet been recognised). Most of us could be forgiven for thinking that miso soup is simply miso paste and water mixed with a bit of tofu and spring onion but it's all about the dashi or stock, made from kombu (dried kelp seaweed) and bonito (a type of dried fermented fish), that forms the foundation of the soup before the miso goes anywhere near it. Just as a Cordon Bleu chef would be judged on the quality of French-style chicken stock, a Japanese chef would be judged by his or her dashi alone.

Kombu is a great ingredient to have at home – just like the Indian asafoetida and Mexican epazote, not only does it create umami flavour but it also helps to break down heavy starches when cooked with food, so it's excellent for making beans more digestible as well as reducing their cooking time. For a quicker, easier miso soup you can replace the dashi stock with about ¾ teaspoon of instant dashi granules – the equivalent, I suppose, of a vegetable stock cube instead of homemade stock. Or you can use bone broth or water. And if you are vegetarian, you can make the dashi stock using double the amount of kombu and no bonito.

Serves 2

Proper miso soup

110g firm tofu (about ¼ pack)
500ml (2 cups) water
5cm (2in) piece of kombu (dried kelp)
6g (½ cup) dried bonito flakes
1 tsp dried wakame

2 tbsp miso paste or to taste
1–2 spring onions, finely chopped

1   Cut off the right amount of tofu in one chunk, and place it on a large plate which is lifted a little at one end to create a slope. Pile a couple of smaller side plates on top of the tofu to add some pressure and squeeze out excess liquid which will gather on the lower side of the plate.

2   Heat the water in a medium saucepan over a low heat. Add the kombu and cook until the mixture just begins to simmer (do not boil kombu, as it makes it bitter). Stir in the bonito flakes until combined. Remove the saucepan from the heat and allow the dashi stock to sit, uncovered, for 5 minutes. Strain and set aside.

3   Transfer the the dashi to a clean saucepan and heat it over a medium heat. Cut the tofu into small cubes and add it to the saucepan with the wakame, stirring to combine. Remove 120ml (½ cup) of the warm dashi to a small bowl and whisk in the miso with chopsticks. Pour the miso mixture back into the saucepan with the remaining dashi. Stir until just warmed through, then serve with chopped spring onions.

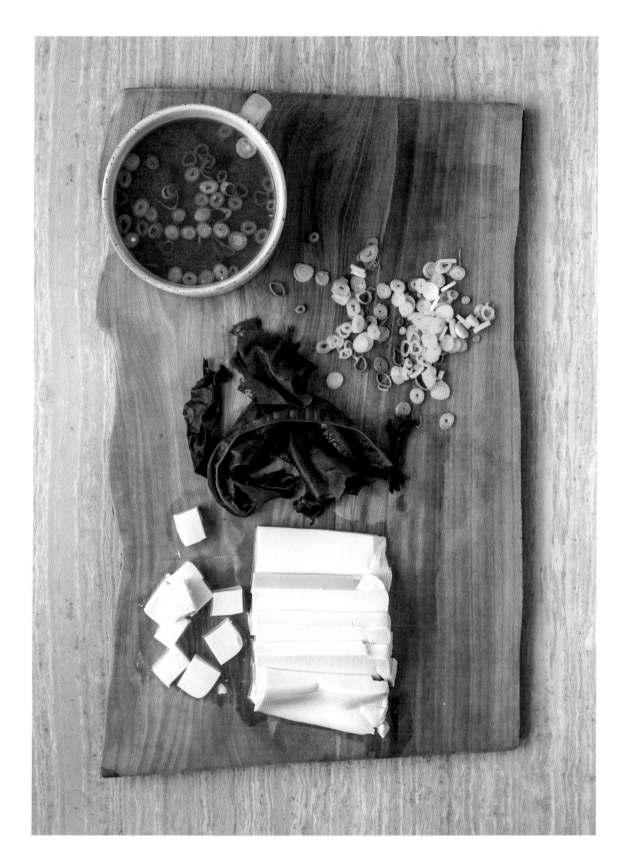

When you see the words lime and coriander together in a recipe name you'd be forgiven for thinking that this was going to be an explosion of Mexican flavours, but not so. This soft and comforting broth is a mild-mannered 'hug in a mug' and a great recipe for anyone in need of a healthy alternative to a coffee for a 4pm pick-me-up. Based on the popular lemon and coriander soup, I've used limes here, which are less harsh and much more cooling. Though they come from the same family, lemons and limes have slightly different characteristics as you can identify from their flavour profiles – limes are slightly more sweet with mild anti-inflammatory properties, whereas lemons can irritate the digestive tract if there is any inflammation already.

In Ayurveda, lime juice and coriander are recommended to improve the appetite and help digestion, making this soup a lovely appetiser. Lime is also useful to aid mineral absorption, help with heartburn and nausea and relieve high blood pressure.

Serves 2

Lime and coriander bone broth

500ml (2 cups) chicken
    bone broth
    (see page 261)
pinch of salt
3 pinches of freshly
    ground black pepper
small handful of fresh
    coriander, chopped
1 tsp lime juice

FEELING
PITTA

Use this to soothe
a hot temper on a cold
day! Or any day, for
that matter.

1 To make the bone broth, follow the instructions on page 261.

2 Heat the bone broth with a pinch of salt and the black pepper and allow to simmer for a few minutes. Add the coriander and lime juice, simmer for a further minute and then serve.

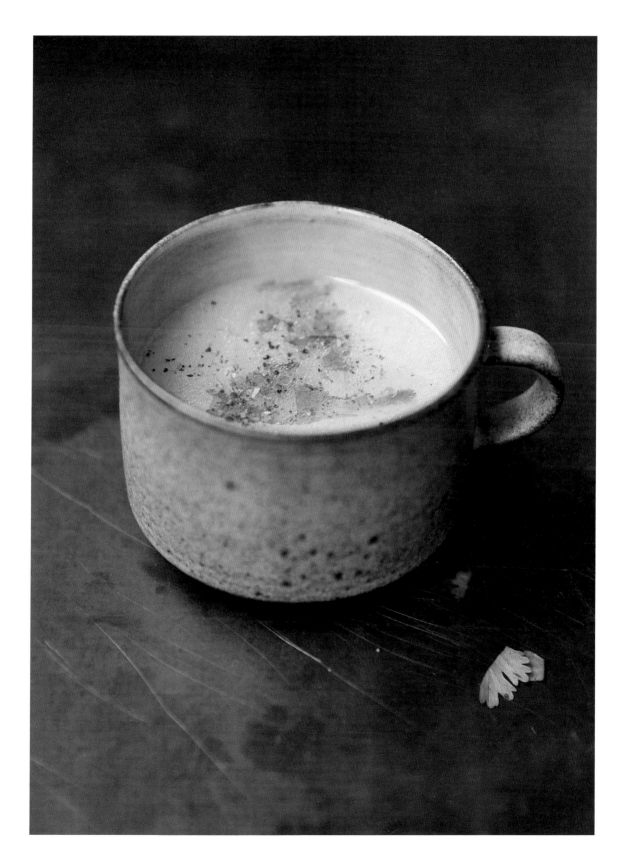

Raita is the cool, creamy herb and vegetable yoghurt condiment served in Indian cuisine to temper the spices, add the all-important sour taste to meals and aid digestion. As a condiment, it is best eaten in small amounts, as yoghurt is heavy and therefore difficult to digest, although the added spices help in this respect. Homemade yoghurt (see page 259) is important for the flavour and in the goodness it imparts. Vegans can use nut milk curds to make raita.

Serves 8

Beetroot raita

1 tbsp ghee
½ tsp black mustard seeds
½ tsp cumin seeds
pinch of asafoetida
150g (1 cup) peeled and
    grated beetroot
250g (1 cup) homemade
    yoghurt (see page 259)
1 tbsp coriander
    or mint leaves,
    chopped
pinch of sea salt

FEELING
PITTA

Raw beetroot aggravates Pitta, so make sure it's well cooked. Add more mint or coriander, if you like, and reduce the spices.

1   Melt the ghee in a small saucepan. Add the mustard seeds, cumin seeds and asafoetida and gently fry until the seeds start to pop. Add the grated beetroot and sauté until just cooked, about 5 minutes.

2   Remove from the heat and allow to cool. Fold in the yoghurt, adding a splash of water if you think it needs it, then stir in the coriander or mint and salt to serve.

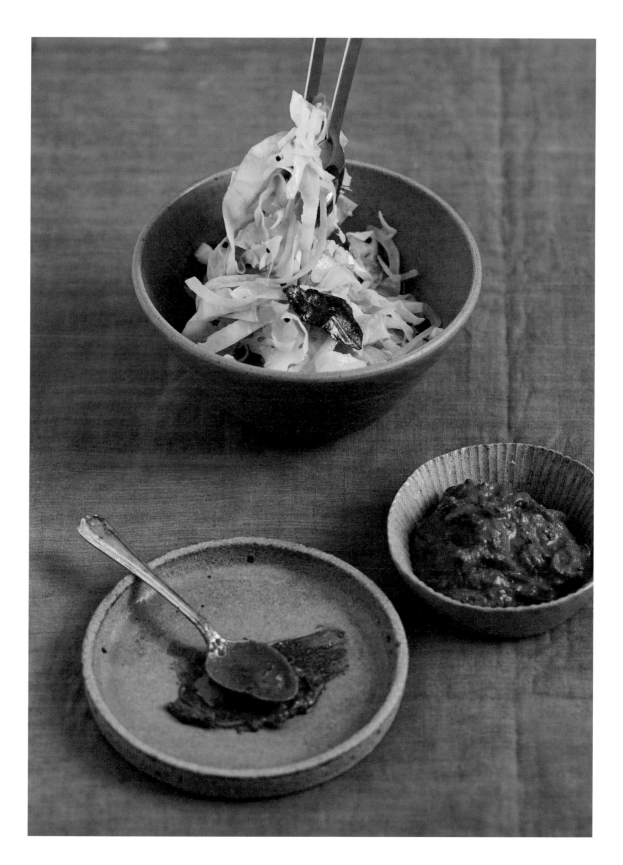

I'd not heard of this dish until midway through the pop-up cafe when I got an email from Christa, a friend who is a journalist. She'd been to the cafe for lunch and had thoroughly enjoyed it and asked whether cabbage thoran, one of her favourite dishes from Goa, could make an appearance on the menu. I love cabbage, and I love a cabbage recipe, so although I've never knowingly eaten this particular dish in India, it's now a staple side dish at home. PICTURED ON PAGE 227.

Serves 2–3

Cabbage thoran

1 cabbage (about 400g), halved, shredded into long 1cm (½ in) slices, washed and drained
1 onion, shredded lengthways into fine slices
1 green chilli, chopped
½ tsp cumin seeds

2 tbsp desiccated coconut
¼ tsp ground turmeric
sea salt, to taste
1½ tsp vegetable oil
1 tsp black mustard seeds
1 dried red chilli, halved and seeds removed
10 fresh curry leaves

1   Combine the cabbage with the onion, green chilli, cumin seeds, coconut, turmeric and salt. Mix thoroughly and leave for about 10–15 minutes.

2   Heat the oil in a saucepan, then add the mustard seeds. When they start to pop, add the dried red chilli and curry leaves and stir until the chilli darkens.

3   Add the cabbage mixture to the pan and stir well. Lower the heat, cover and cook, stirring every so often, until the cabbage is barely limp. Transfer to a dish and serve hot.

WORKS WITH

TIKKA FISH, CARROT, FENNEL AND MUSTARD STIR-FRY
page 159

ZAC 'N' CHEESE
page 139

LEMON, TURMERIC AND BLACK-PEPPER SALMON
page 125

TARKA DAL
page 166

BROWN LENTIL, SPINACH AND COCONUT HOTPOT
page 189

FEELING VATA

Enjoy at lunchtime, making sure this is well cooked and covered in ghee. Try it with a fried egg on top.

FEELING PITTA

Cut out the chilli and add more coconut, to help balance the pungency and heating elements.

Nailed it! This took quite a few attempts to get right, but it was worth the effort. My mum introduced me to dhokla after she enjoyed it with her ex-colleague Dipa; mum reckoned herself such an expert after trying it that she became my harshest critic! These are light as air, sweet-and-sour squares, fashioned out of nutritious gram flour, then steamed and spiked with a tempering of green chillies and mustard. I still don't have a proper Asian steamer – either a Chinese bamboo one or the Indian metal sort – but I loved working out how to turn my existing equipment into one.

Snacks are few and far between for me now, because my main meals are usually supportive enough for my digestion and Agni (see page 278), but this is hands-down one of my favourites, and was also the inspiration for Rosemary Mung Bean Bread (see page 232). Enjoy as a side or starter to any meal, served with green chutney and the tarka. PICTURED ON PAGE 230.

Serves 8

Dhokla with green chutney

½ tsp ground turmeric

½ tsp sea salt

195g (¾ cup) homemade yoghurt (see page 259)

250ml (1 cup) hot water

220g (1¾ cup plus 1 tbsp) gram flour

oil, for greasing

2 tsp bicarbonate of soda (optional – see tip on page 231)

2 tsp apple cider vinegar

FOR THE TARKA

2 tbsp ghee

1 tsp cumin seeds

1 tsp black mustard seeds

10 curry leaves

1 large spring onion or medium onion, sliced

1 green chilli, finely sliced

¾ tsp ground turmeric

¼ tsp asafoetida

1 medium tomato, skinned and deseeded (see page 260), cubed

½ tsp sea salt

2 garlic cloves (or in summer use wild garlic leaves), crushed or finely sliced

FOR THE GREEN CHUTNEY

60g fresh coriander

½ tsp sea salt

1cm (½ in) piece of fresh ginger

juice of 1 lime

2 tsp raw honey

6 tbsp water

30g sunflower seeds, toasted

1 green chilli, chopped (optional)

1   For this recipe, you could use an Asian-style bamboo steamer or steamer with inset pan. Set this up over a high heat. If you don't have one, you can use a pan with a tight-fitting lid that's large enough to accommodate a 20 or 23cm (8 or 9in) cake tin. If you're using the pan method, pour in 750ml–1 litre (3–4 cups) of water and insert a deep cookie cutter or trivet to act as a stand for your tin. The cutter needs to be tall enough so that the water does not touch the bottom of the tin. Bring the water to the boil.

2   In a medium bowl, combine the turmeric, salt, yoghurt and hot water. Stir. Sift in the gram flour and whisk until thick and well mixed. (At this stage you can cover and leave to ferment for overnight or as long as possible – see tip on page 231.)

3   Lightly grease the cake tin. When the water in the saucepan is boiling, add the bicarbonate of soda (if using) and apple cider vinegar to the batter and whisk until the mixture is foamy and bubbly.

RECIPE CONTINUES…

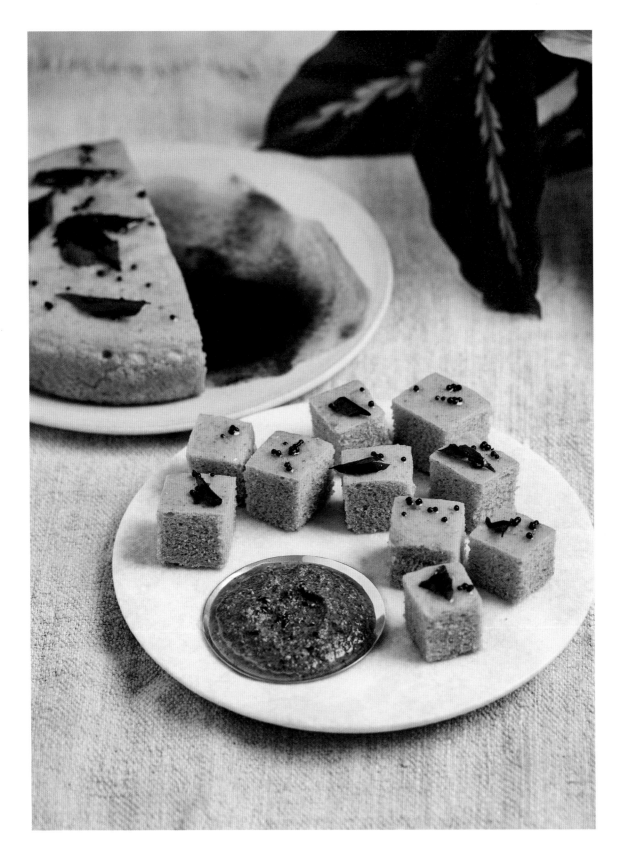

The traditional method of preparing dhokla involves a night of fermentation to make the batter bubbly and light. I speed up the process by using bicarbonate of soda, as if it were a quick bread. But if you want the 'slow food' experience, omit the soda and allow the batter to sit, covered, in a warm spot overnight.

4   Pour the batter into the tin and carefully lower it into the steamer. Cover with the tight-fitting lid and steam for about 20 minutes (or 25 minutes if using the smaller tin) over a medium heat. Test it with a toothpick – if it comes out clean, the dhokla is ready.

5   Carefully remove the tin from the steamer. Place a serving plate upside down over the top of the dhokla and quickly invert the pan, then lift it up, so the dhokla falls onto the plate.

6   To make the tarka, melt the ghee in a pan and toast the cumin and mustard seeds on a medium-high heat until they start to pop. Add the curry leaves, spring onion and finely sliced chilli and stir in the oil for a few minutes. Add the turmeric, asafoetida, tomato, sea salt and garlic and sauté for 2 minutes.

7   Cut the dhokla into pie-style slices or small squares, and pull the pieces apart slightly, so that the dhokla has room to expand as it absorbs the tarka. Pour the tarka in 60ml (¼ cup) measures all over the bread. Allow to cool for 10 minutes.

8   Meanwhile, to make the green chutney, blend all the ingredients apart from the chilli in a blender until smooth. Little by little, add the fresh chilli, if using, until you get the spice level you want. Check the seasoning and add more salt or lime juice if required.

9   Serve the dhokla with the green chutney.

This is one of my triumphs. I don't mind tooting my horn about it because not only do I love it but it's also a total game-changer. Like dipping bread into olive oil? Tick. Like spreading it with butter? Tick. Well, try ghee and a sprinkling of toasted cumin!

I've made so many bread alternatives over the years, and this has got to be one of the easiest to make, and being made with mung beans, easiest to digest. All it requires is delicious, protein-rich, super-cheap mung beans and no flour whatsoever, to make a simple base recipe which you can flavour as you like. Just like the original sourdough breads, this can be fermented overnight for better digestion. Who would have thought that you could get something so fluffy from whole mung beans?

Serves 8

Rosemary mung bean bread

250g (1¼ cups) whole mung beans, soaked overnight

2 tbsp extra-virgin olive oil, plus extra for greasing and to serve

½ tsp garlic powder

1 tbsp chopped rosemary, plus 1 sprig to decorate

½ tsp jaggery

¼ tsp asafoetida

½ tsp bicarbonate of soda

½ tsp sea salt, plus extra to serve

juice of 1 lemon (about 4 tbsp)

120ml (½ cup) lukewarm water

freshly ground black pepper, to serve

1 Drain the mung beans and divide them into two equal portions. Blend one portion to a soft purée with a dropping consistency. Blend the second portion for a few seconds so that you get a rough texture with no whole mung beans remaining. Mix the two portions together in a large bowl. If you can, ferment this paste in a warm spot overnight before continuing to the next step (this makes it better for digestion).

2 Grease a 20cm (8in) cake tin. Preheat the oven to 180ºC (fan 160ºC/gas mark 4).

3 In another bowl, add the oil, garlic, rosemary, jaggery, asafoetida, bicarbonate of soda, salt and lemon juice to the lukewarm water. Mix well, then immediately add it to the mung bean batter and transfer to the tin.

4 Bake the bread in the oven for 20–25 minutes or until lightly brown on top and springy to the touch. Decorate with the rosemary sprig, then cut into wedges and serve with extra-virgin olive oil, salt and pepper.

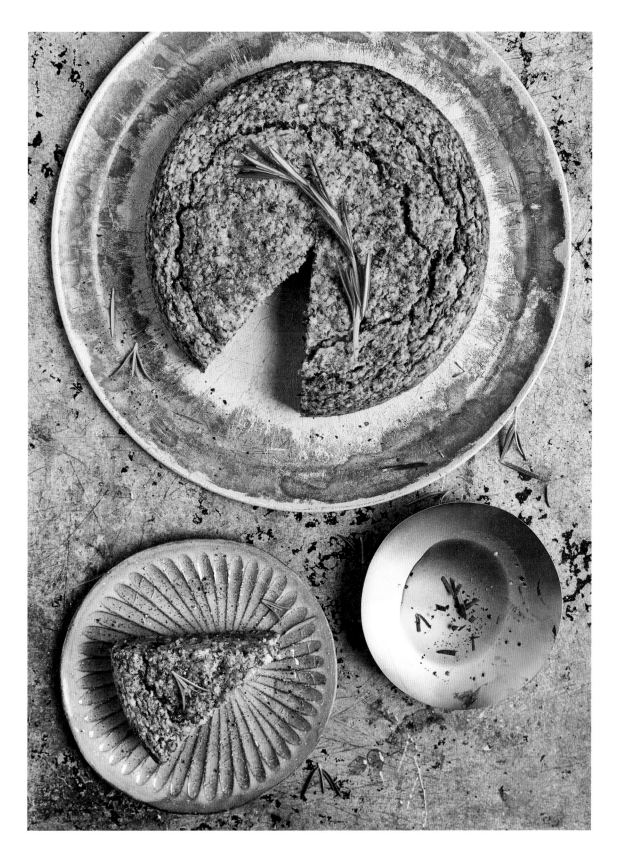

Chutneys and pickles

Whether cooked with spices or chopped and served fresh, chutneys and pickles help to stimulate Agni (see page 278) and therefore promote digestion. Some are quite sweet and some are quite sour, but it's a combination of both within a meal that Ayurveda recommends to cover two of the Tastes (see pages 285–287).

You only need 1–2 teaspoons of chutney to enhance your meal. Serve it directly on the plate or in a small bowl alongside your food for dipping flatbreads or appetisers. You can make and store chutneys in the fridge for several weeks, if they're cooked and preserved properly.

In addition to the famous Sri Lankan Sambal (see page 238), there's another spicy condiment from the same country (see page 237) and two fruit chutneys, which I think also make excellent jams if you leave out the vinegar, reduce the salt and add a touch more sweetness. Two recipes in one!

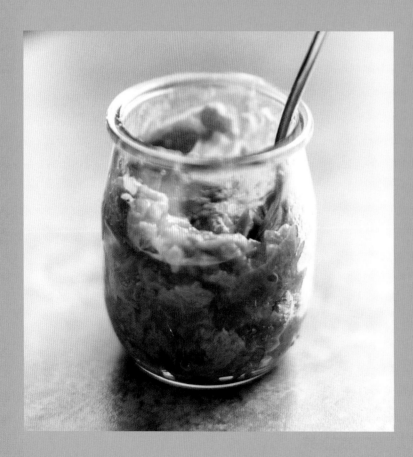

Rhubarb is a vegetable that's usually served as a dessert. Being super-tart in flavour (a subset of 'sour' which has a fruitiness to it), it's usually teamed with lashings of sugar to make it palatable. Here I play on that all-important sour taste to create a chutney that is used in small amounts to bring some piquantcy to a dish. Ginger and rhubarb are a match made in heaven, and this chutney teams beautifully with smoked fish such as mackerel, or grilled fresh fish, ham, cheese, lamb or duck.

To make it into a jam, swap out the vinegar, add only the tiniest pinch of salt and add an extra tablespoon of maple syrup. This won't set like the usual jams, which have a high sugar content, but it will be more of a compote.

Rhubarb is in abundance in late spring and early summer, when it's a nice time o make this – you could even give a jar to a friend who can enjoy it for a few more months to come.

○◑●

Makes 500g

Ginger and rhubarb chutney

500g rhubarb
2 small red onions, finely chopped
50ml (scant ¼ cup) apple cider vinegar
2.5cm (1in) piece of fresh ginger, finely chopped
4 tbsp maple syrup
pinch of chilli flakes
1 star anise
½ tsp sea salt

WORKS WITH

TOASTED BUCKWHEAT
BANANA BREAD
page 60

STEAMED
COCONUT PUDDING
page 112

1 Trim and wash the rhubarb, then slice it, like celery, into fairly fine chunks.

2 Put the onions, apple cider vinegar, ginger, maple syrup, chilli, star anise and salt in a large pan. Bring to the boil and cook for about 5 minutes, then add the rhubarb. Reduce the heat and simmer, lid off, for 15 minutes, until slightly thickened.

3 Remove the star anise and then spoon into a 500ml sterilised jar and allow to cool. Seal and keep in the fridge for up to 1 month.

This arrived in a daydream about a sticky jam that hit my taste buds and kept on giving. Something where sweet balanced salty, something with a punchy heat and umami flavour, something with plenty of texture and a little tang to carry it all through. Enjoy it like a chutney with your thali, spread it on crackers or hot buttered toast or serve with a cheeseboard on festive occasions. It's quite sweet, so if you're looking for more of a sour taste, then add a little more lime, lemon or apple cider vinegar. PICTURED ON PAGE 239.

Makes 250g

Black pepper, prune and sesame seed chutney

250g soft prunes

3 tbsp toasted
   sesame seeds

1 tbsp tahini

1 tsp freshly ground
   black pepper

3 tsp vanilla extract

1½ tbsp lemon or lime
   juice, or apple cider
   vinegar

2 pinches of sea salt

1½ tbsp ghee or sunflower
   oil (optional)

WORKS WITH

TEFF PINWHEELS
page 96

TEFF WAFFLES
page 79

STEAMED
COCONUT PUDDING
page 112

1   Place all of the ingredients in a food processor and process until smooth. Taste and adjust the flavours as needed. Store in the fridge for up to 1 week.

2   Alternatively, you could cook all the ingredients through with a little water in a medium saucepan over a medium heat until the water has evaporated and you get a thick consistency. Allow to cool and store in the fridge in a sterilized jar for up to 1 month.

Pickles are fresh or blanched vegetables preserved in brine or oil to make a chunkier, crisper and fresher condiment than a chutney or relish – although the British do love their quite jammy cooked pickles, which makes things confusing! This pickle is certainly fresh and crunchy and was a recipe taught to me in Sri Lanka for New Year celebrations. I particularly like the name of this recipe – similar to the name of a Filipino pickle called Achara, which is also made from green papaya.

Traditionally this is made in the special clay pots that Sri Lankans use to cook and store food. Because it is fermented, which relies on the natural bacteria, avoid metal equipment, which can adversely affect the bacteria. Instead choose glass or ceramic and use a wooden spoon. Enjoy the many different tastes that the pickle imparts and eat in small quantities with a meal. Make the pickle 2–3 days ahead, to allow it to mature before eating, and store for up to a month. PICTURED ON PAGE 239.

Makes 400g

Achucharu – Sri Lankan celebration pickle

50g red onions, thinly sliced
50g carrots, thinly sliced
50g green papaya, thinly sliced
50g green beans, thinly sliced
1–4 green chillies (about 50g), deseeded and thinly sliced

1 tsp mustard seeds, ground
100ml apple cider vinegar
2 tsp jaggery
1 tsp ground turmeric
¼ tsp chilli powder
1 tsp sea salt, or to taste
60ml (¼ cup) water

1 Place all of the ingredients in a medium pan and bring to the boil over a medium-high heat. Simmer for 1 minute and then allow to cool. Taste and adjust seasoning. Transfer to a sterilised jar and seal.

2 Store in a cool, dark place for 2–3 days to ferment. Keep in the fridge and use within a month as a side to any dish.

FEELING
PITTA

Make this recipe without
chilli, or avoid it until your
Pitta is more balanced.

Also known as pol sambol, coconut sambal is a classic condiment from Sri Lanka. A spicy dry chutney served with everything from rice to string hoppers (rice noodles), it imparts a zesty, tangy and very spicy flavour, thanks to plenty of onion, chilli and lime.

Serves 4

Coconut sambal is one of the most popular side dishes in Sri Lanka – enjoyed with breakfast, lunch and dinner. I have re-created a milder version that uses leek to keep this more Sattvic (see page 14) and has just a tiny pinch of chilli, along with paprika to add colour without too much heat. It is best prepared with fresh coconut, but desiccated coconut is still delicious. If you do manage to find fresh coconut, there's no need to add the hot water. To serve, garnish with a sprinkle of ground paprika and take it straight to the table.

Coconut sambal

60g (¾ cup) desiccated coconut
30g leek, finely diced
1½ tbsp lime juice
pinch of finely grated lime zest
¼ tsp sea salt

pinch of cayenne pepper
pinch of chilli powder
3½ tbsp hot water
2 tsp ground paprika, to serve

1 Toss the ingredients together with the hot water and leave to sit for 10 minutes for the flavours to come together.

2 Garnish with the paprika and serve. This is best eaten on the same day.

FEELING
PITTA

Leave out the
chilli powder and enjoy
the cooling coconut
and lime.

FEELING
KAPHA

Enjoy the chilli,
adding more to taste
if you like.

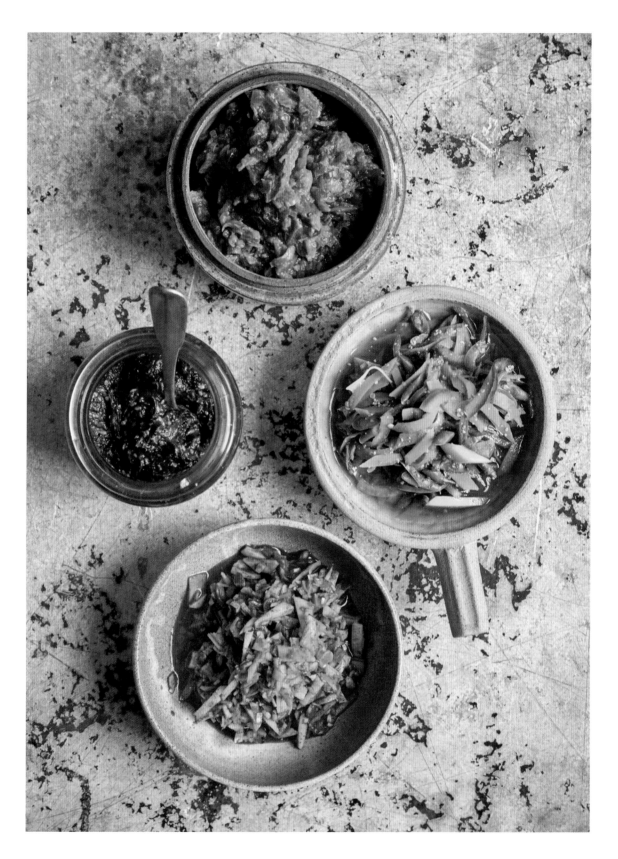

Ideal for sipping after a meal, fennel helps soothe upset tummies and prevent fermentation in digestion. Its diuretic effects also help to flush out impurities. It has anti-inflammatory and carminative properties, as well as a sweet, liquorice flavour.

Serves 1

Fennel tea

1 tsp dried fennel seeds
250ml (1 cup) boiling water

1   Put the fennel seeds into a tea pot or cup with the boiling water. Make sure you do not boil the seeds as this destroys most of the nutrients.

2   Cover, allow to steep for up to 10 minutes and enjoy.

. . . .

Sebastian Pole of Pukka Herbs is a pioneer of Ayurveda in the UK, and his products have gone mainstream – helping to share the wisdom of Ayurveda. The wide selection of Pukka Herbs teas are everywhere, and growing in popularity every day – my friend in New York demands I send her favourite (Three Liquorice) in the post. Sebastian's tea recipe for Natural Balance – a fiery, digestion enhancer – is designed to get Agni going (see page 278), helping you burn fat via a lively digestive fire. Assembling it feels like a proper apothecary session, working with the medicine of nature. It's tangy and pungent with natural caffeine from the green tea. Sip as a morning cuppa or with lunch, but no later. This is also a great pick-me-up – premix it in a jar and take it to work with a little bottle of orange essential oil, swapping the cinnamon stick for ground cinnamon and leaving out the orange zest. The office will smell amazing, so be prepared to share!

Serves 2–3

Natural Balance tea, by Pukka Herbs

4g cinnamon stick
2g ground ginger
2g orange zest
2g matcha tea powder
1g freshly ground
    black pepper

1g ground turmeric
500ml (2 cups)
    boiling water
2–3 drops of orange
    essential oil

1   Put all of the ingredients, apart from the water and the orange essential oil, in a teapot.

2   Add the boiling water. Steep for 10–15 minutes, then strain. Add 1 drop of orange essential oil to each cup.

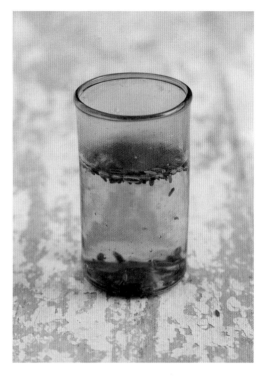

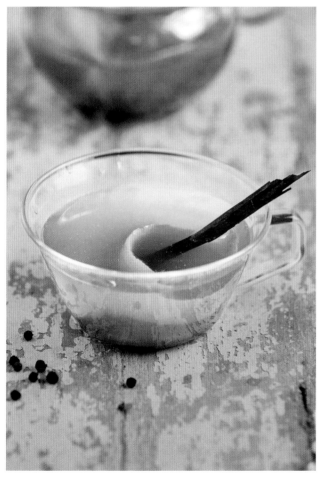

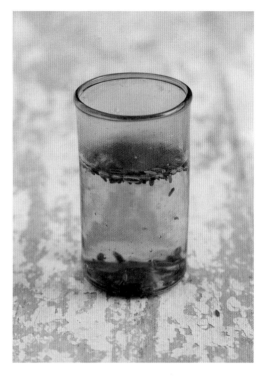

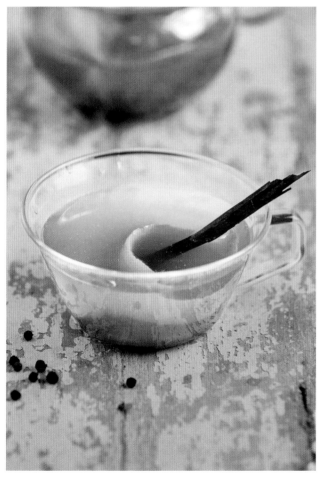

Salabat tea is especially popular during the relatively cool month of December in the Philippines, accompanied by seasonal treats. The hot drink is also recommended for a sore throat.

Generally speaking, we Pinoys (Filipinos) are not huge tea drinkers. In fact, if someone visits your house and you offer them some tea instead of coffee they would respond by saying, 'I am feeling well, thank you' or 'But I am not sick.' That's because tea in the Philippines is usually recommended for when someone is not feeling well.

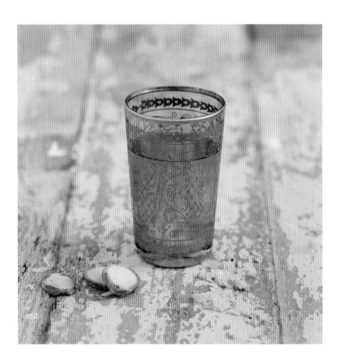

Salabat – Filipino ginger tea

5cm (2in) piece
of fresh ginger
1 litre (4 cups) water
1 tbsp jaggery
juice of ½ lemon,
if desired

FEELING
PITTA

Avoid this tea!

1 Finely slice the fresh ginger and transfer to a small saucepan over a medium heat. Pour in the water and the jaggery and simmer for 8–25 minutes, depending on how potent you want it (you might want to add more water).

2 Strain and serve hot or room temperature.

Tulsi, also known as holy basil, appears in sacred Indian scriptures from 5,000 years ago and has long been used as a folk remedy to support the immune system. It is packed full of antioxidants, and helps reduce inflammation, bloating and digestive gas. It also has antiseptic, anti-ageing and anti-stress properties, helps to regulate sugar and cholesterol levels and is very drying, so is excellent for Kapha.

Holy basil is reputed to have spiritual properties capable of cleansing the body and even spaces (many families have it in their homes), as well as promoting purity and lifting the life-force. This tea has a strong aroma, with an astringent, deep and spicy taste. Choose a white teacup or glass to enjoy the golden colour.

Serves 1

PICTURED ON PAGE 244.

Tulsi tea

FEELING
VATA

Enjoy occasionally.

FEELING
PITTA

Avoid this tea and stick
to fresh mint tea.

1 Add 1 teaspoon of dried tulsi leaves to a tea pot or cup with a teacup of boiling water. Cover and allow to steep for around 5 minutes.

2 Strain and add a little jaggery and whole milk if you wish.

. . . .

Forgetting things? Having trouble concentrating? Remember rosemary. Used to awaken the brain and improve memory, this tea can help you think better, faster, and clearer.

It also helps to calm digestion, detox the liver, relieve indigestion and flatulence, and is used to treat colds and other respiratory problems. Try it to treat depression and anxiety. PICTURED ON PAGE 244.

Serves 1

Rosemary tea

2 sprigs of rosemary
250ml (1 cup) boiling water

1 Place the rosemary in a teapot. Add the freshly boiled water. Cover and leave to steep for 10–15 minutes, then strain.

Normally we hear about flaxseeds because they are packed full of omega-3 essential fats; not so well known is that flax tea is also therapeutic and very hydrating.

Water around our cells is like oil in an engine; without it, they can't function properly. Even if you have a great diet, your body can't take advantage of it if you are dehydrated. The answer is to drink more, but if you are stressed your body can be like a badly watered hanging basket. The water just goes straight through, hardly touching the sides! Flax tea helps, because it is slightly gelatinous – this soothes and relaxes the colon, and allows it to absorb more water.

Makes 1 litre

Super-hydrating flax tea

1 tsp flaxseeds
1 litre (4 cups) water
your favourite tea bag,
    such as ginger, rooibos
    or peppermint

1   Add the flaxseeds and water to a saucepan, bring to the boil and simmer for 20 minutes. Cover the pan and leave the flaxseeds to soak for 12 hours or overnight. Strain – it should be just a bit thicker than water and have a faint nutty taste.

2   To drink, make your usual pot of tea. While it is brewing, fill up your mug with the flax tea until it reaches just under half full and then top up the rest with your hot tea. Stir well and drink fairly quickly as it will not be very hot!

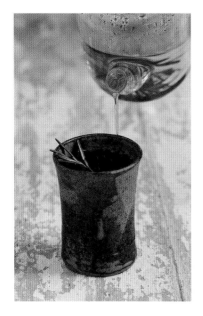
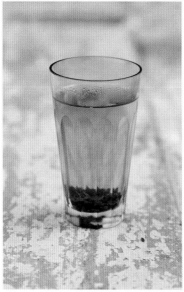
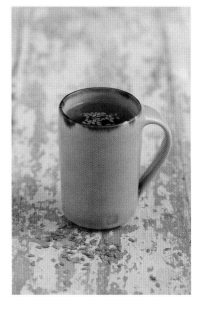

A small dish of these is often found near the exit of Indian restaurants (sometimes with a sugary, coloured coating). Chewing fennel seeds after a meal is a common practice in India for freshening the breath, but it also helps digestion and calms and strengthens the stomach's function. Both toasting the seeds and mixing with sea salt helps to enhance Agni (see page 278).

In Ayurveda, fennel seeds balance all three Doshas. Great for relieving tension, these powerful little seeds can also assist with urinary problems, lung congestion, constipation, flatulence and bloating. Swap your mints for fennel seeds, and get chewing! Your tummy (and breath) will thank you.

Serves 1

Toasted fennel seeds

1 tbsp fennel seeds

1   Toast the fennel seeds in a dry saucepan until golden and fragrant.

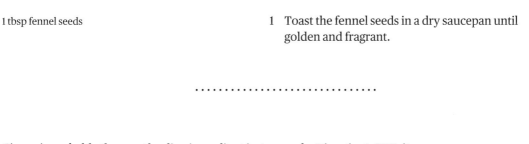

Ginger is probably the most healing ingredient in Ayurveda. Digestion's BFF, it helps to relieve gas and soothe the intestinal tract. Fresh ginger is used for digestion and nausea, while ground ginger is used for colds and respiratory illnesses. Ginger, salt and lime before or after a meal stimulates digestion by increasing Pitta.

For those days when you feel bloated, when you have over-indulged, feel nauseous or in need of a little digestive support, this ginger aid will boost your digestion and increase your metabolism. Eat it 15–30 minutes before lunch and dinner to prepare your digestion for food. Think of it as a healing appetiser.

Serves 1

Raw ginger with salt and lime

5cm (2in) piece
   of fresh ginger
juice of ½ lime
½ tsp good-quality sea salt

1   Peel the ginger. Cut it into thin slices and squeeze the lime juice over the top. Sprinkle with the salt and mix.

2   Allow the ginger to marinate for 1–1½ hours, if desired, or enjoy immediately. Eat a few slices of the ginger before your lunch and dinner.

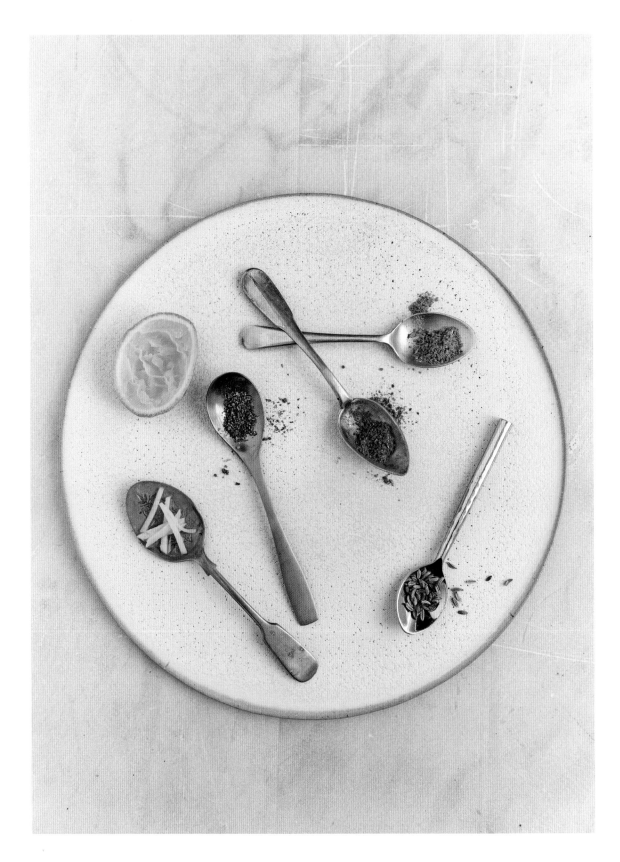

Using the wisdom of Ayurveda, a well-formed spice mix contains all six Tastes (see page 285–287), helping to bring nutritional balance as well as satisfaction to a dish. Pack some up and take it on your travels to sprinkle over everything.

Makes 100g (½ cup)

Kiss goodbye to the stale spices in your cupboard and make your own fresh spice powders, known as churnas or choonas. These medicinal spice mixes are your 'get out of jail' cards, helping to make sure your Agni (see page 278) is burning nicely. I mostly need to manage my Vata Dosha, so often make two batches – one with asafoetida and salt for savoury dishes and one without for sweet dishes. I'd recommend this, unless you like to bring garlic- or onion-like flavour to your puds!

Dosha churna spice mix

FOR VATA

2 tbsp fennel seeds
1 tbsp coriander seeds
1 tbsp cumin seeds
1 tbsp ground turmeric
2 tsp ground ginger
2 tsp sea salt
1 tsp asafoetida
1 tbsp jaggery

FOR PITTA

2 tbsp fennel seeds
2 tbsp coriander seeds
2 tbsp dried mint
seeds of 20 cardamom
   pods
½ tsp saffron strands
¼ tsp ground ginger
1 tbsp cinnamon

FOR KAPHA

2 tbsp coriander seeds
1 tbsp cumin seeds
1 tbsp fenugreek seeds
1 tbsp ground ginger
1 tbsp ground turmeric
1 tbsp ground cinnamon
1 tsp ground cloves
¼ tsp freshly ground
   black pepper
¼ tsp chilli powder or
   cayenne pepper

TIP

·

You could make a quick tarka to enhance your dals, veggie and lentil soups, baked casseroles, curries and stews. Simply heat up some ghee or hot oil, take off the heat and then stir in the churna spice mix. Quickly pour over your dish.

1 Grind all of the whole seeds in a pestle and mortar, then gently toast the spices in a dry frying pan over medium heat until fragrant, stirring frequently.

2 Leave to cool completely, then store in an airtight container somewhere dark for 6–8 weeks. It's best to make spice mixes in small batches to keep the potency of the spices, so halve the mixture if you think you'll need less in that time.

This is a cough syrup and cold-relief remedy made from just two ingredients and a jar. The old-school remedy was given to me by one of my best friends, who is Polish – she loved this cough medicine so much that even if she didn't have a cough she used to sneak into the kitchen for a spoonful or two. Very simply slices of onion layered with sugar and left to marinate, this remedy is best enjoyed every few hours for coughs and colds. I leave it out overnight to create even more of a syrup and then store it in the fridge for the next 24 hours. After that it's best to make a fresh batch.

Onion contains a milder form of some of the active components in garlic, but both strengthen the immune system, work as natural antibiotics, anti-inflammatories and expectorants, which means they loosen mucus so you can cough it up. I've updated this recipe with raw honey, which is a great natural antiviral, antibacterial, antifungal that's also soothing for itchy and irritated throats. For a thicker syrup and for young kids, use jaggery in place of the honey.

This is cheaper, tastes better than it sounds and is healthier (and probably more effective) than over-the-counter cough medicine. PICTURED ON PAGE 252.

○◐●

Makes 1 jar

Honey and onion cough syrup

1 medium red or white
    onion (red is less harsh
    in flavour)
340g (about 1 cup) raw
    honey or jaggery

1 Slice the onion into rounds. Place a round in the bottom of a 500ml (2 cup) airtight jar with a layer of honey over the top. Continue alternating these layers until you've used up all of the onion.

2 Cover tightly and allow to sit overnight or for 8–12 hours. There will now be liquid in the jar: take a spoonful as needed to control your cough (aim for three spoonfuls an hour, up to four times a day).

TIP
.

If you're coughing up mucus, avoid suppressing it. The action of coughing is important to loosen phlegm or mucus and get it out of your lungs.

This deep purple, clear broth is a rejuvenating blood-builder, rich in potassium, which helps to flush out toxins and replace electrolytes. A long, slow simmer helps to draw out the goodness from these carefully chosen vegetables to deliver microminerals to the body with barely any digestion required. Unlike the usual Ayurvedic recipes, this one can be made in bulk as it is more of a medicine than a meal and is focused less on the Prana (see page 16) and more on medicinal values. If you're unwell, have a small bowl of this instead of dinner, and when you're back on your feet try this as a remedy 30 minutes before meals, so as not to dilute its effect. It's a medicine, so don't eat this every day – instead, freeze in portions so that you can access it whenever you need to.

You could turn the leftover vegetables/pulp into another dish, flavoured with a tarka (see page 265). PICTURED ON PAGE 252.

Serves 10

Potassium broth

3 medium potatoes, scrubbed but not peeled

3 medium carrots, scrubbed but not peeled

1 large onion, peeled

1 medium beetroot, peeled

2 sticks of celery, halved

50g (½ cup) shredded red cabbage

7.5g (¼ cup) parsley stalks

1 bay leaf

2.4 litres (10 cups) water

1   Roughly chop the vegetables and combine everything in a large pan. Bring to the boil and simmer, lid on, for 2 hours on a very low heat.

2   Carefully strain the broth using a large slotted spoon or a colander to remove the large pieces of vegetables and then either allow the broth to settle and ladle from the top or further strain through a muslin or cheesecloth to remove the tiniest pieces for a clear broth. The broth should be as clear as possible for easy digestion.

3   Pour the broth into several jars which you can keep in the fridge and enjoy over 2 days, or freeze in portions.

TIP
.

Storing the broth in the fridge in smaller portions means you don't disturb the nutrients as much as if you were to keep pouring from the same pot. You can also freeze the broth as ice cubes and store for 3–4 weeks for use post-workout, remembering not to do it every day.

This is a great go-to recipe for warm weather, or days when you're just not feeling yourself. The ingredient combination is particularly cleansing and refreshing on the palate – calming for your digestive system, and a great way to ensure a joyful belly! You can also enjoy this with Dosha Churna Spice Mix (see page 247) instead of the ginger apple juice – it makes a lovely refreshing drink for guests as an alternative to wine in the summer. PICTURED ON PAGE 252.

Serves 6–8

Fennel, mint, salt and grape refresher

600g red or black grapes
200g fennel
25g fresh mint leaves
150ml (⅔ cup) water
large pinch of salt

TIP
·
Cook the pulp and use
to top porridge.

1 Place the grapes, fennel and mint in a blender and roughly blend, adding 60ml (¼ cup) of the water. Retain a little texture, rather than blending until smooth, so that the grape seeds don't get blended and go brown. (Alternatively, use green seedless grapes and blend until smooth.)

2 Place a fine-mesh sieve over a large jug and pour in the pulp. Add a weight if you like, or pound with a rolling pin, to press through as much juice as possible.

3 Set the pulp aside and stir the remaining water and the salt into the liquid. Serve.

A South Indian soup made with pungent spices and sour tamarind, Rasam or 'king soup' is an Ayurvedic hug in a mug. It's the Indian chicken soup for the soul and food to feed a cold, opening up the sinuses and melting away the mucus. I learnt how to make it at Vana Ayurveda Retreat in northern India. Being mostly Vata Dosha, which loves sour and salty, I had one taste of this hot, peppery, tangy soup and was hooked. Its Agni-boosting qualities stir the appetite and revitalise, which also makes it a good starter at Indian weddings to aid the feasting.

Serves 2

There are different ways to make and enjoy Rasam. Some are just broths flavoured with the essential oils of the aromatic spices and others include lentils to make it more nourishing. If digestion is compromised by illness, then those made with lentils are gently strained so that the broth remains clear while taking on the extra nourishment from the dal. Otherwise, it is served as a soupy dal over a bowl of hot basmati rice. I love this recipe in the winter as a suppertime staple to combat the wet and cold, and to add balance when we are gearing up for holiday festivities.
PICTURED ON PAGE 252.

Rasam

80g toor dal or split
    mung dal, soaked for
    at least 2 hours
1 tbsp ghee
1 tsp black mustard seeds
2 bay leaves
2 cinnamon sticks
1 tsp coriander seeds
4 cloves
5 black peppercorns
6 curry leaves

1 clove garlic, crushed
2.5cm (1in) piece of fresh
    ginger, crushed
1½ tsp tamarind paste (see
    page 260)
1 litre (4 cups) water
25g fresh coriander, stalks
    and leaves, chopped
sea salt, to taste

1 Rinse the dal two to three times and drain. Melt the ghee in a medium saucepan over medium-high heat, then add the mustard seeds and cook until they start to pop. Add the remaining spices and curry leaves and fry for 2 minutes.

2 Add the garlic and ginger and fry for another 2 minutes, then add the tamarind paste and cook for 5 minutes. Add the dal and water and bring to the boil. Reduce the heat and simmer, lid on, for 30 minutes.

3 Taste and adjust the seasoning. Strain gently without pressing to get a thin broth, otherwise enjoy as a soup or over rice. Garnish with the coriander and add a pinch of salt to taste before serving.

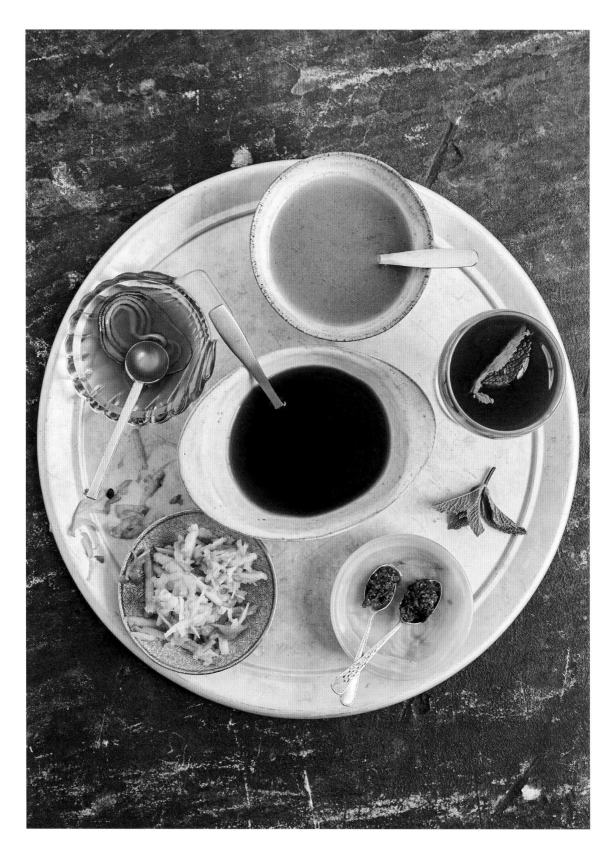

Made from Kapha-pacifying pungent spices and honey to heat and detoxify the body, this coarse thick paste is the Ayurvedic remedy for coughs, head colds and sinus infections... and it tastes delicious. You'll need a taste for pungent spices, but combining them with a little cinnamon and honey makes the medicine go down. I've used whole peppercorns, cloves, cinnamon sticks and fresh ginger here to ensure the active ingredients of these spices are as fresh as possible but otherwise go for the ground spices.

Serves 2

Respiratory remedy

12 black peppercorns
8 cloves
1cm (½in) piece of fresh
   ginger, chopped, or
   1 tsp ground ginger

1 cinnamon stick, broken,
   or ½ tsp ground
   cinnamon
1 tsp raw honey

1 In a pestle and mortar, crush and grind the peppercorns, cloves, ginger and cinnamon as finely as possible.

2 Transfer to a bowl and stir in the honey to make a paste.

. . . .

In Ayurveda, diarrhoea is said to be the result of weak digestive fire causing the accelerated movement of food through the digestive system. This super-simple recipe has come in handy over the years, especially during my travels as it's usually relatively easy to find apples.

Serves 1

This is a great example of an Ayurvedic remedy making its way into other cultures, with this one being known as a classic household cure for an upset stomach. There are two main types of upset stomach: infection from parasites or bacteria; or a reaction to stress, emotional upset or poor food choices. Since the diarrhoea is a natural response by the body – an attempt to flush out toxins – we should if possible honour this natural purification and support our body by staying at home and resting, abstaining from food but making sure we stay hydrated by drinking hot water with a pinch of salt and a teaspoon of honey every now and then. The second stage is to eat light soups, such as watery Kitchari (see page 184), plain Lassis (see pages 118–121) and this simple remedy.

Brown apple

1 Grate 1 apple, then leave it for 20 minutes–1 hour to go brown. Eat it slowly, chewing well.

In India, paneer, a type of fresh cheese, comes in two forms – soft and firm. Soft paneer is just like whole-milk ricotta and the methods for making both are very similar. All you need is a decent sieve and muslin or cheesecloth – or a clean chef's hairnet, which also does the trick!

Here is an oh-so-easy (and quick!) recipe for super-fresh homemade ricotta or soft paneer and then instructions on how to turn it into firm paneer. Ricotta is much lighter to digest than other cheeses because it has less milk fat in it. Traditionally it's made from the whey that's left over after making other types of hard cheeses, but since we're not cheesemakers we make it with whole milk for a creamier ricotta.

Delicious when seasoned and flavoured with herbs, ricotta and paneer make lovely protein additions to many meals. Try ricotta with olive oil on toast (see page 53) or in place of the cottage cheese in Saffron Cardamom Cheesecake with a Millionaire Crust (see page 212). Use paneer in the Golden Paneer with Tomato-y Green Beans and Carrots (see page 152).

Whey is a cheesemaking by-product and contains all the water-soluble proteins, vitamins and minerals that didn't make it into the cheese. Add the leftover whey from your ricotta or paneer to smoothies, use it for Light Lassis instead of yoghurt and water (see pages 118–121) or best of all, make my mum's Wahay Soup, which is delicious with dumplings (see page 202).

TIP
·

Some people leave the curds until they become really tight before straining but this makes a very grainy ricotta. I prefer to strain the curds earlier when they are still pillowy and soft.

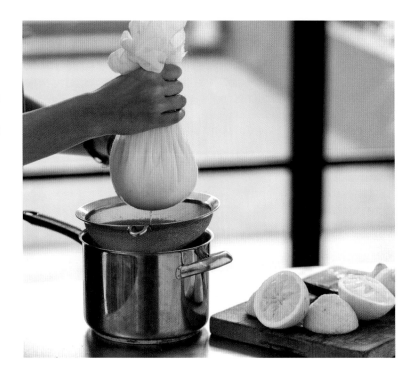

Ricotta and paneer

2 litres (8 cups) whole
   organic milk
   (preferably
   unhomogenised)
75ml (⅓ cup) lemon juice
   (from 1–2 lemons) or
   apple cider vinegar
1–4 tsp sea salt

FEELING
KAPHA

Avoid eating paneer,
or too much ricotta, due
to its sticky quality.

1   In a large saucepan, heat the milk gradually until it comes to the boil, then boil it for 20 seconds.

2   Remove the milk from the heat. Gently stir in the lemon juice and 1 teaspoon of the salt and leave to sit undisturbed for 10 minutes. The milk will start to separate into milky white curds and pale yellow watery whey. If the curds do not separate then return the pan to the heat and bring gently up to the boil again and simmer for a few minutes – the curds should separate at this point. If you're making paneer, stir in another 3 teaspoons of salt.

3   Set a sieve or strainer over a bowl and line with a muslin, cheesecloth or clean tea towel. Gently pour the mixture into the bowl – transferring some of the bigger curds with a slotted spoon first can help reduce the splashing.

4   Let the cheese strain for 10–30 minutes if you're making ricotta, depending on how wet or dry you prefer your ricotta – I prefer it after 10 minutes. If the ricotta becomes too dry, stir some of the whey back in before using or storing it. The ricotta is now ready to eat.

5   If you're making paneer, prepare it as above but leave it to strain for 1 hour. Then, keeping the paneer fairly tight in its cloth, place it into a wide shallow tray, folding the cloth over the top of the paneer.

6   Take a heavy-bottomed pan (a cast-iron skillet or a griddle pan is ideal) and place it on top of the paneer and leave to stand for 30–40 minutes or until it is flattened into a firm block. Cut into cubes or crumble, depending on how you want to use it.

7   Fresh ricotta and paneer can be used right away or refrigerated in an airtight container for up to a week, but it is best to use it within 1–2 days so that it's fresh, easy to digest and therefore Sattvic (see page 14).

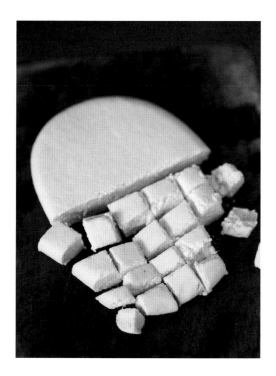

Here is an easy egg substitute which works well in many recipes, including the Chestnut, Carrot and Ginger Muffins (see page 72) and Teff Waffles (see page 78). Freshly ground flax works best to make it as thick as possible – you'll need a spice grinder, coffee grinder or a powerful blender. Just mix and leave to set, moving it to the fridge if it needs help with thickening.

Flax egg

1½ tbsp ground flax
2½ tbsp cold water

1 Mix the ground flax and cold water together in a small bowl. Allow to sit for 5 minutes.

. . . .

Ayurveda has long considered almond milk to be very nourishing, Sattvic nuts that help to produce Ojas (see page 16). Almonds are packed with protein and nutrients, and are rejuvenating and strength-building. They are also believed to nourish the bones and the deeper tissues of the nervous and reproductive systems. I recommend removing the skin from the almonds, which not only makes them more digestible, but also makes the milk snow-white and oh-so pretty. Try it, you will never go back!

Makes 150ml
(⅔ cup)

Almond milk

10 almonds, soaked
    overnight
150ml (⅔ cup) water
pinch of sea salt

1 Rinse and drain the almonds and squeeze or peel the outer skin off. Put the nuts in a powerful blender and add the water. Add the salt and blend until smooth. Strain the milk, if desired.

3 Use immediately or keep in the fridge and consume within 3–4 days. Since there are no preservatives or fillers, this milk may separate once stored – shake or stir before using.

A powerful blender will make short work of this – just be sure to make sure the rice is as soft and cooked as possible. White rice is easier to work with to make it smooth. This makes a thick milk which you can then adjust yourself with a bit more water. Keep it this thick if you're using it to make the Coconut Creams (see page 114).

Makes 500ml
(2 cups)

Rice milk

50g (¼ cup) brown basmati rice soaked overnight, rinsed and drained, or 50g (¼ cup) white basmati rice, rinsed thoroughly

575–620ml (2⅓–2½ cups) water
1 tsp jaggery, or to taste
tiny pinch of salt

TIP
.

To strain these milks, use a fine-mesh sieve first to get most of the solids out, and then squeeze through a clean tea towel or several thicknesses of muslin or cheesecloth.

1 Place the rice in a saucepan and add 100ml (generous ⅓ cup) water if you're cooking basmati rice and 150ml (⅔ cup) water if you're cooking brown rice. Bring to the boil and then simmer until very overcooked.

2 Transfer to a blender with another 250ml (1 cup) water and blend until as smooth as possible, before adding another 250ml (1 cup) water, plus the jaggery and salt. Blend again. Taste and add more jaggery and water if needed. Strain the milk, if desired. Use immediately or keep in the fridge and consume within 1–2 days.

. . . .

Coconut milk is another easy-to-make dairy alternative. Find several methods below – tinned coconut milk is the easiest option but the BPA used to line the tins makes it the least favourable. Although they are wrapped in plastic, creamed coconut bars are the better choice, but they can make a slightly grainier milk unless you strain it.

Drinking coconut milk

USING DESSICATED
MAKES 750ML
125–160g (1½–2 cups) desiccated coconut or fresh coconut flesh plus 1 litre (4 cups) hot water

USING TINNED
MAKES 250ML
60ml (¼ cup) full-fat coconut milk plus 175ml (¾ cup) water

Thicker texture: 75ml (⅓ cup) coconut milk plus 150ml (⅔ cup) water

USING CREAMED
MAKES 100ML
20g creamed coconut plus 80ml (just over ⅓ cup) water
Or for thicker:
25g creamed coconut plus 75ml (⅓ cup) water

1 Add the ingredients to the blender and blend on high for several minutes until thick and creamy. Strain the milk, if desired. Use immediately or keep in the fridge and consume within 1–2 days.

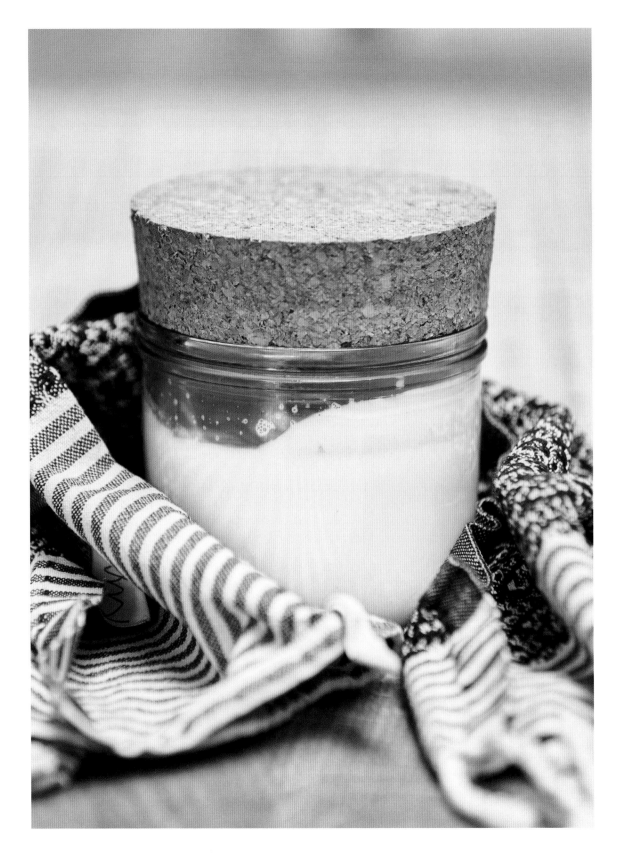

Freshly made yoghurt is wonderfully nourishing in small amounts. It aids the digestion of other foods and replenishes the good bacteria in the body, and is also an effective remedy for indigestion and upset stomachs, which is why you'll find it used throughout the book as a condiment (see Beetroot Raita, page 226) and a digestive aid (see Lassis, pages 118–121). Sweet and sour in taste and slightly heating in quality, it's great for pacifying Vata and Pitta. However, eaten in large amounts or with the wrong foods, yoghurt is not a digestive aid at all! Avoid eating it every day, in cold weather and cold seasons, or for breakfast and your evening meal, and do not mix with fresh fruit, milk, cream, cheese, eggs, hot drinks, nightshade vegetables, lemons, meat or fish (see food combining information on page 22).

Homemade yoghurt is super-easy and quick to make, and if you can find non-homogenised or raw milk you are getting an even more natural product. I eat yoghurt every other day at most, which means I usually only make it a couple of times a week and eat it fresh the next day. I make it at the same time as my evening milk, and only in small quantities at a time unless I'm expecting guests.

Makes about 250g
(1 cup)

Yoghurt

250ml (1 cup) milk
1 tbsp live-culture yoghurt

1 The day before you wish to serve, bring the milk to the boil. Pour into a heatproof glass jar or insulated flask and allow to cool to room temperature.

2 Mix in the live-culture yoghurt. If you are using a glass jar, wrap it in a towel. Otherwise, screw on the thermos lid. Store overnight in a warm place, such as the airing cupboard or the oven with the light on.

3 The next morning you will have fresh yoghurt. Store it in the fridge and eat at room temperature within 1–2 days, saving 1 tablespoon to make the next batch.

FEELING
PITTA

FEELING
KAPHA

TIP

Homemade yoghurt that is left to ferment and go sour beyond 48 hours can aggravate Pitta. Avoid eating it when it is too cold or in large amounts.

Avoid eating in large amounts, especially at breakfast or dinner when the digestive fire isn't as strong.

The tablespoon left over from the last batch will keep well in the fridge for up to a week to use for your next batch. You can also mix this up with full-fat coconut milk, which is nice and cooling for summer.

Tomato is beloved of many cuisines and adds sour and stimulating taste, but is highly acidic so is considered Rajasic (see page 14). It is good for Kapha, but should be kept to a minimum for Vata and Pitta. The skins and seeds are irritating for some, so Ayurveda recommends skinning and deseeding them.

Skinning and deseeding tomatoes

1 For tomato chunks: score an 'X' into the base of each tomato and place in a bowl. Cover in boiling water and leave for a minute. Peel off the skin, cut in half and use a teaspoon to scoop out the seeds.

2 For tomato sauce: roughly blend, then pour into a sieve, using the back of a spoon to push through the tomato juices leaving behind the skins and seeds.

. . . .

Sour is an essential taste in Ayurveda, usually added with limes, tomatoes or tamarind – a sweet-sour Asian fruit. Tamarind is usually sold as blocks of the dried fruit or as a ready-made paste. The paste is convenient but varies in taste, strength and additional ingredients, so if you like tamarind and want the true flavour it's worth knowing how to work with the blocks, which last for ever in the cupboard and are cheap to buy. Tamarind pulp is very fibrous so you need to soak and separate it, which also catches any rogue seeds that are in the block.

Makes about 60g (¼ cup)

Tamarind paste

50g (¼ cup) tamarind block (a piece about the size of a lemon)
120ml (½ cup) hot water

TIP
·
Save the soaking water to add to dals, curries, stews or broths or to make a refreshing drink with a little jaggery. Avoid if you're feeling Pitta, though!

1 Cover the tamarind with the water. Roughly speaking you'll get just over half the volume of paste from the pulp.

2 Allow the pulp to sit for 15 minutes until softened. Use your fingers or a fork to mash it up a bit, then press the soaked tamarind a little at a time through a fine-mesh sieve, using a stiff spatula to work it against the mesh, leaving behind a smooth thick tamarind paste with an apple sauce-like consistency. Use the tamarind paste in your recipe.

I've been a huge fan of bone broth for years. I love its hot, clear, sweet, umami qualities, not just for the flavour it imparts and the easy-to-digest nutrition it delivers, but also for its soothing and healing capacities. A traditionally made, long-cooked bone broth can help strengthen your immune system and improve digestive health, and just as like increases like, it supports the joints and bones. It's during the long cooking process that more vitamins, minerals and proteins are drawn from the bones, including the amino acids that make collagen, the most healing nutrient found in bone broth – and one that is evident by the gelatinous texture that forms when it cools.

Makes about 1 litre

Choose organic fish, chicken, turkey, duck, lamb or venison bones, to avoid added hormones, antibiotics, chemicals and pesticides. Ask the butcher or use leftovers from your meals and simmer for up to 24 hours – the bigger the bones, the longer the simmering time.

The cooking time will also vary, depending on the cooking method you use. You can make bone broth on the stove or in a slowcooker. A slowcooker is the easiest as well as the most cost-effective way of making broth, and it means you can keep the slowcooker running if you like to enjoy fresh broth over a couple of days.

Bone broth

bones from 1 chicken
1 tbsp apple cider vinegar
    or lemon juice
6 black peppercorns
2 bay leaves

1.5–2.25 litres (6–9 cups)
    filtered water,
    depending on size
    of pot

1   Place all the ingredients in a slowcooker or large saucepan. Cover and cook on low heat for 6–8 hours, bringing the water to the boil first and then reducing to a simmer if cooking on a stovetop.

2   Remove the lid and take out the vegetables and chicken bones with a slotted spoon or run the broth through a sieve. Strain the broth through a fine-mesh sieve and use. If it is particularly fatty, skim the surface with a slotted spoon or allow to cool completely to make skimming easier – the fat will solidify on top of the stock as it cools.

TIP

Chicken feet help create a gelatinous and nutritious broth. Don't worry, you will remove them before consuming the broth. If you can't find chicken feet, ask your butcher for a few chicken neck bones.

For a more concentrated broth you can also simmer, with the lid off to further reduce it, but be prepared for a steamy kitchen!

3   Alternatively, continue to cook on a low heat, adding ladlefuls to your recipes as you go.

Using spices

Ready to spice up your life? Stocking up on spices can help you turn your pantry into your medicine cabinet. Disease-fighting, immunity-building, capable of lowering blood-sugar levels, effective as painkillers and for weight-loss, those jars lurking in your cupboards were considered more valuable than gold during the Roman Empire. Such are their therapeutic powers that they are said to have been the cause for numerous invasions of India over the centuries.

The fun part is experimenting with spices: adding a little spice to everything – from the usual curries, soups and stir-fries to sweets, hot drinks and cakes. I refer to fresh herbs and spices throughout, but I also include some dried herbs, which are great to fall back on. To substitute dried herbs for fresh, the general rule is that 1 teaspoon of dried is equal to 3 teaspoons of finely chopped fresh herbs.

Whether it's just the one or two spices singing out or a medley of mingling flavours, the trick is to cook the spices just right for both flavour and digestive effect, being careful not to overcook or burn them. If they do burn, make sure you start again, as they can completely ruin your dish.

Through the wisdom of Ayurveda we know that spices must be as fresh as possible, prepared in a certain way, and used in the right amounts and of course in balance to each other. As you can see from the Qualities (see page 283–284) and Tastes (see page 285–287), most spices are pungent in flavour and therefore heating (for instance turmeric, ginger and cayenne), and they require balancing with bitter or astringent spices, such as fennel, coriander and cumin, which are cooling – unless of course you need to use their heating or cooling properties to remedy an aggravated Dosha (see pages 274–275).

Since freshly ground spices are always more flavoursome and nutritious, throughout this cookbook you will find various fresh spice combinations to make on the spot. For everyday cooking, and for spicing up veg dishes or cooking into porridges and soups, you can use a recipe known as a 'churna' or spice blend – either a shop-bought garam masala or a homemade Dosha-specific blend that keeps for weeks (see page 247). I love making my own spice blends and having a stash in my bag to sprinkle over food when travelling or eating out. These spice mixes are also very important when cooking dals, most of which are gas-producing – the spices make the dish easier to digest and alleviate the gas.

The correct sourcing of spices is important to avoid chemicals and fillers. To find out more about the properties of each spice, turn to the pantry on pages 24–29, or visit my website.

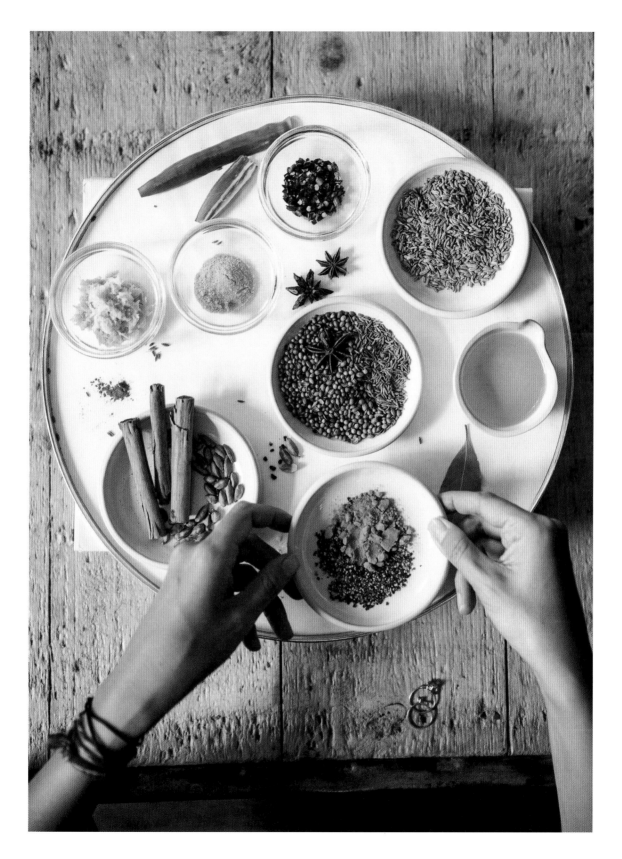

Cooking with spices

To get the most from your spices, it is best to heat them, as this activates their nutrients, which are mostly fat- and water-soluble. This is why it's usually best to cook them into your food, rather than to take them as a supplement. They also need to be broken down, so you will find that most of the spices used here are either freshly ground or, if whole, left to cook for a long period of time to soften up and infuse into the dishes. In order to protect the aroma and infuse flavours into your food, leave the lid on during cooking.

TIP

·

Such is the power of spices that Ayurveda recommends that if you are having intense treatment of any kind – for instance recovering from illness, diarrhoea, suffering poor digestion or doing a cleanse – no spices should be added to your food which should be as plain and well cooked as possible at this time.

TIP

·

If you're slow-cooking a dish with fat in it, you don't need to fry the spices in ghee before putting the ingredients together. They will naturally cook and release their properties with the available fat.

TIMINGS

There are no set rules regarding when to add the spices in cooking. if you're cooking them into the dish you can add them before or during the cooking process – the longer they cook for, the more mellow the flavour will be – or if you want to add them at the end for a flavour punch (some churna spice mixes are even added at the table), make sure you toast or fry them first to activate them.

To add spices at the start, toast or fry ground or whole spices for a very mild flavour.

To add during cooking, use whole unground herbs and spices when only a hint of flavour is wanted. If you are simmering food for a long time, add the spices 15 minutes before you remove the dish from the heat. Otherwise, the aromatic oils will slowly evaporate, and the flavour will go with them.

To add just before serving, sprinkle the spices over the top or stir in freshly toasted and ground churna spice mixes. You could also make a tarka, by frying spices in ghee or oil, and then pouring it over the food. Place the lid on the pan, take it off the heat and leave for 5 minutes to infuse.

TOASTING – TO MAKE A CHURNA

1   Heat a dry pan on a low heat. Once it's hot (but too hot) add the whole spices – one type at a time. If you are using ground spices, you can toast them together as they are all the same shape and size.

2   Keeping an eye on the pan, dry-toast the spices until fragrant, stirring frequently (don't walk away!).

3   Allow to cool completely, then grind in a spice grinder or in a pestle and mortar. Store in an airtight glass jar in a cool, dark place for 6–8 weeks.

FRYING – TO MAKE A TARKA

You can fry ground spices or seeds in a small amount of oil or ghee, known as a 'tarka', before adding other ingredients. This releases the oil-soluble components and activates their flavour and effects, making sure their medicinal properties are fully released. This method is good for pouring over foods that won't be further cooked and for recipes with no fat or oil in them, such as rotis, steamed veggies or salads. Ghee also helps transport the healing properties of spices to the different parts of the body. Spices that especially benefit from being activated in ghee or oil are mustard seeds, cumin seeds, coriander seeds, fennel seeds, fenugreek seeds, onion, garlic, asafoetida and whole peppercorns.

1   Heat a dry pan on low-medium heat.

2   Add the ghee and once it's hot (but not smoking) add the whole or ground spices in the order the recipe recommends, stirring frequently and removing the pan from the heat as soon as they release their aroma. They cook quickly in hot oil, so keep an eye on them.

This spice mix is used for the South Indian Moong Sambhar (see page 182). The secret is to roast the spices and lentils individually or in similar groupings so that you can get them perfectly toasted before grinding. Don't be tempted to rush this stage or walk away from the pan at any time, otherwise it won't taste anywhere near as good. For more on toasting spices, see page 265.

Makes 200g

Sambhar powder

40g (½ cup)
   coriander seeds
2 tbsp cumin seeds
8 dried red chillies,
   stalks removed
1½ tsp fenugreek seeds
1 tbsp black peppercorns
2 tbsp chana dal

or toor dal
1 tbsp urad dal
6–8 fresh or dried
   curry leaves
½ tbsp mustard seeds
½ tbsp asafoetida
½ tbsp ground turmeric

1　Heat a dry frying pan over a low heat and toast the coriander and cumin seeds, stirring for 1–2 minutes until they become fragrant and change colour. Transfer to a large plate and set aside.

2　Wipe the pan clean and toast the red chillies, stirring until they change colour and release a pungent smoky aroma. Transfer to the same plate.

3　Add the fenugreek seeds and toast, stirring until they turn brown. Transfer to the same plate. Repeat the process with the black peppercorns, stirring until aromatic. Add the chana dal to the pan and toast, stirring frequently. The chana dal takes longer to cook and should turn a uniform golden brown colour. Transfer to the same plate. Add the urad dal to the pan and repeat as above.

4　Add the curry leaves and toast until the leaves become crisp. Transfer to the same plate. Last but not least, add the mustard seeds and toast until they have finished popping. Transfer to the same plate.

5　Take the pan from the heat and add the asafoetida, stirring quickly – the colour just needs to change and the aroma to be released. Remove and set aside.

6　When the plate of spices has cooled to room temperature, transfer to a spice grinder or powerful blender with the turmeric and grind or blend to a coarse powder, not too fine. You may need to do this in several batches.

7　Allow the sambhar powder to cool again if it got hot in the blender, then mix thoroughly and store in a clean airtight jar in your cupboard, ready for sambhar recipes. It keeps for up to 3 months.

The aisles in our grocery stores are lined with a multitude of rice options but in Ayurveda, basmati is the golden grain, and believe it or not white basmati is considered the most Sattvic. Not only is it the easiest to digest and therefore delivers the best nutrition, it also has a much higher GI than other white rice.

The bran layer on brown rice has more nutrients but also contains phyto-nutrients, which can be troublesome for mineral absorption as well as tougher to digest. Enjoy brown rice occasionally if your digestion is strong – make sure to soak, then rinse well and slightly overcook it to make it easier to chew and break down.

For such a simple ingredient, cooking rice is definitely a bit of an art, so don't be discouraged if the first few attempts aren't quite right! You'll soon get a feel for it. Follow the instructions below, and don't be tempted to stir while it cooks.

Cooked rice should be soft rather than al dente, and brown basmati takes a lot longer to cook so will need more water. A little ghee and sea salt to season can be added at the end, depending on what you're serving it with. Always choose organic rice where possible. Some people soak white rice or fry it first in oil or ghee to stop the grains sticking together, but I find a good rinse works well. Most recipes call for one part rice to two parts water, but since we are rinsing, we need less. The serving below is 100g (½ cup) of uncooked white rice per person with 175ml (¾ cup) of water, but you may find you only need 70g (⅓ cup) of rice, in which case try 120ml (½ cup) of water – with much more water for brown rice. If using a rice cooker, make sure that it is not lined with aluminium.

Cooking rice

200g (1 cup) white
    basmati rice (or brown
    basmati rice, soaked for
    8 hours or overnight)
375–500ml (1½–2¼ cups)
    water

1   Rinse the rice three times. If you're using brown rice, soak for at least 8 hours or overnight. Drain.

2   Place the rice in a saucepan. Pour over 375ml (1½ cups) water if using white rice or 560ml (2¼ cups) water if using brown rice. Bring to the boil, lower to medium and then cook, lid on, until soft and fluffy – about 10–15 minutes for white rice, and up to 45 minutes for brown rice.

TIP
·

Towards the end of cooking, test a grain between your fingers and then finish cooking with the lid off if you feel that there is still a bit too much moisture in the pan. If you need to add more water once the rice has started cooking, use hot water.

AYURVEDA
EXPLAINED

Meet the Doshas

You could easily go ahead and create any of the dishes in this cookbook and enjoy delicious Ayurveda-inspired meals without reading on. However, it's fascinating to learn ways to identify and articulate how you're feeling, and what to eat and do to bring your body back into balance for optimal health. This is where the three Doshas come in: Vata, Pitta and Kapha. You will have seen these little symbols throughout the recipe chapter (see right).

Ayurveda recognises that all of creation – including us! – is made up of a unique ratio of Elements: Space, Air, Fire, Water and Earth. These are the building blocks of life and are therefore present in me as I write this, in the chair that I'm sitting on and in the mug that I'm sipping from. They are all around us and within us: in our minds and bodies; in nature; colours; sounds; in the senses; and in the foods we eat.

At every level of life – from the seasons, your age, to the time of day – these five physical Elements are present. For example, our tissues and bones have a great amount of Earth because they are made of minerals found in the earth, the body fluids represent Water, the metabolism is a manifestation of Fire, and all movement in the body is carried by Air. In a poetic sense, the human body is Earth, Water, Fire and Air moving through channels of Space. Just like the world around us, we move and flow in a rhythm – and moving with the flow makes us feel less stressed.

Doshas are the three vital energies that relate to the specific combinations of these five Elements. Known as Vata, Pitta and Kapha, which loosely translate as Air, Fire and Earth, they are 'the language' that describes the ratio in which the Elements flow within the universe and therefore in and around our bodies, governing our thinking and behaviour and guiding our bodily intelligence in one direction or another. The Doshas create and govern many layers within the body, from physical through to psychological. Each Dosha contains two Elements (see illustration opposite), giving each their own characteristics: Vata is a mixture of Space and Air, which is found within all forms of 'movement'. Pitta is a mixture of Air, Fire and Water and is found within all 'transformation'. Kapha is a mixture of Water and Earth and is found within 'structure'.

The physical characteristics of the Doshas are understood to some degree in the West, where the body shapes are recognised: Ectomorph as Vata, Mesomorph for Pitta and Endomorph for Kapha. Ayurveda takes this idea further, to encompass mental and emotional traits, too.

FEELING
VATA

FEELING
PITTA

FEELING
KAPHA

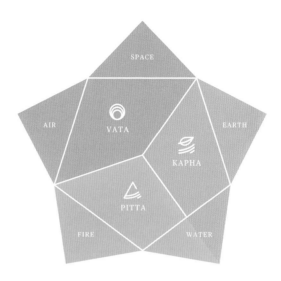

DOSHA COMBINATIONS

Our own unique blend of all three Doshas makes up our individual constitution, usually with one or two dominant Doshas. When we're referring to mind–body types (sometimes referred to as 'body type' or 'my Dosha' in the West) we usually cite our dominant Dosha at that moment (for example, I'm Vata or I'm Pitta). If two of your Doshas are more dominant, with just a little bit of the third Dosha, you might say 'I'm Pitta–Kapha', stating whichever is the slightly more dominant first, and if you have the rare mix of all three Doshas in equal measure, you are Tridoshic.

TWO DOSHA TYPES

1 PRAKRITI, OR BASIC MIND–BODY TYPE Known as your Ayurvedic constitution, your Prakriti is akin to your inherent genetic type. Think of it as 'Nature' – the characteristics that we are born with: hair, stature, eye colour, etc., which never change. This is our state of optimum balance where we want to get back to when things go out of whack, and it becomes our guiding light when we want to find our own unique equilibrium. This is also commonly known as 'body type', but I prefer 'basic mind–body type', because of your Vikriti (see below).

2 VIKRITI, OR CURRENT MIND–BODY TYPE: This is more about the here and now – think of it as 'Nurture', or what's affecting us at this moment. Vikriti can fluctuate yearly, monthly, daily, or even minute to minute. It is influenced by the environment we're in and the foods we eat.

If our Prakriti is out of balance, we will be experiencing imbalances in the first instance along the lines of bloating, rashes, spots, hot flushes, itchy skin, sore gums, farting, tummy upsets, bad temper, tiredness or anxiety. These are the precursors to the long road that leads to disease. We can identify which Dosha is playing up according to symptoms (see the Dosha test on my website – jasminehemsley.com) and bring ourselves into balance. Often your dominant Dosha type is the one that becomes imbalanced, since we tend to lean towards what we are already predisposed to.

PROFILES OF THE DOSHAS

One of my Vaidyas (Ayurvedic practitioners) explained that you can spot which Dosha is at play by observing people waiting on a station platform for a late train to arrive. Vata types will be pacing up and down, anxious for the train, thinking over and over again about the consequences of being late and wondering what to do next. Pitta types will be on the phone, not wanting to waste a moment of their time, while simultaneously extracting answers from the station guard. Kapha types will be sitting on the bench, chilling with a book or newspaper, or listening to music.

All three Doshas are within us, so most people exhibit characteristics of several Doshas simultaneously.

 VATA TYPES

Usually slim with bony limbs and straight body shapes, Vata types gain weight in the middle. Their skin is fine and dry, they feel the cold more than others and have difficulty sweating. They have an irregular and erratic appetite. Vata types are prone to feeling 'wired' and stressed, and may feel tired come late afternoon. They are creative, enthusiastic, active, alert and restless, jumping from one idea to the next.

Despite not having a great memory, Vata types are quick to learn, spiritually perceptive and are happiest when in contact with nature and the outdoors. They have a heightened sense of touch and an appreciation for beauty. You might recognise them as having their head in the clouds and talking at a million miles per hour.

IN BALANCE	Vata personalities are energetic, vivacious, joyful, friendly, open-minded, free in spirit, embrace change and learn easily, are clear and alert, sleep long and lightly, have balanced digestion, good circulation and an even body temperature.
OUT OF BALANCE	Vata personalities can be tired or fatigued, forgetful or spaced-out, anxious and frazzled with a lack of focus, have difficulty falling asleep, suffer occasional constipation and poor circulation.

 PITTA TYPES

With a moderate, athletic physique, Pitta types gain weight evenly or on the bottom half. They have soft, lustrous, warm skin and get hot easily. They have a strong metabolism, good appetite and digestion. Pitta types are determined, competitive, ambitious and highly intelligent, with good insight and keen discrimination. They like to be in control and at the centre of attention, they are highly focused innovators with energy levels to match and can be likened to a 'Type A' personality. Pitta types, although nocturnal, are deep sleepers and prone to vivid dreams and nightmares.

IN BALANCE	Pitta personalities are perfectionists, have strong intellect, strong digestion, are radiant, have glowing skin, sleep through the night and have inner peace and happiness.
OUT OF BALANCE	Pitta personalities can be controlling, irrational, judgemental, fiery-tempered, irritable, workaholic, overheated, and prone to rashes and acne. They may experience interrupted sleep, acid reflux, headaches and loose bowel movements.

DOSHAS AND YOU

Dosha means 'that which spoils or disturbs' in Sanskrit. I like to think of the Doshas as three little cups – each filled to the level determined by your Prakriti at birth. As life's experiences come in, depending on how efficiently they are dealt with, the cups can start to fill up, or occasionally go down. We start to feel 'out of sorts', and it's at this point that we can rebalance our cups. Like increases like, so in removing the excess of each cup on a regular basis we can manage our health. It's when those cups really fill up (or empty) that it is hard to balance. Making healthy choices can feel futile, unappealing or even impossible. Ayurveda helps to support you, so eat a good meal, have a good night's rest, then refocus on the task of getting back to balance. If those cups spill over and everything gets jumbled, that's when Ayurveda says that disease becomes prevalent. It's a massive clean-up act that's needed, but it can be done.

 KAPHA TYPES

With well-developed bodies, broad shoulders and soft, oily and lustrous skin, Kapha types enjoy a regular appetite with a relatively slow-burning digestion. They are naturally deep sleepers. Akin to mother earth, Kapha types are patient, grounded, caring, stable and supportive of family and loved ones.

Kaphas have an appreciation for art, dance and music. They have an innate sense of taste and smell and love to eat. They can be very attached to material possessions, and have difficulty in recognising the difference between essentials and luxuries. Despite being hard-working people, they also have a tendency to be lazy and are capable of sleeping for longer than others. They strongly dislike the cold and adore warmth.

IN BALANCE	Kapha personalities have a stable temperament, good long-term memory, good strength and stamina, a healthy and robust physiology, are team players, are reliable and enjoy sound sleep, are compassionate and affectionate.
OUT OF BALANCE	Kapha personalities can gain weight easily, have slow digestion, may be prone to sinus and respiratory problems, feel lethargic, find it difficult to wake-up and can experience food cravings and depression.

DISCOVER YOUR TYPE

Your Prakriti and Vikriti (see page 271) can only be accurately worked out by a Vaidya, who will expertly assess everything about you, but you can also have fun getting an indication of both by using the Dosha quiz on my website (jasminehemsley.com) – however, there is one condition! When you use this test, don't judge yourself against other people, because we are all our own unique blend, and it's more about where we are now, i.e. which Dosha(s) are dominating and how we can stabilise within the environment in which we're living. A natural Kapha type, raised by a Vata – or educated in a Vata style – could be very Vata. Likewise if you're born a Vata type, who tends to be cold and dry, but you're living in a hot humid country, you might not need to worry as much about keeping warm or moisturising your skin.

Western interpretations of Ayurveda have often focused on 'What's your Dosha?', usually referring to your Prakriti. The most important thing to remember in all this is not to get into the Western mindset of 'x = x'. Your needs are not set in stone, and you should not think that one body type is better than another or label yourself as an absolute, because everything ebbs and flows. Although your Prakriti remains constant, outside factors may completely override the ratios of your Doshas.

Knowing what pacifies and aggravates the Doshas is not only fun and insightful but also helps you identify the ingredients, Tastes and behaviours that create balance. We need to be friends with all the Doshas – all three are within us and have effects at different times of life, specific seasons and even in each day. Giving attention to Vata in particular, which very quickly affects the other two Doshas, makes it easier to respond to imbalances. Once you know which Dosha it is you're feeling, you can use the Balance Finder, Meal Planners and Shopping Lists on my website to help get back to your basic mind–body type, which is where true balance lives.

The great news is that in Ayurveda we can draw on Elements around us as 'medicine'. There is a window in time to make the easiest adjustments – we can look to herbs, foods, colours, drinks, environments, smells and lifestyle choices to create equilibrium. For example, if you are feeling hot, take off your jumper; if you are cold in your bones, have a hot bath; if you want a salad rather than a stew in the summer, or to follow a large heavy meal with something light, or want something stimulating like a coffee or a spicy dish when you're feeling sluggish – we do all of these things naturally all of the time. Ayurveda takes things one step further, understanding the qualities of food and lifestyle habits that can help or hinder us. This is really important for those of us living in a climate where we experience all of the seasons – from blistering summer days to snowy winters, wet springs and windy autumns – sometimes all in one day!

BRING BALANCE

When you understand the Doshas, you understand Ayurveda. Balancing the Doshas is the key to your health, and to do this it's important to identify the characteristics of your prevailing dominant Dosha(s) – using your Senses (for example 'taste' when it comes to food). You can then find balance by seeking the 'opposite' characteristics in your food and lifestyle choices. Focus on what makes you feel your best, taking it one day and one season at a time. In Ayurveda, foods or actions are not labelled good or bad, they are simply either aggravating or pacifying to your health in the right amounts. This is where the phrase 'everything in moderation' rings true. However, only if that is true to you – one person's poison is another person's cure!

There are many subtleties in caring for your Prakriti (basic mind–body type) and any imbalances in your Vikriti (current mind–body type). That is why this book is less focused on telling you what to eat according to Dosha type and more about how you are feeling today. This table gives an at-a-glance idea of the kind of foods and activities you can employ in order to pacify and therefore balance the Doshas.

	VATA	PITTA	KAPHA
AGGRAVATING QUALITIES	Light, dry, rough, clear, active, cold, mobile, subtle	Oily, sharp, hot, light, fleshy, liquid	Heavy, solid, cold, smooth, slow, soft, oily, dense
PACIFYING QUALITIES	Heavy, oily, smooth, cloudy, stagnant, hot, static	Dry, dull, cold, heavy, solid	Light, sharp, hot, dry, rough, porous, hard
AGGRAVATING TASTES	Bitter, pungent, astringent	Sour, salty, pungent	Sweet, sour, salty
PACIFYING TASTES	Sweet, sour, salty	Sweet, bitter, astringent	Pungent, bitter, astringent
EAT LESS	Raw, leafy greens, chilli, coffee, stimulants, cold salads, too many greens.	Spicy, sour, salty food, such as chips and salsa. Coffee, red meat. Deep-fried, garlicky and tomato dishes.	Sweeteners and sweet foods such as ice cream, fruit, grains, root vegetables, milk, ghee, yoghurt, eggs, nuts, seeds, dairy fats/oils and meat.
EAT MORE	Warming spices, heavy meats, legumes and grains, calming fats, sweet fruits and root veg, hot milk. Hot soups and well-cooked dishes with fats and some animal proteins.	Cooling, fresh raw veg, salads and herbs – especially in summer – sweet juicy fruits, water. Raw foods and a few animal proteins.	Stimulating herbs and spices, bitter greens, airy legumes and fruit and vegetables such as apples, broccoli. Lightly steamed or cooked veggies, light vegetarian dishes.
AVOID	Cold/fizzy drinks, skipping meals, eating when stressed, salt baths, cold showers.	Alcohol, tobacco, over-exercising, over-heating, sunbathing, hot baths.	Napping, hoarding, snacking, heavy meals, eating late, lie-ins.
PACIFYING MOVEMENT	Hatha yoga, pilates, weight training, pranayama (breathwork).	Yoga, walking, long-distance running, swimming.	Vinyasa flow, high-intensity interval training, weight training, running and sprinting.
MOTTO	Get grounded, slow down, connect with Fire and Earth. Take care of yourself.	Keep cool, connect with Water and Earth. Be understanding of others.	Let go, get active, connect with Air and Fire. Shake things up.

The star of Ayurveda

I have designed this little star for anyone who needs a visual. It really helped me 'see' everything as a whole. It gives you an overview of how the Elements, Doshas, Tastes, Senses and Qualities sit together and relate to each other. Life is built on opposites in order to maintain balance.

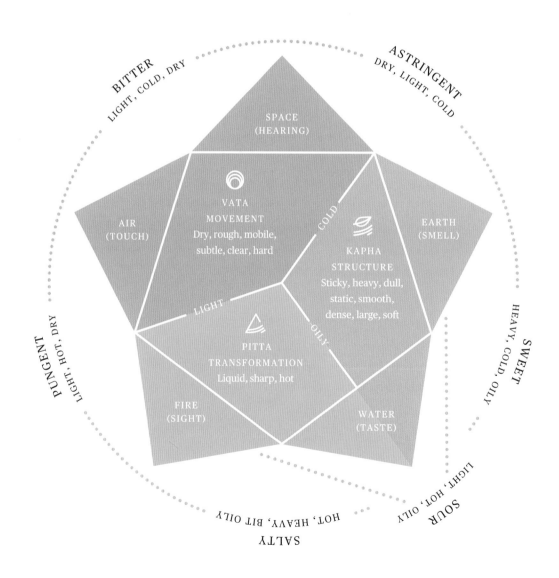

HOW TO READ THE STAR OF AYURVEDA

This may all seem quite complicated in the beginning but it's actually a more simple – some might say poetic – way of looking at life and, more importantly, it makes sense.

The star shows:
1 The role specific Doshas play in the body (Movement, Structure or Transformation).
2 The Qualities of each Dosha (such as dry, rough, sticky, heavy, liquid, sharp – see page 283 for more on this).
3 The five Elements that make up each Dosha (Space, Earth, Water, Fire, Air).
4 The Senses of those Elements (hearing, smell, taste, sight, touch).
5 The Tastes (astringent, sweet, sour, salty, pungent, bitter – see page 285 for more on this).
6 The Qualities of each Taste (such as dry, heavy, light, hot, cold, etc).

Using this visual we can see that the Qualities, Senses and Tastes that govern Pitta are orange, therefore everything that is not orange (the Qualities, Senses and Tastes of Vata and Kapha) are opposites, which can balance Pitta. Since the five Elements are unequally weighted between the three Doshas you will see that there is some crossover in Qualities, Senses and Tastes. Therefore, to balance Pitta we require a little of what it already is (Fire Element, salty Taste, liquid, sharp and hot Qualities), a medium amount of what it is partially made of (Water Element, pungent and sour Tastes, and light oily Qualities), and a lot of what it is not (Air, Space and Earth Elements, bitter, astringent and sweet Tastes, and cold, dry, heavy, rough, mobile, subtle, clear, hard, sticky, heavy, dull, static, smooth, dense, large and soft Qualities). See the box below for another example.

I AM PITTA	TO BALANCE PITTA I NEED TO
The Qualities of Pitta are liquid, sharp, hot and a bit oily	Look for Qualities of cool, dry, rough, mobile, subtle, clear, hard, sticky, heavy, dull, static, smooth, dense, large, soft
The Elements that govern Pitta are predominantly Fire with some Water	Find calm in Air, Space and Earth Elements, which stimulate touch, hearing and smell
The Senses that govern Pitta are sight and taste	Seek out bitter, astringent and sweet Tastes, which hold opposite Qualities of dry, light and cool
The Tastes that govern Pitta are pungent, salty and sour	Limit lifestyle choices and foods that have Pitta properties

Agni, or digestive fire

Above all else, Ayurveda recognises that your digestive fire or Agni is EVERYTHING. The strength of your Agni is key to good health, and if you focus on stoking that fire and keeping it lively with your lifestyle choices – for example making time to cook real, fresh, seasonal foods and balancing out the effects of a busy life with meditation and proper rest – you won't need to fixate on your Dosha type but rather you can balance your ever-fluctuating Doshas as they move with you.

There are thirteen different Agnis, or biological fires, at work throughout your body, including the tiny metabolic processes that take place in every single cell. Here we focus on the main Agni that lies in your stomach, filled with the enzymes and hydrochloric acid that break down your meal and begin the conversion of it into a nourishing energy that your body can use.

If we are the sum of our experiences, and we are what we assimilate, our digestive fire is responsible for our overall health and wellbeing – digesting emotional, mental and physical experiences, as well as our food. If we look after our digestive fire, it looks after us. A lively fire can reduce negative experiences into the basic information that we need to get us through life without having to drag it around with us and allowing it to 'become us'. A lively fire gets the best from both nutritious food and nutrient-poor food. It protects us from bad bacteria and viruses and 'cooks down' raw and indigestible foods into something that our bodies can use. It has the power to transform everything it digests into 'us' and everything that we are. It takes the energy of the universe and converts it into forms that we can immediately use.

As I have heard over and over again from my Vaidyas and vedic meditation teachers: 'It is better to have good digestion and a bad diet, than to have bad digestion and a good diet.' While Ayurveda recommends eating wholesome, healthy and nutritious meals that are prepared appropriately for our Dosha and the season, digestion is so important that it pushes the importance of the actual food that we are eating down to third place, behind how we digest and how we eat.

While the actual quality and type of your food is important, the simplicity of your plate is even more so. As Vaidya Dr Avilochan said, 'Don't make a meal out of a meal' – which basically means, the simpler the dish, the easier it is on the system. That doesn't mean boring food, it just means that we should try to balance out our crazy eating days with a bit more, or maybe a lot more, zen.

HOW WE DIGEST

According to the principles of Ayurveda, our overall health and therefore our happiness, radiance and longevity rests on the health of our Agni. A happy, functioning in-balance Agni equals a happy, functioning in-balance you. On the flip side, a defective Agni will most likely present as illness, discontent and imbalance. The intake of food should be regulated by the condition of the Agni, the digestive fire in the body. If you feel hungry, your digestive fire is enkindled.

That means if your digestive fire is firing at the right level – not raging too quickly, which will destroy the food, nor too slowly that the food depletes your energy – your body can effectively get a decent amount of nutrients from any meal without too many problems. It's also a bit of a vicious cycle, though, as the taste of your meal depends upon your Agni. You will not taste the food properly if your Agni is impaired, which leads to you making the wrong kind of choices to balance you.

Digestive fire works on the food mass that has been swallowed and liquefied, separating the nutrients from the waste material to produce a nutrient-rich nectar that flows freely and easily through the body. Imagine Agni as the fire in a wood-burning stove. The more efficiently the fuel (our food) burns in the stove, the more heat (energy) is produced. When the fire only smoulders, black soot builds up in the pipes and chimney, which can metaphorically be likened to toxins produced by an Agni that is not strong enough to burn cleanly. In Ayurveda this is known as Ama, a general term for the internal toxic residue produced by improper metabolic functioning – either as a result of poor digestion and/or poor dietary choices (or a reflection of an imbalance somewhere else in the gastro-intestinal system). This thick, black fluid is the opposite to the rich, nutritious nectar produced by a well-functioning Agni. The reason we're all up in arms about a poorly operating Agni is because Ama is understood to to be the root cause of all disease.

Agni and Ama are opposite in properties. Agni is hot, dry, light, clear and aromatic, whereas Ama is cold, wet, heavy, cloudy and malodorous. To treat Ama, it is necessary to increase Agni. Symptoms of Ama are similar to those that we understand in the West of 'feeling toxic' – bogged down with unhelpful substances that quash our vitality, including loss of taste and appetite, indigestion, tongue-coating, loss of strength, insomnia, heaviness, lethargy and a dull or heavy pulse. Other common symptoms include bad breath, body odour, congestion, constipation, lack of attention and clarity, and depression. Ama is also perpetuated by foods that don't work together in the stomach, and one cause of this is eating inappropriate food combinations (see pages 21–22).

HOW WE EAT

There's so much more to eating than just chucking food into our mouths and swallowing it down, believing that our work is done. We have to take pleasure in eating it, which is surely why we want to do it in the first place, and why we're all crazy about cookbooks, restaurants and TV cooking shows!

Pay attention the next time you eat a meal calmly and in a good mood and compare it to how you feel when eating whilst upset and stressed out or in a busy place with lots of distractions. Note how your system feels. It's always better to take some time out, digest your environmental situation first, then when you've done that, return to the process of eating. For some people, life moves quickly and is very varied. Implementing the above goes a long way to recalibrating your nervous system, and this is the power of being mindful or 'in the moment'.

Agni is also linked to the sun, 'Surya'. Think of it as a bigger picture: without the heat of the sun, nothing can live. Let's go to an even bigger picture. Think of the planetary system: too much heat from the sun, no life; too little heat, no life. The higher the sun is in the sky, the stronger the Agni, which is why in Ayurveda we eat our biggest meal of the day at lunchtime, which I refer to as Surya Agni ('Sun Fire'), to fit this state.

THE FOUR TYPES OF AGNI

BALANCED AGNI – This is a lively Agni, known as 'Sama Agni', which belongs to the happy-go-lucky types. Few and far between, these types seem to sail through life, making clear decisions, right or wrong. They don't get swept up in any bad luck and are very easy with themselves and others. They don't suffer mental irritations or physical blockages, they don't seem to get 'hangry' if a meal is late, and even if they are sleep-deprived they appear to get by with barely a grumble. Everything seems effortless for them, and that's because they are not suffering conflicting internal agitations and toxic build-up. Balanced Agni is a result of a life in balance, one where stress is dealt with quickly and life is lived in alignment.

VATA AGNI – This is irregular or erratic, because Vata fire is wavering. Think of the movement of air on a fire – sometimes it fans the flames, sometimes it blows the embers away. Irregular and erratic in nature, it can change in a heartbeat. The waste material resuting from this type of fire is often dry or hard to pass.

PITTA AGNI – Fast-burning, Pitta fire is a well-built furnace. However, an overactive Agni is just as detrimental because the digestive process burns away, through combustion, the normal biological nutrients in the food, which results in emaciation. The waste material resulting from this type of fire is often oily and runny, and it burns.

KAPHA AGNI – Slow-burning, Kapha fire is as if built with wet branches on cold, damp soil. Too much moisture, too much cold and the fire doesn't work. The waste material resuting from this type of fire is usually large, heavy and soft.

I can't tell you how many times while writing this book that ideas of 'hunger' popped up and sparked cravings as my digestive fire responded to the tantalising details. It was the kind of feeling that makes you head straight for the biscuit tin, but is it a reason to eat?

Those of us who are fortunate enough to live in the West are surrounded by food – cheap and abundant, it stares us in the face on a regular basis. If we're not eating, someone next to us is. If we're not cooking food, someone else is selling it. I love food, and I've always been pretty lucky to be able to 'put it away' at will. From the outside, my skin was good, my frame was small, but my digestion wasn't happy with me, and when I fed that kind of hunger I never felt satisfied, only craved more until I was pushed over the edge and regretted it. We've all been there – eating when you're full, staying up late when you're tired and taking on more than you can do. In the past it was a challenge not to do something that I 'impulsively' wanted to do, but now I understand more about my Agni, so my reasoning kicks in. If I get a craving: I ask myself, am I just procrastinating? Is the nostalgia of my mum's cooking or a holiday dish calling my name? Even simpler is to say – would I drink a lassi right now, or eat a carrot or a bowl of dal? If not, guess what? It probably isn't hunger.

There are so many variables that dictate the amount of time it will take you to digest a meal; as a minimum you're looking at two hours for a smaller meal, so if you're hungry only two hours after eating, when the food has only just left your stomach, you're probably not actually hungry (unless your Pitta is off-balance) and it's just a case of waiting 30 minutes or so for the next stage of digestion. Sip hot water and wait for the earlier food to become the nutritious nectar that will soon nourish you and provide energy. Keep calm and carry on until you feel true hunger.

Our stomach is the size of two fists. When your guts bloat out, it's in reaction to the food you're eating and/or the way you've eaten it. When you overeat, the food ferments and putrifies, not only wasting its goodness but taxing your body. Aim to fill only one-third of your stomach with food and leave one-third for liquid and one-third empty, to allow enough space for the action of digestion to take place.

Overeating can be caused by stress (in an effort to placate feelings), eating too fast and not wanting to waste food. I was brought up to always over-cater but never to waste food, so this has been a challenge for me. I try to cook what I need for the day and any leftovers go to my three dogs, which serves them better than me! If you keep chickens, or have a compost bin or food collection bins, use these for the leftovers – in the grand scheme of things, that food is going to do better for the world recycled that way. Meanwhile, work on cooking just what you and your family need.

SECRETS OF A LIVELY DIGESTIVE FIRE

Too little digestive fire produces Ama (see page 279), which toxifies the body, and too much produces nothing so that the body has no material to repair, build and grow with. Here are tips to protect and promote a lively digestive fire.

HOW TO EAT

1 Chew your drink, and drink your food.

2 Go slow. You can't read the signs if you rush life, and eating a meal should be done with grace.

3 Fill the stomach with one-third food, one-third liquid and leave the last third empty.

4 Bless your food. Gratitude helps you feel happy and keeps you in the moment.

5 Sit down to eat, and avoid using the TV, computer, mobile phone, or even reading.

6 Chew your food thoroughly and taste it; focus your mind on and be aware of the Tastes.

7 Sip hot water throughout the day to stoke your digestive fire and to prevent the accumulation of Ama. Avoid drinking more than three herbal teas per day, and preferably with meals (though just plain hot/room-temperature water is fine too), otherwise it's something else for your body to digest between meals.

8 Take time to enjoy your food – usually you'll feel full with less. Practise mindful eating and stop at the first burp! It will most likely be subtle, but this air bubble is the signal that your body has had enough food, so tune in to notice it.

9 Sit back and relax for a few minutes after finishing your meal and then take a short, brisk walk.

WHAT TO EAT

1 Simple is best. Balance out restaurant-style fare with plenty of peasant food. Too many ingredients (and courses!) make harder work for your digestion.

2 Enjoy plenty of slow-cooked one-pot meals, such as soups and stews, where Tastes and ingredients have a chance to mingle and are easier to digest.

3 It's better to enjoy hydrating food, rather than drowning your stomach fire with too much water with meals. Avoid cold and carbonated drinks.

4 Spice it up! Cook with pungent spices to aid digestion, and add sour Tastes with pickles and chutneys (see pages 234–239).

5 To regulate digestion, get your digestive juices flowing and your Agni firing, enjoy fresh ginger or Ginger Anise Chews (see page 103) and bitter, pungent herbs.

6 Eat foods filled with Prana ('life'): rather than processed, packaged, fast food and frozen food, or even reheated/leftover foods. Whenever possible, eat freshly prepared.

7 Avoid certain food combinations that will weaken your fire (see page 21).

8 Cook wholesome, nutritious meals to keep your digestive fire lively.

9 Tweak your cooking to bring balance and harmony to your Doshas and eat fewer foods that cause imbalance.

WHEN TO EAT

1 Do not eat unless you feel hungry, to make sure your digestive fire is awake, and do not drink unless you are thirsty.

2 At the same time, do not eat when you feel thirsty, and do not drink when you feel hungry.

3 Aim for regular meal times, 2–3 times a day is best, and establish a routine.

4 Avoid snacking between meals (including too many herbal teas!) – let your hunger and Agni build.

5 Leave adequate time between meals to properly digest food (at least 3 hours after a light meal and 4–6 hours after a full meal).

6 If you can, make lunch the most important (and biggest) meal of the day, because your digestion is strongest at midday (or between 10am and noon Pitta time, see page 288). Avoid heavy breakfasts or evening meals, which is Kapha time. Think of breakfast as easing yourself into the day and dinner as easing yourself out.

7 Watch your stress levels: don't eat when you're stressed or upset; eat with a sense of calm.

8 Eat a light supper and eat it early, 2–4 hours before bed, so that you can digest before sleeping.

9 Do a cleanse and reset (see pages 290–291) a few times a year, ideally at the change of the seasons.

20 Qualities
and 10 opposites

According to Ayurveda, everything you can see, hear, smell, taste and touch is experienced as a mixture of 20 Qualities. These Qualities represent two ends of a spectrum, with 10 on one side and 10 on the other – positives and negatives, yin and yang. They are used to describe the way we feel and understand the world.

These co-existing opposites are how nature keeps a balance, and in being able to identify them, and then work with them, we can help our health stay on course – this points the way to effectve diagnosis and treatment of illness in Ayurveda. The premise is simple: like increases like, and only an opposite Quality can combat it to bring balance. So, if it's hot then add some cold, and if it's smooth then add something rough.

Ayurveda has identified the 10 pairs of opposites that are most useful as medicine. Notice that sometimes a few words are used – trying to find the perfect translation for Sanskrit, which is such a rich language, is like trying to simplify Shakespeare! Start to get into the language of describing your world through these adjectives to help you view life as nature – it's a much more romantic and in-tune approach.

These Qualities are all found within the Elements and are the descriptors of all things: from the five Elements to their corresponding Doshas (including the mental, emotional and physical aspects); for food (its texture and its six Tastes); and for the seasons.

	BUILDING QUALITIES	LIGHTENING QUALITIES
1	Heavy	Light
2	Dull/slow	Sharp/quick
3	Cold	Hot
4	Oily/unctuous	Dry/brittle
5	Smooth	Rough
6	Dense/solid	Liquid
7	Soft	Hard
8	Static	Mobile
9	Gross/large	Subtle/small
10	Cloudy/sticky	Clear

Those in the left-hand column are called the building Qualities because they are anabolic, bringing weight, warmth and structure. In food they are the comfort foods such as hot milk, root vegetable soups, porridges and meat. Opposite to those are the lightening Qualities (they lighten the body, rather than being a fork of electrical energy!) which reduce, eliminate and enliven – think of the steamed vegetables, salads, broths and fresh fruit. As you can imagine, if you are feeling overweight, eating more lightening foods can help, but if you go too far you tip the balance and are left with reduced energy and immunity. We need both building and lightening foods, in the right amounts. By understanding the Qualities you can intuitively go about your day-to-day life knowing what you need less or more of.

For example, an oil massage on a regular basis is grounding and therefore extremely beneficial for Vata types, who are generally flighty, dry and light from all that Air and movement. The oil helps to pacify those Qualities of Vata because the Qualities of oil are opposite. Since those Qualities are similar to Kapha (for example, oily, heavy, slow and cold), oil will only serve to aggravate Kapha and make them more congested and lethargic if used on a regular basis. Heating the oil first would go some way toward helping, but even better is a dry powder massage, which increases light, dry and hot Qualities.

In a broader sense, when we are feeling unloved or under the weather, we crave a soft bed to to cradle us, in a foetal position, surrounded by pillows. When we are feeling hot and bothered, or our personal space has been invaded, we crave an open space with a cool breeze or fresh air.

THE QUALITIES OF FOOD

All foods can be described using these 20 Qualities. For example, heavy foods include grains, cheese, yoghurt, salty processed food and red meats, whereas light foods include leafy veggies and spices and herbs like turmeric and coriander. Cold foods include cucumber, watermelon and fennel, which also happen to be wet, while hot foods include ginger and chilli peppers. Dry foods include millet, barley, dry fruits and toast, whereas oily foods include butter, oils, nuts and seeds, and fried foods. It is helpful to start thinking of food in this way, in order to know which foods to eat to balance Qualities that prevail in your everyday life.

For example, toasted or raw oats every morning, which have Vata Qualities of 'dry, light and airy', would aggravate Vata in time, yet well cooked as a soupy porridge with a dollop of ghee would lubricate, hydrate and pacify Vata. Another example, is the different preparations of dairy – the Qualities of milk are very different to those of butter, ghee and yoghurt, and hot, cooked milk is very different (much easier to digest) than raw or fridge-cold milk.

As you consume these Qualities, they come together in the body to form a ratio. Since trying to work out these Qualities from the meals you eat can be quite a job and a subtle art, we can look to the smell and taste of foods, which handily combine these 20 Qualities into six Tastes. For example, foods that have heavy, oily, cool and sticky Qualities of Water and Earth Elements taste sweet (think of milk and cream). Foods that have dry, cool, light qualities of Space and Air taste bitter (think of kale). It's the subtle Tastes that we're also tuning into.

The six Tastes

It's not just the Qualities of the food we eat that matter, but also the Tastes. There are six defining Tastes (known as Rasas) in Ayurveda: sweet, astringent, sour, salty, pungent and bitter. In Western cuisine, only five of these Tastes are recognised. The sixth one, which may seem unfamiliar, is 'astringent', which is more of a sensation of dryness than a flavour. Think of the tannins in tea, the taste of broccoli or the feeling of a green banana or orange or lemon pith on your tongue.

There's much more to the Tastes than flavour. Just as for the Doshas, each Taste is composed of two of the five Elements, and therefore each Taste corresponds to one or more Doshas. Any Taste eaten in excess will aggravate its relative Dosha, and in the same vein, opposing Tastes can help to pacify each Dosha. As all the Elements have specific Qualities too (for example, Air is mobile, cool, light, dry, rough) knowing the Elements of the six Tastes makes it easy to understand their influence on our mental and physical state. See the Star of Ayurveda on page 276 to find out which Qualities and Tastes pertain to each Dosha, and then note which Qualities and Tastes are opposites.

The concept that taste is important to health might seem strange, but through the pleasure of eating foods we are able to assess better whether they are suited to us and in what amounts they are needed. Just as we might have cravings for the wrong foods, with the knowledge of Ayurveda we can intuitively seek out those that we need to bring balance. With your tastebuds tuned in, you will be able to discern the Elements in foods and can distinguish what you need, how much and when.

Below you will find a chart detailing which of the two Elements can be found in each of the six Tastes. Consequently you can see which Tastes should be eaten frequently according to the Doshas, as well as which should be enjoyed in lesser amounts in order to bring or maintain balance. By understanding the taste of foods you can work out what should make up the bulk of your day-to-day diet. For example, if your dominant Dosha is Vata or your Vata is aggravated, you should enjoy sweet, salty and sour foods in the majority of your meals – one example might be salmon or rice (sweet) with seaweed (salty) and a squeeze of lime (sour), avoiding large amounts of leafy greens and spices in order to keep pungent, bitter and astringent foods on the down-low. Using this as a guide, you can then adapt any of the recipes in the book to suit you.

Every Taste is important in satisfying our overall health – from how much a meal hits the spot to how good we continue to feel a long time after eating it. That's where cooking comes in, and the art of putting a meal together to make sure that every Taste is satisfied in the ratios that are personal to you – not just for your basic mind–body type (see page 271) but for your current type at any given time. You might think that cooking is complicated enough without having to worry about including every Taste and in varying amounts, but that's the beauty of the Ayurvedic intuition that you will come to inhabit. And even if you have to keep checking at first, it becomes a very useful tool for self-diagnosis, while giving you the means to tackle the problem. The basic rule is to vary the ingredients to make your meals so that you don't overeat foods and to team them with a selection of pickles and chutneys to add pronounced Tastes where necessary. Overall, one of the easiest ways is the regular use of 'masalas' or spice mixes, which can be created to suit each Dosha (see page 239) and if you really like cooking, you can experiment with the real Taste showstopper: the Thali (see page 208).

A 'complete and balanced meal' should not only consist of all six Tastes to suit an individual's balance, but ideally also these Tastes should be eaten in order, starting with sweet, then salty, sour, pungent, bitter and finally astringent. That's right, a meal should begin with sweet! As you'll see below, it's the most nourishing, as well as the heaviest, food to digest, and therefore you will feel satisfied by a meal much earlier. Consider how we usually start a meal with something salty and end with something sweet; that's why we can be left feeling overly full after a meal with pudding, yet not quite satisfied if we go without it. Try eating a small amount of dessert, pudding or simply a ladoo (see pages 84–87) before a meal and see how this changes your overall eating experience. At my pop-up cafe we served a ladoo, digestive Lassi (see pages 118–121) and main course for lunch as the 'Surya Agni Trio'.

| SWEET | | | Most fruit, milk, cream, honey, liquorice, most nuts, cinnamon, cardamom, |
| EARTH + WATER | | | rice and other heavy complex carbs, fats and oils including ghee, meats. |

| BALANCES: | ◎ | △ | The sweet Taste of foods is the most nourishing of all, which explains why we are so drawn to it. It's body-building, gives us energy, enhances fertility and helps us feel love, happiness and satisfaction. Too much causes congestion, sluggishness |
| AGGRAVATES: | | ⌇ | indigestion, obesity, diabetes and oily skin, and can make us feel greedy, needy, lethargic and lazy. |

| SOUR | | Citrus fruit, cheese, vinegar, wine, raisins, tamarind, miso, wine, fermented foods, |
| EARTH + FIRE | | yoghurt and strawberries. |

| BALANCES: | ◎ | The sour Taste boosts digestion and elimination, wakes you up and helps to clarify thoughts and emotions if dosed correctly. Too much results in acidity, ulcers, heartburn, rashes and muscle weakness, and can quickly lead to aggression, |
| AGGRAVATES: △ ⌇ | | jealousy and resentment. |

SALTY
FIRE + WATER

Seafood, celery, seaweed, tamari, salt.

BALANCES:

The salty Taste adds flavour, stimulates digestion and aids circulation. Rounding and hydrating, it brings solidity and structure, giving you mental ease, confidence and a zest for life. Too much promotes addiction, attachment and greed.

AGGRAVATES:

PUNGENT/SPICY
FIRE + AIR

Onion, leek, garlic, turnips, horseradish, asafoetida, cayenne, cumin, paprika, black pepper, cocoa, coffee, chilli and ginger.

BALANCES:

The pungent Taste is is an appetiser; it clears phlegm, has antifungal and antibacterial properties, stimulates digestion, and helps motivate us and make sense of complicated matters. Too much causes infections, intense perspiration, diarrhoea, acid indigestion, dehydration and ulcers and makes us irritable, angry and aggressive.

AGGRAVATES:

ASTRINGENT
AIR + EARTH

Pasta, broccoli, potatoes, parsley, apples, pomegranates, pears, unripe bananas, artichokes, lettuce, Brussel sprouts, cabbage, cauliflower, rosemary, nutmeg, beans, lentils and green and black tea.

BALANCES:

Astringent Taste increases nutrient absorption, stops bleeding, shrinks pores, reduces sweating and leaves you feeling optimistic, helping you feel stabilised, centred and unified. Too much causes slow digestion, gas, constipation and dryness, and can leave us fearful, insecure, anxious and depressed.

AGGRAVATES:

BITTER
AIR + SPACE

Bitter greens such as dandelion, dark leafy greens, mustard seeds, neem, green tea and aubergines.

BALANCES:

The bitter Taste is physically and mentally purifying, anti-inflammatory, detoxifying, skin toning and liver cleansing; it encourages weight loss and brings insight and mental clarity. Too much can deplete bodily tissues, cause constipation, insomnia, low blood pressure, premature wrinkles and provoke feelings of loneliness, dissatisfaction and cynicism.

AGGRAVATES:

Living la vida 'veda

Ayurveda is a 360 approach, so it's reassuring to know that not everything is about getting the food right – and that when you can't, there are so many other ways to bring balance. From routines to rituals, meditation to yoga, intention-setting and even putting your world to rights with positive thoughts before bed, we can help look after our mental, spiritual and emotional health, which will revive us and take care of our Agni so that we are better equipped to digest life.

There is a wealth of information from 5,000 years of Ayurveda and this book certainly can't hold the half of it! Here, I've shared a taster of the lifestyle knowledge of Ayurveda – techniques that can become your everyday tools and examples of what, in time, can become intuitive knowledge. For more details about living la vida 'veda, please go to my website (jasminehemsley.com), where there is a wealth of information to enlighten and guide you.

THE DAY ACCORDING TO THE DOSHAS

2–6AM: Rise before 6am to cash in on the energising and creative energy of Vata.

6–10AM: Balance Kapha with exercise and a light, warming breakfast to ease you into the day.

10AM–2PM: The most productive time to work. Eat your main meal at midday when the body's digestive fire is at its most intense.

2–6PM: This is a creative time to tackle problems and make plans.

6–10PM: Balance Kapha with exercise and a light, easy-to-digest supper eaten early to wind down. Sleep before 10pm, or Pitta will get you active (and hungry) again!

10PM–2AM: Time to sleep, rest and rejuvenate, processing food and thoughts from the day.

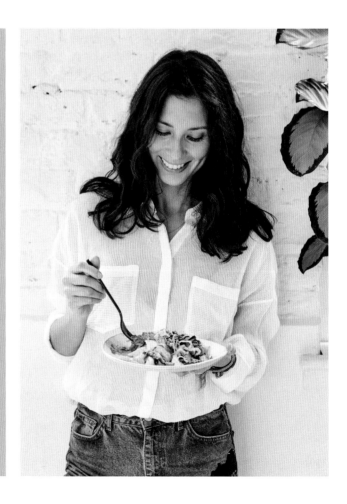

YOUR TIME OF DAY, YEAR AND LIFE

The Doshas not only influence our body types and environments, they also govern different stages of the day, seasons and the cycles in every person's lifetime. By understanding these influences, Ayurveda teaches that you can work with them to your advantage.

For example, Kapha qualities of cold, wet, static, slow and heavy govern the time of day when breakfast and dinner happen. With digestive fire burning low, aim to eat light, warming breakfasts that don't leave you feeling more heavy. Midday is when Pitta is at its peak and when your digestion is strongest, so it is the best time to eat your main meal, which requires the full strength of your Agni. Pitta also governs adulthood – a time when you get things done, are ambitious and at your most productive. The Vata time of life is old age, and just like its time of year – autumn to winter – it is cold, light and dry, so nourishing soups and stews made with plenty of fats and root vegetables will help nourish, hydrate and ground.

Working your day according to the rhythm of nature helps you gain energy as you go with the flow. Going against the flow means we expend energy, and we can only do it for so long before we exhaust ourselves.

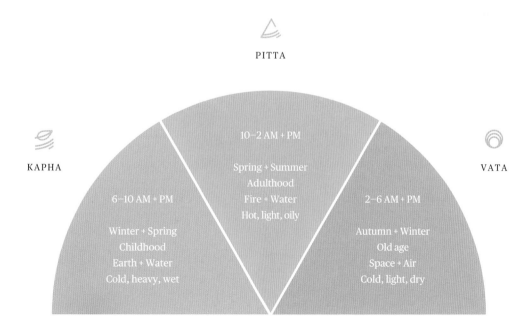

PITTA

KAPHA

VATA

10–2 AM + PM

Spring + Summer
Adulthood
Fire + Water
Hot, light, oily

6–10 AM + PM

Winter + Spring
Childhood
Earth + Water
Cold, heavy, wet

2–6 AM + PM

Autumn + Winter
Old age
Space + Air
Cold, light, dry

ROUTINES AND RITUALS

'Ritual is a necessity, a human need – use this to always come back to mindfulness of what you're doing.' Dzongsar Jamyang Khyentse Rinpoche

Over the years I've worked in the everyday practices and routines that make up an Ayurvedic lifestyle, from oil-pulling and tongue-scraping, to meditation, yoga and breathwork, as well as little rituals of awareness that I've found helpful, such as blessing my food, taking a break from the digital world, mindful working, clearing my space and taking an attitude of gratitude to bed with me.

As a sister science of Ayurveda, yoga has been a vital part of the daily Ayurvedic routine for thousands of years. Where Ayurveda is the 'knowledge', yoga is said to be the practice of this knowledge and the unification of the mind, body and spirit.

When you feel your environment is having unfavourable effects on your mind and body, here are some of the practices I swear by – I call them my toolkit. Find out more details about all of these rituals on my website (jasminehemsley.com).

GET INTO NATURE – Turn off your phone, grab a flask of hot water and get yourself to a park, forest or garden and breathe.

THE POWER POSE – Standing tall, heart open and shoulders back, brings you back into alignment and into your body before meetings or difficult situations.

DOSHA BREATHING – Bee breath (Bhramari Pranayama) grounds and pacifies Vata, Alternate nostril breathing (Nadi Shodhana) cools and calms Pitta, and Breath of fire (Bhastrika Pranayama) stimulates and energises Kapha.

YOGA ASANAS – Pacify your dominant Dosha: from slow and steady Hatha yoga to ground Vata, and opening and cooling Yin yoga to calm Pitta, to fast flowing Ashtanga yoga to stimulate Kapha.

WHITEBOARD WORRIES – Address your fears by miming writing them in front of you and wiping them away; replace with positive affirmations.

FOOT SOAKING AND FACE MASSAGE – Sit on the edge of the bed and soak your feet on for 10 minutes while giving yourself an aromatherapy face massage to help you unwind and get back into your body. Keep a basin, towel and essentials oils under the bed so that you can soak your feet and whip them under the covers, then drift off to sleep.

SOUND BATHING – The ultimate antidote to the buzz of a busy life – find a class or session where you can finally fully relax, with no investment other than getting yourself there and onto a mat.

THE TREAT OF A RETREAT – Create a home retreat (see opposite) where you can rest your body and mind.

CLEANSE AND RESET

Who doesn't want to feel their best? No matter what our best intentions, life gets in the way and things slip. With vices such as drinking, late nights and junk food at our fingertips, it's too easy to numb pain, anxiety or tiredness and disrupt our natural rhythm and state of consciousness, leaving us in an energy-draining cycle.

The old way of dealing with this is to make a punishing pact with ourselves, hitting the gym after a long day at work, coupled with another diet – but this is not sustainable or healthy. Not only does it make you exhausted and hungry, but also you feel defeated and turn to the old vices you were trying escape in the first place ... and so the vicious cycle continues.

You don't have to be having a hard time to schedule a reset for yourself – there are also more subtle reasons to do this. You might feel that your life is on track and you're managing everything quite well, yet you suffer with some of the following niggles: perhaps you're noticing a little anxiety bopping around in the background, a lack of patience or increased irritability, a more emotional outlook, a lack of focus on certain tasks or some fogginess when it comes to making decisions. Maybe you're in an exciting phase of your life yet your 'number twos' have not been fun, your skin is in a spot of bother, your periods are a pain, your sleep is interrupted by too many thoughts, and cravings have kicked in. Most of the time, over-the-counter remedies can numb these symptoms effectively and we continue on. But wait – what exactly is our body telling us here? What is it inviting us to learn about ourselves? Observing subtle changes allows you to step in quickly with the things you need, bringing you back to the balance we all seek.

Sleep! Go to bed at 9.30pm. A good night's sleep, during the optimal time, is the natural way to cleanse and reset. Wind down and give yourself a night off. You deserve it! Even if you can't sleep, or don't think you can, just being in bed sends the signals to your brain and body that all is done for the day and now is the best time for rest.

Have Golden Milk (see page 34) for dinner. Not only will it help make you sleepy, it takes 15 minutes to make and it's quickly digested in time for bed.

Do a restorative yoga class – find a local one or look online. This gives you enforced time-out from social media, reset your breathing and get you back into your body. Even if I'm not 'feeling it' to begin with, I always float out in a better headspace.

Once you've had a decent night's sleep or two, and feel more up to making a plan, put aside a long weekend to indulge in a thorough reset. Nothing fancy or gruelling; this is about nurturing yourself and giving yourself time and space to feel better.

TAKE A THREE-DAY BREAK

In ancient civilisations and other social practices, fasting is observed at various times of year, usually during a change in seasons. Fasting doesn't have to mean out-and-out eliminating food, but rather abstaining from certain foods and activities to give your digestion, and therefore your entire body, a break.

This is a three-day break based on eating plenty of comforting, yet light and easily digestible soups, kitchari and herbal teas – full of detoxifying fluids and warming, pungent herbs and spices such as ginger and cayenne, to support and rekindle your Agni. Not only are you giving your body what it needs, you are also getting out of its way by not loading it with the social, digital and food stimulation that we typically ingest each day, allowing it to repair itself while encouraging the body's natural mechanisms of detoxification. It can also be profoundly clarifying for the mind and the tissues. In just three days you will likely notice an enhanced sense of taste, as well as marked improvements in your appetite, digestion, elimination and mental clarity. Even if you can only stick to a day, or half a day, it will be time well spent. I like to save a lovely book to dip in and out of during this time – and by lovely I mean nothing thrilling or harrowing!

WHAT TO EAT

You could opt for Stewed Apples (see page 76) or Fig, Cinnamon and Cardamom Congee (see page 50) for breakfast, Kitchari (see page 184) for lunch and Golden Milk (see page 34) for dinner – this adds variety throughout the day and is good for anyone looking for something sweet for breakfast. Another option is to make one batch of Kitchari (page 176) to last you the day – this means you only need to cook once each day, leaving more chill time, plus giving you a break from dairy. Another benefit is that if you know that all you can eat is Kitchari, you'll soon know if any 'hunger' that pops up is truly hunger or simply cravings! Keep your lunch and dinner portions in insulated flasks or make them in a slowcooker the night before and set it to warm once it's cooked, then you can help yourself throughout the day. Make it as soupy as you like and add the appropriate Dosha churna spice mix (page 239) according to how you're feeling. If your digestion is struggling or you are feeling unwell, cut back on the herbs and spices and keep the food as simple as possible. For best Prana, make sure the food is made fresh every day and is not reheated.

Sip hot water throughout the day – I find it useful to fill a flask rather than boiling the kettle every 20 minutes – and enjoy a herbal tea mid-morning, mid-afternoon and before bed. Avoid continually drinking herbal tea, which will involve your digestion to some extent. Try Fennel, Tulsi, Rosemary or Salabat tea (see pages 232–235) if you have any digestive discomfort, and a fennel tea if you are feeling constipated.

ENFORCED REST

Take this time to pamper yourself with Abhyanga massage (see page 294) and gentle walks in nature. Listen to your body and tune in to what it's trying to tell you, with thoughts and emotions and aches and pains. You might find that your symptoms get louder, now that you're giving them airtime, or they may subdue as your body is more at ease and your innate bodily wisdom is able to start addressing them. You will most likely find yourself very sleepy during this time – try to meditate or do restorative yoga, as although sleep is a good thing, lie-ins or naps won't help your circadian rhythm! You may find yourself agitated and anxious, feeling that you should be doing something all the time – notice how your body is defaulting to stress mode and how society has shaped that. This is a good time to question and consider anything in your life that is draining or hindering you, and also what you need more of. This is not a time for brainstorming big ideas, but if they flow in, enjoy drawing them out to help release and materialise them.

Experiment with aromatherapy and fill your home with scents of nature. Try frankincense (Indian, if you can get it) in a diffuser or vaporiser during the day, with a dash of ylang ylang to give your home that spa feel, or lavender and Roman chamomile in the evening (do not use these essential oils directly on the skin without diluting with carrier oils). By establishing these scents now when you are fully conscious and committed, you can aid better sleep practices when you go back to your busy life. Scent is one of the most powerful triggers for memory, so using the same 'sleep' essential oil will train your body to respond to it accordingly.

BE PREPARED

Make sure that you have prepared everything you need so you can avoid going shopping. Have yoga videos and guided meditations at the ready if you need them to avoid searching on your phone or laptop. This is also a good time to put the secrets to a lively digestive fire into practice (see page 282) and begin to incorporate routines and rituals (see page 290) into your day-to-day life, allowing the mind and body to cleanse. Use other gentle recipes, such as Spring Clean Vegetable Brown Rice Soup (see page 196) and Vegetable Soba Noodle Soup (see page 171) to ease out of your cleanse.

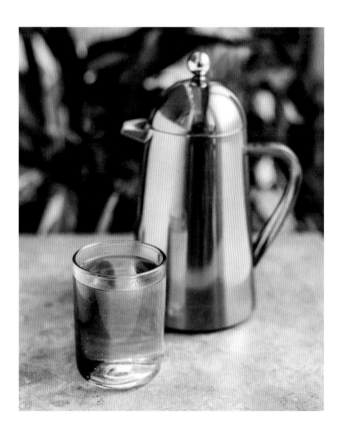

BEAUTY

I love the saying 'beauty from the inside'. Our skin is the physical reflection of everything that happens within the body: the way we eat and breathe, as well as our thoughts and emotions. Our dominant Dosha(s) also play a part in determining our skin type, so every time we look in the mirror we can recognise any imbalance we might be experiencing. Maintaining good overall health is key to beautiful skin – it's all about learning to de-stress your insides in order to de-wrinkle the outside!

You can also use the power of lotions and potions from nature to help from the outside in: aromatherapy, massage, Ayurvedic herbs and spices such as neem, turmeric and tulsi, and honey and milk preparations to nurture the skin. Stick to gentle and natural skincare and make-up which is absorbed into our body via our largest organ – the skin. Such natural products are both good for us and our environment. Not only is the variety of natural beauty products improving, but so too is their performance power, as more and more companies look into feeding this new appetite. Pay special attention to lipsticks and lipbalms, since most of this ends up getting eaten! As a make-up remover I like to use coconut oil, almond oil or ghee (yes, ghee!), massaged into dry skin and then removed with a hot wet flannel.

ABHYANGA 'OIL MASSAGE'

Frazzled nerves can be quickly calmed with a relaxing warm-oil Abhyanga self-massage, which also balances the Prana (see page 16) in the body. Warm the oil first and use long strokes to push it into the skin for 10 minutes, relaxing afterwards for up to 40 minutes before rinsing off with just warm water and a flannel. Customise your massage to balance the Doshas while increasing circulation, stimulating your internal organs, aiding in detox and helping with sleep.

**FEELING
VATA**

Use warming oils such as (untoasted) sesame or almond oil, 4–7 days a week.

**FEELING
PITTA**

Use cooling oils such as coconut or sunflower oil, 3–4 days a week.

**FEELING
KAPHA**

Use sesame oil only occasionally. Even better, focus on dry massage (Udvartana) or dry body brushing.

TAKING AYURVEDA INTO YOUR HOME

We all know the emotional aspect of turning a house into a home, but what about turning it into a spiritual haven? I'm not talking about church or anything religious here, but rather a space that supports and nourishes you. Fill it with plants and natural elements and materials, and throw open the windows as often as possible. And don't forget the powerful effect of a good spring clean!

1   Create a relaxing playlist or tune your radio to classical or chilled stations so you can immediately set the mood when you come home from work.
2   Make your bedroom a sanctuary: fill it only with the things you love and remove the digital technology.
3   Regularly declutter your space of anything that you don't need or love, so that the energy can flow easily and avoid clogging up your creativity.
4   Simmer citrus peels or herbs in a little water for some instant aromatherapy and a nice tisane – see recipe for Rosemary Tea on page 243.
5   Dedicate an area to eating – if you have to work on the same table, use a box or tray to quickly and easily clear everything.
6   Earmark a comfy space for meditating, so you are more inclined to use this effective tool. As my sofa is not particularly supportive, I use a bolster.
7   Bring nature in with a plant or two. The very presence of nature is relaxing and comforting, while helping to detox any impurities from the environment.
8   The right lighting does wonders for your mood: low-level, warm-toned lighting will trigger relaxation at the end of the day and help you sleep better.

AYURVEDA ON THE GO

There is no doubt that the key to optimal health is being prepared, and of course this takes time. I truly believe that this time and effort is all relative to experiencing the benefits of eating well consistently. For a long time now, I've dedicated a few hours on a Sunday for prep to get me ready for the week ahead, putting in place a few simple time-savings strategies such as soaking pseudocereals, re-stocking the pantry and putting something in the slowcooker. Treat yourself to an insulated flask to take your home-cooked hot lunches to work.

PACKING FOR A TRIP

Flying and crossing time-zones at such a fast rate is quite an unnatural shift for the body. Before you travel, eat well and look after yourself, to build your stamina and immunity for your trip. Breathwork, meditation and Abhyanga are also very helpful to counter the travel, as is meditating on take off and landing. Don't forget to pack an eye mask and scarf for the flight to keep your ears and neck covered.

DIGESTIVES – Pack your Dosha spice mix (see page 247) and some of the Ginger Anise Chews on page 103 (also good for nausea) to help stimulate the appetite and aid digestion when you are between time-zones and your body isn't sure what's going on. Vata spice mix (see page 247) is especially good for anyone flying long-haul to help ground and combat the extreme movement of this type of travel.

AYURVEDIC SUPPLEMENTS – There are many effective Ayurvedic supplements of perfectly proportioned herbs and spices available, which can be a real help for travelling. Try Ashwagandha, Triphala and Chyawanprash.

NON-PERISHABLES – Take herbal teabags such as liquorice to pacify Vata caused by the airy nature of flight, plus Millet Flake Travel Mix (see page 67), to enjoy on the journey, or in your room.

Resources

For the most up-to-date information on Ayurvedic resources, stockists and applications to your daily life, visit jasminehemsley.com. Here you'll find articles, shopping lists, meal plans, techniques and tips for the recipes and all of the above, as well as recommended meditation teachers, retreats and products to help you on your Ayurvedic journey.

Sign up to my website for all the latest releases including my up and coming Living La Vida 'Veda series in the form of a monthly newsletter exclusive to friends of Jasmine Hemsley where we will introduce you to ways of integrating Ayurveda into your life and support you on your journey to a natural equilibrium.

If you want to find out more firsthand, then it's better to see a qualified practitioner; in the UK try the Ayurvedic Practitioner Association at apa.uk.com.

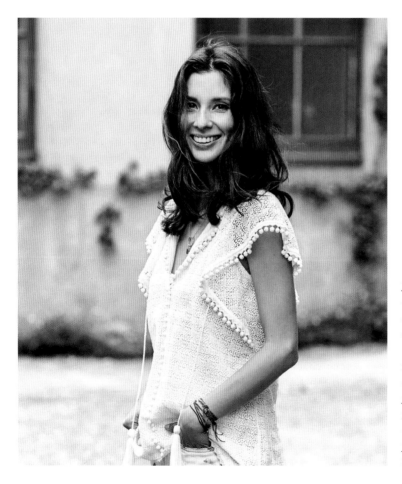

JASMINE HEMSLEY is the co-founder of the Hemsley + Hemsley brand and cafe at Selfridges, and bestselling co-author of *The Art of Eating Well* and *Good + Simple*. Based on her passion for eating well to feel good and driving change through healthy, conscious and joyful living, Jasmine has inspired a global audience to shift their perspectives on food. Inspired by her personal journey, Jasmine's mission is to make a holistic and healthier life accessible to all.

Acknowledgements

To Nick, the man that makes things happen – turning my visions into reality every time. For all your creativity, love, support and freedom – balancing my creative energies with your steadfastness and relaxed approach to life. Thank you for joining me in this life – and all the other ones ;) Oh, and for all the beautiful photos yet again!

To my mum for her love and support, and for making everything okay, no matter what. And to my dad who I miss every day – I know you would have been just as fascinated as I am to understand the world with this new language, and I'm sure you would have been able to inspire me with many of the dishes you enjoyed around the world, which would also have had such rich wisdom.

To the wise old owl – great (and my greatest!) aunt Joan – I didn't inherit you as my birthright but you must have been in my dharma.

Lot of special people have helped me on this journey and have become like family – supporting and sharing their love, wisdom and passion unconditionally. Beginning with Gary Gorrow who really propelled and nurtured me on this journey. Susie Pearl, my big sister, who has been holding my hand throughout and telling me how it is! Can't wait to collaborate with you on *True You*. And Will Williams, who helped me shake things up and get on with it with his insights.

To my brilliant and very zen editor Carole, for fully embracing this – I knew you were the one! And Martha, who has been a bastion of patience and hard work, and my right-hand woman on the job. To the rest of the incredible team at Bluebird, including my PR team, Jodie, Jess and Tom for helping to convey the beautiful message of Ayurveda.

My design team at Imagist, Colm, Rose and Lucy, for your can-do approach to everything, and of course all your creative and design brilliance in interpreting my visions. You've done it again.

My shoot team, for bringing my ideas to life – Lizzie and Bianca, Jenna, Jess, Rosie and Jenna for the styling; Linda for the props; and Nick Hopper, the man behind the lens, for capturing it all on camera.

To the Ayurvedic Vaidyas of the Raju family, and Dr Avilochan Singh and Dr Dhanraj Shetty of Vana Retreat for always sharing their invaluable wisdom. Dr Deepa Apte of Ayurveda Pura and Dr Shijoe Mathew Anchery, of The Alternative Healthcare.

To the brilliant support of Chris Davies (Mayarishi AyurVeda), Dr Charlotte Bech, Dr Donn Brennan, Jess Cook, Sebastian Pole (Pukka Herbs) Mahesh Natarajan (Ananda Spa Hotel), Rob Verkerk (Alliance of Natural Health).

To some real stars and East By West team players: Jeanine, Kate, Claire and Poppy, with special thanks to Libby Nixon – thank you all for coming into my life at exactly the right time.

Emma and Alfie Pye, for letting us take over your beautiful home more than once.

To my book agent, Valeria Huerta, for doing things the right way and always open-heartedly. My sound sister Toni Dicks for always keeping it real and knowing me inside out from the star. And to all my other friends – too many to name! – who have supported me in so much over the years. I'm very lucky.

To George and Nikki Shehadah and Paul Van Zyl of Maiyet for all your help in making the pop-up cafe a success and Taylor and Britt, my Aussie dream team.

To my restaurant team at the East by West London pop up: Veronica, and Alex and the rest of the gang at Caiger and Co.

To the incredible PR team at Liz Matthews PR: Liz, Jordan and Naomi for all your hard work in helping me share the philosophy of Ayurveda.

To the recipe testers: Jessica Malik, Alina Buyko and Emma Pye who are always game to test my recipes! And a few new ones Ive picked up along the way – thanks Naomi Denziloe and Nikki Saunders for getting involved and Jenna Leiter for double checking!

Khreena Dhiman for bringing me curry leaves and ragi flour whenever she sees me and Sjaniel Turrel for all her last minute checks.

Tom Dixon, for superior style and all the support, and beautiful ceramics from Billy Lloyd and Iva Polachova.

Finally, to my wolf pack! My dogs, Arjuna, Bheema and Julie, who teach me life lessons everyday and keep me laughing whatever the world decides to throw at me.

Index

First published 2017 by Bluebird an imprint of Pan Macmillan
20 New Wharf Road, London N1 9RR Associated companies
throughout the world www.panmacmillan.com

ISBN 978-1-5098-5812-5

9 8 7 6 5 4 3 2 1

A CIP catalogue record for this book is available
from the British Library.

Printed and bound in Italy.

PUBLISHER Carole Tonkinson
SENIOR EDITOR Martha Burley
SENIOR PRODUCTION CONTROLLER Ena Matagic
ART DIRECTION & DESIGN Imagist
PROP STYLING Linda Berlin
FOOD STYLING Lizzie Harris and Bianca Nice

Visit www.panmacmillan.com to read more about all our books and
to buy them. You will also find features, author interviews and news
of any author events, and you can sign up for e-newsletters so that
you're always first to hear about our new releases.

Please note that the advice in this book
is for general information only, and
should not be taken as a substitute for
qualified medical advice. If you have
a medical condition, are pregnant, or
suffer from allergies, please consult
your doctor before changing your diet
or taking herbal remedies.